The Handbook of

Surgical
Intensive Care

The Handbook of
Surgical Intensive Care

**Practices of the Surgical Residents
at Duke University Medical Center**

FIFTH EDITION

EDITED BY

Bryan M. Clary, M.D.
Assistant Professor of Surgery,
Department of Surgery,
Division of General Surgery,
Duke University Medical Center,
Durham, North Carolina

Carmelo A. Milano, M.D.
Assistant Professor of Surgery,
Department of Surgery,
Division of Cardiothoracic Surgery,
Duke University Medical Center,
Durham, North Carolina

with 34 illustrations

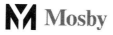

A Harcourt Health Sciences Company

St. Louis   Philadelphia   London   Sydney   Toronto

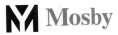
Mosby

A Harcourt Health Sciences Company

Editor: Judith Fletcher
Senior Managing Editor: Kathryn H. Falk
Project Manager: Carol Sullivan Weis
Senior Production Editor: Rick Dudley
Designer: Mark A. Oberkrom
Cover Art: Duke University/Butch Usery

FIFTH EDITION
Copyright © 2000 by Mosby, Inc.

Previous editions copyrighted 1984, 1989, 1992, 1995

NOTICE
Pharmacology is an ever-changing field. Standard safety precautions must be followed, but as new research and clinical experience broaden our knowledge, changes in treatment and drug therapy may become necessary or appropriate. Readers are advised to check the most current product information provided by the manufacturer of each drug to be administered to verify the recommended dose, the method and duration of administration, and contraindications. It is the responsibility of the treating physician, relying on experience and knowledge of the patient, to determine dosages and the best treatment for each individual patient. Neither the publisher nor the editor assumes any liability for any injury and/or damage to persons or property arising from this publication.

Mosby, Inc.
A Harcourt Health Sciences Company
11830 Westline Industrial Drive
St. Louis, Missouri 63146

Printed in the United States of America

International Standard Book Number ISBN 0-323-01106-3

01 02 03 04 CL/FF 9 8 7 6 5 4 3 2

CONTRIBUTORS

Unless noted, all contributors are from the Department of Surgery, Duke University Medical Center, Durham, North Carolina.

Shahab A. Akhter, M.D.
Chief Resident, General Surgery

Hartmuth Bruno Bittner, M.D.
Assistant Professor of Surgery,
Department of Surgery,
Division of Cardiovascular and Thoracic Surgery,
University of Minnesota,
Minneapolis, Minnesota

Lisa A. Clark, M.D.
Senior Assistant Resident, General Surgery

Bryan M. Clary, M.D.
Assistant Professor of Surgery,
Division of General Surgery

Larkin J. Daniels, M.D.
Senior Assistant Resident, General Surgery

Joseph M. Forbess, M.D.
Instructor of Surgery,
Harvard Medical School;
Associate in Cardiovascular Surgery,
Children's Hospital,
Boston, Massachusetts

Charles W. Hoopes, M.D.
Cardiothoracic Surgery Fellow,
The University of Michigan Medical Center,
Ann Arbor, Michigan

G. Chad Hughes, M.D.
Senior Assistant Resident, General Surgery

Paul M. Kirshbom, M.D.
Resident, Cardiothoracic Surgery

Alan P. Kypson, M.D.
Chief Resident, General Surgery

Jeffrey H. Lawson, M.D., Ph.D.
Assistant Professor of Surgery,
Assistant Professor of Pathology

R. Eric Lilly, M.D.
Resident, Cardiothoracic Surgery

Andrew J. Lodge, M.D.
Chief Resident, General Surgery

Carmelo A. Milano, M.D.
Assistant Professor of Surgery,
Division of Cardiothoracic Surgery

Eugene W. Moretti, M.D.
Associate, Department of Anesthesiology;
Attending Physician, Surgical Intensive Care Unit

Robert B. Noone, M.D.
Chief Resident, General Surgery

R. Anthony Perez-Tamayo, M.D., Ph.D.
Cardiothoracic Surgery Fellow,
Department of Cardiovascular and Thoracic Surgery,
Loyola University Medical Center,
Maywood, Illinois

Scott C. Silvestry, M.D.
Resident, Cardiothoracic Surgery

Lynne A. Skaryak, M.D.
Assistant Professor of Surgery,
Division of Cardiothoracic Surgery,
University of Massachusetts Medical School,
Worcester, Massachusetts

James D. St. Louis, M.D.
Resident, Cardiothoracic Surgery

J.E. (Betsy) Tuttle-Newhall, M.D.
Assistant Professor of Surgery,
Divisions of Transplant Surgery and Critical Care

Bryan C. Weidner, M.D.
Surgical Intensive Care Unit Fellow

John C. Wellons III, M.D.
Senior Assistant Resident, Neurosurgery

Kirsten Bass Wilkins, M.D.
Senior Assistant Resident, General Surgery

PREFACE

The Duke Surgical ICU Handbook was first compiled in the mid-1980s by David C. Sabiston, Jr., M.D. and H. Kim Lyerly, M.D. for residents at the institution. Due to its popularity within the institution, it was expanded and published. Now as we submit the new fifth edition of this handbook, there are many changes relative to the original edition. The goal of the handbook, however, remains the same: to provide ICU practitioners with a insightful and functional reference to assist them in the care of their critically ill patients. In addition to providing a reference to practitioners with experience, this manual is designed for residents and other trainees with limited ICU experience.

ICU patients represent perhaps the most challenging of patients for new trainees. ICU patients frequently present complex problems with ventilator management, inotropic support, renal, and metabolic issues. While medical students often receive formal lectures regarding the pathophysiology related to these topics, residents may still find the actual clinical management of these patients difficult or even overwhelming. Furthermore, management decisions often need to be executed quickly or at odd hours, making reference to a formal textbook impractical. We have tried to limit the discussion of physiology and pathophysiology in order to focus on clinical management. We have shortened the text to provide a more user-friendly format. Four new chapters have been added, three of which address the important topics of nutrition, anesthesia, and the management of burns and wounds. A chapter focusing specifically on the techniques of common ICU procedures has also been added. Lastly, the chapter on medications has been greatly expanded and updated to include those medications that have been incorporated into clinical practice since the release of the last edition.

This book has been written predominantly by senior surgical residents at Duke University Medical Center who have recently completed or are near completion of their surgical training. We feel this has helped to focus the content away from theoretical aspects toward practical ICU management issues that younger residents face on a daily basis. Furthermore, while ICU management is becoming a subspecialty itself, the authorship of this handbook reflects our program's continued emphasis that surgeons remain not only involved in the management of their ICU patients but leaders in the field.

We thank Dr. David C. Sabiston, Jr. and Dr. Robert W. Anderson, our Chairmen, for their continued support and guidance on this project. The editors are indebted to our contributing authors for their dedication and perseverance in maintaining the quality of this manual. We also thank our wives and families whose constant support facilitated the completion of this project.

Bryan M. Clary
Carmelo A. Milano

LIST OF ABBREVIATIONS

AAA	abdominal aortic aneurysm
ABI	ankle-brachial index
ABG	arterial blood gas
ACE	angiotensin-converting enzyme
ACLS	advanced cardiac life support
ACT	activated clotting time
ACTH	adrenocorticotropic hormone
ADH	antidiuretic hormone
AHA	American Heart Association
AIOD	aortoiliac occlusive disease
APTT	activated partial thromboplastin time
ARF	acute renal failure; acute respiratory failure
ARDS	adult respiratory distress syndrome
ATN	acute tubular necrosis
AVo_2	arteriovenous O_2 content difference
BLS	basic life support
BP	blood pressure
BSA	body surface area
BUN	blood urea nitrogen
CABG	coronary artery bypass graft
CAD	coronary artery disease
CAVHD	continuous arteriovenous hemodialysis
Cao_2	arterial oxygen content
CBC	complete blood count
CCR	creatinine clearance
CDH	congenital diaphragmatic hernia
CHF	congestive heart failure
CI	cardiac index
CK	creatine kinase
CMV	cytomegalovirus; controlled mechanical ventilation
CNS	central nervous system
CO	cardiac output
COPD	chronic obstructive pulmonary disease
CPAP	continuous positive airway pressure
CPB	cardiopulmonary bypass
CPK	creatine phosphokinase
CSF	cerebrospinal fluid
CT	computed tomography
CVA	cerebrovascular accident
Cvo_2	mixed venous oxygen content
CVP	central venous pressure
CXR	chest x-ray
DIC	disseminated intravascular coagulation
Do_2	oxygen delivery
DVT	deep vein thrombosis
EBV	Epstein-Barr virus
ECG	electrocardiogram
ECMO	extracorporeal membrane oxygenation
EEG	electroencephalogram
EMD	electromechanical dissociation
ERCP	endoscopic retrograde cholangiopancreatography
ERV	expiratory reserve volume
FDP	fibrin degradation product

FENA	fractional excretion of sodium
FEV	forced expiratory volume
FFP	fresh frozen plasma
Fio_2	fractional concentration of oxygen in inspired gas
FRC	functional residual capacity
GABA	γ-aminobutyric acid
GE	gastroesophageal
GFR	glomerular filtration rate
GH	growth hormone
GHIF	growth hormone inhibiting factor
GHRF	growth hormone releasing factor
GI	gastrointestinal
HATT	heparin-associated thrombotic thrombocytopenia
Hct	hematocrit
HPLC	high performance liquid chromatography
HR	heart rate
HRS	hepatorenal syndrome
HSV	herpes simplex virus
IABP	intraaortic balloon pump
IC	inspiratory capacity
ICP	intracranial pressure
I : E	inspiration to expiration ratio
IFR	inspiratory flow rate
IL	interleukin
IMA	inferior mesenteric artery
IMV	intermittent mandatory ventilation
IPPB	intermittent positive pressure breathing
IRV	inspiratory reserve volume
ITP	immune thrombocytopenia purpura
JVD	jugular venous distention
KUB	kidney, ureter, bladder
LA	left atrium/atrial
LAP	left atrial pressure
LDH	lactate dehydrogenase
LDL	low-density lipoprotein
LFT	liver function test
LUQ	left upper quadrant
LV	left ventricle
LVEDP	left ventricular end-diastolic pressure
MAP	mean systemic arterial pressure
MAS	meconium aspiration syndrome
MAST	medical antishock trousers
MB	muscle-brain
MI	myocardial infarction
MIBG	metaiodobenzylguanidine
MOF	multiple organ failure
MUGA	multigated
MVo_2	myocardial oxygen consumption
NG	nasogastric
NS	normal saline
NSAID	Nonsteroidal antiinflammatory drug
NTG	nitroglycerin
O_2ER	oxygen extraction ratio
OI	oxygen index
PA	pulmonary artery
Pao_2	arterial oxygen partial pressure
$Paco_2$	arterial carbon dioxide partial pressure

PCWP	pulmonary capillary wedge pressure
PE	pulmonary embolism
PEEP	positive end-expiratory pressure
PIP	peak inspiratory pressure
PPHN	persistent pulmonary hypertension of the newborn
P_{osm}	plasma osmolality
PRBCs	packed red blood cells
PSVT	paroxysmal supraventricular tachycardia
PT	prothrombin time
PTCA	percutaneous transluminal coronary angioplasty
PTHC	percutaneous transhepatic cholangiography
PTT	partial thromboplastin time
PVC	premature ventricular contraction
RA	right atrium/atrial
RATG	rabbit antithymocyte globulin
RBC	red blood cells
RIA	radioimmunoassay
RIND	reversible ischemic neurologic deficit
rt-PA	recombinant tissue plasminogen activator
RV	right ventricle/ventricular; residual volume
Sao_2	arterial oxygen saturation
SGOT	serum glutamic-oxaloacetic transaminase
SIADH	syndrome of inappropriate secretion of antidiuretic hormone
SIMV	synchronized intermittent mandatory ventilation
SLE	systemic lupus erythematosus
SNP	sodium nitroprusside
SV	stroke volume
Svo_2	mixed venous oxygen saturation
SVR	systemic vascular resistance
T_3	triiodothyronine
T_4	thyroxine
TCT	thrombin clotting time
TE	tracheoesophageal
TIA	transient ischemic attack
TLC	total lung capacity
TNF	tumor necrosis factor
TPN	total parenteral nutrition
TSH	thyroid stimulating hormone
TTP	thrombotic thrombocytopenia purpura
UGI	upper gastrointestinal series
U_{osm}	urine osmolality
UPJ	ureteropelvic junction
URI	upper respiratory infection
VC	vital capacity
V_d	ventilatory dead space
V_E	minute volume ventilation
VMA	vanillylmendelic acid
V/Q	ventilation/perfusion
Vo_2	oxygen consumption
VSD	ventricular septal defect
V_T	tidal volume
vWD	von Willebrand's disease
vWF	von Willebrand's factor
VZV	varicella zoster virus
WBC	white blood cells
WDHA	watery diarrhea hypophosphatemia acidosis

CONTENTS

The Handbook of

Surgical
Intensive Care

PART I

Fundamental Principles of Surgical Intensive Care

HEMODYNAMIC MONITORING

R. Eric Lilly

I. NONINVASIVE HEMODYNAMIC MONITORING

A. INDICATIONS

1. **Used in all intensive care unit patients** with frequency of measurements determined by the clinical situation
2. **Typically, measurements are recorded every 1 to 2 hours**

B. TYPES OF MEASUREMENTS

1. **Continuous ECG:** Useful for early detection of arrhythmia or ischemia and determination of heart rate
2. **Cuff blood pressure:** Automated systems are commonly used
3. **Pulse oximetry**
4. **Temperature**
5. **Respiratory rate**

II. SYSTEMIC ARTERIAL CATHETERS

A. INDICATIONS

1. **Frequent blood gas determinations**
2. **Need for continuous blood pressure monitoring**
   a. Patients receiving inotropic or vasoactive drugs
   b. Patients on high levels of ventilator support
   c. Presence of shock
   d. Any hemodynamic instability
   e. Intraoperative monitoring in high-risk patients

B. TECHNICAL ASPECTS

1. **Collateral blood flow distal to the insertion site must be adequate to prevent ischemia**
   a. Presence of a pulse oximetry signal distal to the insertion site confirms pulsatile blood flow.
   b. Allen's test is useful to determine dual circulation to hand.
2. **Insertion sites**
   a. Radial artery is the most common insertion site.
   b. Dorsalis pedis, femoral, and axillary arteries are other common insertion sites.
3. **Measurements**
   a. The measuring system consists of fluid-filled tubing connected to the arterial line with a transducer inline.
   b. Air within the system alters the natural frequency and increases damping, which will lead to inaccurate pressure recordings.
   c. The transducer is a strain gauge that should be positioned optimally at the level of the midaxillary line or alternatively at the level of the artery.

C. COMPLICATIONS

1. **Ischemia**
   a. Infarction of an extremity distal to an arterial catheter should be a rare event provided the patient is carefully monitored.

b. If distal ischemia does develop, the arterial catheter should be promptly removed and consideration be given to systemic heparinization.

c. Although radial artery thrombosis occurs in as many as 38% of patients with radial arterial lines, few patients develop ischemic complications.

d. Distal embolization from the catheter is possible.

2. Infectious

a. Infectious complications are dependent on the duration of arterial cannulation.

b. Multiple studies have demonstrated a low incidence of catheter-related infections at less than 4 days of cannulation.

c. Catheter infection rates of 9.5% to 18% have been reported after 4 days.

d. Systemic sepsis secondary to arterial catheters is an infrequent complication.

III. CENTRAL VENOUS LINES

A. INDICATIONS

1. Vascular access for vasoactive drugs, fluid therapy, or parenteral nutrition

2. Hemodynamic monitoring

a. In normal patients, CVP correlates well with left ventricular (LV) filling pressures.

b. Abnormal airway pressures, such as in the case of underlying lung disease, or high levels of ventilator support will falsely elevate CVP with respect to LV filling pressures.

c. In states of right heart ischemia/infarction, valvular heart disease, cardiac tamponade, or pulmonary hypertension, CVP may not correlate with LV filling pressures.

B. TECHNICAL ASPECTS

1. Cannulation sites: Include the subclavian, internal jugular, external jugular, and femoral veins

2. Normal central venous pressure: 0 to 8 mm Hg

3. CVP: Measured with a fluid-filled catheter system as described above for arterial lines

C. COMPLICATIONS

1. Associated with catheter insertion—overall rates of 7.7% have been reported.

a. Pneumothorax—occurs in approximately 1%

b. Hemomediastinum/hemothorax

c. Air embolization

d. Chylothorax

e. Neurologic injury

2. Infectious complications are related to duration of cannulation. A prospective study found that catheter infections occur in 6.9% of patients with triple-lumen central venous catheters. Positive blood cultures occurred only when the duration of cannulation exceeded 10 days. Routine exchanges of central venous catheters should be performed after 10 days of cannulation.

IV. PULMONARY ARTERY CATHETERS

A. INDICATIONS

1. Absolute indications

a. Myocardial infarction with hypotension, shock, mechanical complication (e.g., ventricular septal defect [VSD], mitral regurgitation), or right ventricular failure

b. Intraoperative for patients undergoing high-risk vascular or cardiac surgery

c. Severely injured and elderly trauma patients

d. Patients with severe coronary artery disease or severe valvular heart disease undergoing major noncardiac surgery

2. Relative indications

a. Congestive heart failure

b. Pulmonary hypertension

c. Shock or hemodynamic instability

d. Neurosurgical procedures

e. Sepsis/septic shock

f. To aid in achieving and monitoring supranormal oxygen delivery

g. High-risk surgical patients

h. Respiratory failure

3. Not indicated

a. Routine coronary artery bypass surgery

b. Geriatric patients undergoing surgery

B. MEASUREMENTS AND CALCULATIONS

1. Pulmonary artery occlusion pressure (PAOP)

a. Estimates LV filling pressure by assuming an unbroken column of blood between the site of occlusion and the left ventricle.

b. PAOP does not correlate with LV filling pressures when a mechanical obstruction exists between the pulmonary artery (PA) and LV, such as in cases of mitral stenosis, pulmonary venoocclusive disease, or atrial myxomas.

c. Positive end-expiratory pressure (PEEP) increases intrathoracic pressure, which, in turn, increases PAOP independent of actual changes in LV filling pressures.

d. PAOP can be used in most clinical situations as an index of LV preload.

e. LV preload is best described by LV end-diastolic sarcomere length (i.e., chamber volume). Although the relationship between LV end-diastolic pressure and end-diastolic volume is quite variable and dependent on a number of factors (e.g., LV ischemia, pericarditis), in most clinical situations PAOP-estimated LV filling pressure is a useful index of LV preload.

2. **Cardiac output (CO)**
   a. PA catheters actually measure right ventricular (RV) cardiac output, which must equal LV cardiac output as long as no intracardiac shunt is present.
   b. CO is calculated as the product of stroke volume and heart rate.
   c. CO may be determined by the PA catheter using a thermodilution technique. Ice-cooled saline (usually 10 ml) is injected through the right atrial port of the PA catheter located 4 cm proximal to a thermistor. Integration of the area below the thermodilution curve recorded by this thermistor allows calculation of the cardiac output using the Stewart-Hamilton equation:

$$CO = \frac{VI(TB - TI)K1K2}{\int TB(t)dt}$$

Where: CO = cardiac output (L/min)
        VI = injectate volume (L)
        TB = blood temperature
        TI = injectate temperature
        $K1$ = density factor
        $K2$ = correctional constant

   d. Continuous cardiac output PA catheters are also currently available. These catheters utilize a thermodilution technique to determine CO. Rather than an intermittent cold bolus as in the standard catheters, continuous catheters repeatedly heat the blood and measure the resultant small temperature change distally. Continuous cardiac output catheters have been shown to be equivalent to standard PA catheters for determination of cardiac outputs. Continuous cardiac output systems require manual entry of the blood hemoglobin level. Online, automated cardiac output determination allows easier data integration.

3. **Mixed venous oxygen saturation**
   a. PA catheters are also available with fiberoptic capabilities for continuous pulmonary arterial oxygen saturations (Svo_2).
   b. Svo_2 can be used for calculation of oxygen consumption by the systemic circulation (Vo_2) as follows:

$$Cvo_2 = 1.36 \times Hgb \times Svo_2$$
$$Cao_2 = 1.36 \times Hgb \times Sao_2$$
$$Vo_2 = (Cao_2 - Cvo_2) \times CO$$

Where Cvo_2 = mixed venous oxygen content
    Hgb = hemoglobin (g/dl)
    Svo_2 = mixed venous oxygen saturation
    Cao_2 = arterial oxygen content
    Sao_2 = arterial oxygen saturation
    1.36 = the amount of oxygen bound to 1 g Hgb at full saturation (ml O_2/g Hgb)

CO = cardiac output (L/min)

V_{O_2} = systemic oxygen consumption (ml/min)

Normal values for V_{O_2} are 225 to 275 ml/min, at rest.

c. Systemic oxygen delivery (D_{O_2}) is calculated as follows:

$$D_{O_2} = Ca_{O_2} \times CO$$

Normal values for D_{O_2} are 800 to 1200 ml/min at rest.

d. The ratio of systemic oxygen consumed to oxygen delivered (V_{O_2}/D_{O_2}) is normally 15% to 20%. Randomized clinical studies have demonstrated improved patient outcomes when supranormal oxygen delivery is achieved. The goal of this supranormal oxygen therapy is to render V_{O_2} independent of D_{O_2}, which occurs at a D_{O_2}-to-V_{O_2} ratio of 4:1.

e. Sv_{O_2} alone is an extremely useful clinical parameter.

  (1) Decreasing Sv_{O_2} indicates increased oxygen extraction by the systemic circulation, decreased arterial oxygen content, or a decreased cardiac output. Therapeutic intervention should be directed at restoring D_{O_2} either by increasing oxygen content (i.e., administer blood or improve Sa_{O_2}) or by improving cardiac output (i.e., increase inotropic state, LV preload, or heart rate).

  (2) Increasing Sv_{O_2} indicates increased D_{O_2} (e.g., increased cardiac output or hemoglobin) or decreased systemic oxygen extraction. Decreased systemic oxygen extraction can occur secondary to sepsis, with its resultant metabolic uncoupling, or to single-system organ failure (e.g., hepatic failure).

C. COMPLICATIONS

1. Catheter-related sepsis occurs in 2% of patients

2. Arrhythmias

a. Self-limited ventricular arrhythmias occur commonly during insertion of PA catheters.

b. Sustained ventricular tachycardia necessitates removal of the PA catheter.

c. Atrial fibrillation has been reported.

d. Self-limited, asymptomatic right bundle branch block can occur with PA catheter placement. In patients with underlying left bundle branch block, a prophylactic temporary pacing wire should be inserted via the PA catheter.

3. Pulmonary artery rupture

a. A very rare complication

b. Possible mechanisms include overinflation of the balloon or catheter tip perforation of the pulmonary artery

c. Hemoptysis may be an associated clinical finding

d. If hemoptysis develops, the PA catheter should be removed

4. Vascular injury, including chamber perforation or valvular apparatus injury

5. PA catheter knotting

V. ALTERNATIVES TO PA CATHETERS

A. GASTRIC TONOMETRY

1. **Gastric mucosal pH (pHi) measurements** have been shown to predict morbidity and mortality in both postsurgical and severely traumatized patients.

2. **A prospective randomized trial** demonstrated that critically injured patients with a pHi maintained at 7.35 had a significantly greater survival than those with pHi < 7.35 (58% vs. 42%, $P < 0.01$).

3. **Measurement of pHi** can be accomplished using a tonometer balloon inserted into the stomach that is then allowed to equilibrate, with subsequent analysis of the balloon contents by a blood gas analyzer. This process is slow and can delay therapy.

4. **Fiberoptic intramucosal Pco_2 sensors are under investigation.** These devices have been shown to correlate well with pHi.

B. OTHER DEVICES

1. **Thoracic electrical bioimpedance**

2. **Transesophageal echo-Doppler:** Allows direct assessment of both right and left ventricular volumes and wall motion; this technique also allows assessment of mechanical problems, such as cardiac tamponade or valvular dysfunction

SUGGESTED READINGS

Gutierrez G, Palizas F, Doglio G, et al: Gastric intramucosal pH as a therapeutic index of tissue oxygenation in critically ill patients, *Lancet* 339:195-199, 1992.

Manglano R, Martin M: Safety of triple lumen catheters in the critically ill, *Am Surg* 57:370-372, 1991.

Pulmonary Artery Catheter Consensus Conference: consensus statement, *Crit Care Med* 25:910-925, 1997.

Reid KR, Leasa DJ, Sibbald WJ: Postoperative monitoring of the thoracic surgical patient, *Chest Surg Clin North Am* 2:317-335, 1991.

Shoemaker WC, Appel PL, Kram HB, et al: Prospective trial of supranormal values of survivors as therapeutic goals in high-risk surgical patients, *Chest* 94:1176-1186, 1988.

Taylor DE, Gutierrez G: Tonometry, a review of clinical studies, *Crit Care Clin* 12:1007-1018, 1996.

SHOCK

James D. St. Louis

I. INTRODUCTION

A. DEFINITION

Shock is a syndrome of derangement in oxygen delivery or utilization, leading to cellular hypoxia and organ dysfunction.

B. PATHOPHYSIOLOGY

The derangement in oxygen delivery or utilization is preceded by a single event that is the basis for classification. Regardless of the initiating event, the end result is a decreased adenosine triphosphate (ATP) production via the respiratory chain and a near-total reliance on the anaerobic production of energy.

C. DIAGNOSIS

Early diagnosis remains difficult because early symptoms and physical findings are frequently nonspecific (Table 2-1).

1. **Symptoms**
   a. Shortness of breath
   b. Altered mental status (from minimal agitation or anxiety to obtundation or coma)
2. **Signs**
   a. Hypotension
   b. Tachycardia
   c. Tachypnea/respiratory distress
   d. Decreased urine output

D. TREATMENT

Requires defining and treating specific causes.

II. CLASSIFICATION

Shock is classified based on etiology. It must be emphasized that patients may have any combination of causes, making the diagnosis and resultant treatment plan difficult to determine.

A. HYPOVOLEMIC SHOCK

1. **Subtypes** (Table 2-2)
   a. Pure hypovolemic
      (1) Hemorrhagic
      (2) Other fluid loss: vomiting, diarrhea, bowel obstruction
   b. Traumatic
      (1) Associated tissue edema
      (2) Burn injuries
2. **Pathophysiology:** Decreased preload secondary to plasma volume loss
   a. External (e.g., laceration)
   b. Internal (e.g., gastrointestinal)
   c. Interstitial (e.g., increased vascular permeability)

TABLE 2-1

CLINICAL PRESENTATIONS OF THE VARIOUS TYPES OF SHOCK

Etiology	Skin	Urine Output	JVD	Cardiac Index	PCWP	SVR	Svo$_2$
Hypovolemic	Cool, pale	↓	↓	↓	↓	↑	↓
Traumatic	Cool, pale	↓	↓	↓	↓	↑	↓
Cardiogenic	Cool, pale	↓	↑	↓	↑	↑	↓
Early sepsis	Warm, pink	↓↑	↓ ↑	↑	↓↑	↓	↑
Late sepsis	Cool, pale	↓	↓	↓	↓	↑	↓↑
Neurogenic	Warm, pink	↓	↓	↓	↓	↓	↓
Anaphylactic	Cool, pale	↓	↓	↓	↓	↑	↓

TABLE 2-2

CLASSIFICATION OF DEGREES OF HYPOVOLEMIC SHOCK

	Class I	Class II	Class III	Class IV
Blood loss (ml)	<750	750-1500	1500-2000	>2000
Blood loss (%)	<15	15-30	30-40	>40
HR (beats/min)	<100	100-120	120-140	>140
BP	Normal	Normal	Decreased	Decreased
Pulse pressure	Normal	Decreased	Decreased	Decreased
Capillary refill ,	Normal	Delayed	Delayed	Delayed
Respiratory rate	14-20	20-30	30-40	>40
Urine output (ml/hr)	>30	20-30	5-15	Negligible
Mental status	Slight anxiety	Mild anxiety	Confusion	Lethargy
Fluid replacement	Crystalloid	Crystalloid	Crystalloid and RBCs	Crystalloid and RBCs

3. **Diagnosis**

a. The clinical presentation depends on the degree of hypovolemia.

  (1) Patients with advanced hypovolemic shock (>40% loss of blood volume) manifest the following symptoms:

    (a) Tachycardia

    (b) Orthostatic hypotension

    (c) Supine hypotension

    (d) Oliguria

    (e) Obtundation

b. Patients who have lost 15% of their blood volume may have normal or mildly abnormal vital signs.

4. **Treatment** (see Table 2-2)

a. Volume replacement:

  (1) Class I and II shock: Initial replacement with crystalloid (normal saline) until heart rate, pulse pressure, and urine output normalize.

  (2) Class III shock: Initial replacement with crystalloid with immediate preparation of type-specific packed red blood cells (PRBC) and administration when available.

(3) Class IV shock: Initial replacement with crystalloid and immediate administration of uncrossed match (type O negative) PRBC. Pressor agents are absolutely contraindicated.

b. Noninvasive assessment: Preevent medical conditions (e.g., cardiac function) will dictate the amount of volume given using only noninvasive monitoring:

(1) Urine output

(2) Heart rate

(3) Pulse pressure

(4) Skin turgor

c. Invasive assessment: If no response after the initial 2 L of crystalloid or if the patient will not tolerate large fluid challenges, additional invasive monitoring is indicated:

(1) Central venous pressure

(2) Pulmonary artery catheters: CI, PCWP, SVR, Svo_2

d. Autotransfusion maneuvers: Designed to shift blood from the legs and increase venous return, thereby improving the cardiac output

(1) Trendelenburg's position

(a) Never proven to increase the volume of blood in the central circulation or improve cardiac output

(b) May increase intracranial venous sinuses pressure, resulting in diminished carotid flow

(c) Not recommended as a safe or effective therapy

e. Goal

(1) Heart rate <120 beats/min

(2) Urine output = 0.5 ml/kg/hr

(3) CVP = 15 mm Hg

(4) PCWP = 10 to 12 mm Hg

B. CARDIOGENIC SHOCK

1. Subtypes

a. Primary (pump failure)

(1) Cardiomyopathy

(2) Ischemia/infarction

(3) Arrhythmias/heart block

(4) Congenital heart defects

(5) Coronary air embolism

(6) Valvular heart disease

b. Secondary

(1) Pulmonary embolus

(2) Pericardial tamponade

(3) Mechanical ventilation

(4) Pulmonary hypertension

(5) Aortic dissection

2. Pathophysiology of primary cardiogenic shock: Decreased cardiac output resulting from contractile dysfunction of the myocardium

3. **Diagnosis** (see Table 2-1)
a. The clinical presentation depends on the degree of myocardial dysfunction:
   (1) Tachycardia
   (2) Jugular venous distention
   (3) Oliguria
   (4) Pulmonary edema: rales
   (5) Peripheral edema: pitting
   (6) Hepatomegaly
b. Invasive assessment: Pulmonary artery catheters are often required to assess the degree and side of failure.
   (1) Increase PCWP and CVP
   (2) Decrease stroke volume (SV)
   (3) Decrease CO because tachycardia no longer compensates for SV
   (4) Right heart failure: CVP > PCWP
   (5) Left heart failure: PCWP > CVP
4. **Treatment:** See Chapter 6.

C. SEPTIC SHOCK

1. **Subtypes**
a. Gram-positive organisms
b. Gram-negative organisms
c. Fungal organisms

2. **Pathophysiology**
a. Sepsis is a syndrome resulting from the inflammatory response to an infectious focus. The systemic manifestations result from the production of mediators and may lead to dysfunction of the renal, pulmonary, and central nervous systems.
b. Numerous mediators of inflammation (cytokines) are released during sepsis, which may contribute to the cellular dysfunction (Box 2-1).

3. **Diagnosis** (see Table 2-1)
a. Clinical features are nonspecific and variable:
   (1) Fever or hypothermia
   (2) Leukocytosis or leukopenia
   (3) Tachypnea and tachycardia

BOX 2-1	
MEDIATORS OF THE SEPTIC RESPONSE	
Prostaglandins	Leukotrienes
Bradykinin	Histamine
Endotoxin	Endogenous catecholamines
Oxygen free radicals	Interleukin-1
Tumor necrosis factor	Interleukin-6
Complement	Endothelin
Nitric oxide	β-Endorphins
Platelet activating factor	

     (4) Organ dysfunction
       (a) Altered mental status
       (b) Hypoxia
       (c) Oliguria
b. Gram-positive sepsis is associated with normal urine output, sensorium, and serum lactic acid and has a significantly better prognosis than does gram-negative sepsis.
c. The earliest manifestations of gram-negative sepsis are hyperventilation, respiratory alkalosis, and altered sensorium. A high index of suspicion must be present to make the diagnosis at this stage.
d. Late manifestations of gram-negative sepsis include anuria, hypotension, coma, and multisystem organ failure. At this stage the chance of progressing to multisystem organ failure is high.
e. Lactic acidosis
     (1) Reliable indicator of inadequate tissue oxygenation and survival.
     (2) Levels greater than 2 mm/L are associated with increased mortality.
f. Hemodynamic patterns
     (1) Pulmonary artery catheter (Table 2-3)
     (2) Oximeteric pulmonary artery catheter
       (a) Mix venous saturation >75%
       (b) Increase oxygen delivery (Do_2)
       (c) Increase oxygen uptake (Vo_2)
       (d) Decrease extraction ratio

4. Treatment

a. Eradicate the infectious source
     (1) Appropriate antibiotics
       (a) Broad spectrum initially
       (b) Selective with culture results
     (2) Drain all purulent collections
     (3) Remove necrotic tissue
b. Hemodynamic support
     (1) Supranormal levels of oxygen supply may improve outcome from septic shock
       (a) Cardiac index >4.5 L/min
       (b) Oxygen delivery >600 ml O_2/min $\cdot$ m^2
       (c) Oxygen uptake >170 ml O_2/min $\cdot$ m^2
     (2) Intervention
       (a) Volume loading
       (b) Vasoactive agents (dobutamine, dopamine, epinephrine)

TABLE 2-3

HEMODYNAMIC PATTERNS IN SEPTIC SHOCK

	PCWP	CO	SVR
Early sepsis	Low	High	Low
Late sepsis	High	Normal	Normal
Terminal stage	High	Low	High

D. NEUROGENIC SHOCK

1. Subtypes include the following:

a. Spinal cord injury

b. Regional anesthesia

c. Autonomic blocking agents

2. Pathophysiology: Loss of sympathetic tone causes venous pooling.

3. Diagnosis (see Table 2-1)

a. Precipitating event

b. Blood pressure low

c. Heart rate low

d. Dry, warm, flushed skin

4. Treatment

a. Volume resuscitation

b. Vasoactive agents

    (1) Ephedrine

    (2) Phenylephrine

E. ANAPHYLACTIC SHOCK

1. Etiology

a. Occurs in 1 of every 10,000 hospitalized patients, with a mortality of 10%

b. Remove precipitating agents

    (1) Drugs: antibiotics

    (2) Contrast material

    (3) Plasma products

2. Pathophysiology: The exposure of a sensitized individual (i.e., one with immunoglobin E [IgE]-bound mast cells and basophils) to antigen results in the release of large quantities of histamine and other vasoactive substances

3. Diagnosis (see Table 2-1)

a. Clinical manifestation routinely occurs within minutes of exposure

b. Signs and symptoms

    (1) Hypotension with vascular collapse

    (2) Laryngeal edema

    (3) Bronchospasm

    (4) Angioedema

    (5) Urticaria

    (6) Flushing

    (7) Pulmonary hypertension and edema

    (8) Hemolysis

4. Treatment

a. Remove antigen

b. Endotracheal intubation to secure airway: stridor

c. Intravenous fluids: colloid preferred to crystalloid

d. Pharmacologic therapy

    (1) Epinephrine

        (a) Load: 0.1-1.0 mg IV

        (b) Maintenance: 0.1 μg/kg/min IV

(2) Glucocorticoid: methylprednisolone 100-250 mg IV
(3) Diphenhydramine 25-50 mg IV
(4) H_2 antagonist: cimetidine 300 mg IV or ranitidine 50 mg IV

III. MULTIPLE-SYSTEM ORGAN FAILURE

A. GENERAL

1. **Mortality relates to number of organ systems involved**
   a. One system: 30% to 50% mortality
   b. Two systems: 50% to 60% mortality
   c. Three systems: 60% to 80% mortality
   d. Four systems: 100% mortality
2. **Lungs, kidneys, and liver most commonly involved**
3. **No change in mortality rates since its original description**
4. **Affects 8% of multiple trauma patients and 11% of patients undergoing emergency surgery**

B. TREATMENT

1. **Treat the underlying pathology as described above.**
2. **Restore microcirculatory perfusion.**
3. **Support affected dysfunctional organ system.**
   a. Respiratory system
      (1) Treat hypoxia and hypercarbia while minimizing barotrauma (pressure control ventilation)
      (2) Early identification of pneumonia
   b. Cardiovascular system
      (1) Provide adequate oxygen delivery
         (a) Volume replacement
         (b) Vasoactive agents
      (2) Prevent myocardial sacrifice
   c. Hematologic system
      (1) Maximize oxygen-carrying capacity: normalize hematocrit (30% to 40%)
      (2) Treat coagulopathy
   d. Renal system
      (1) Maintain cardiac output and renal perfusion
      (2) Avoid nephrotoxic agents
         (a) Contrast agents
         (b) Aminoglycosides
      (3) Hemodialysis and continuous arteriovenous hemofiltration
   e. Nutrition
      (1) Enteral preferred to parenteral nutrition
      (2) Use antacids/H_2 blockers to avoid stress gastritis/GI bleeding
      (3) Use pro-motility agents (cisapride, metoclopramide [Reglan], erythromycin)

2

SHOCK

SUGGESTED READINGS

Astiz ME, Rackow EC, Weil MH: Pathophysiology and treatment of circulatory shock, *Crit Care Clin* 9:183, 1993.

Carrico CJ, Meakins JL, Marshall JC, et al: Multiple-organ-failure syndrome, *Arch Surg* 121:196, 1986.

Dantzker D: Oxygen delivery and utilization in sepsis, *Crit Care Clin* 5:83, 1989

Fiddian-Green RG, Haglund U, Guttierres G, et al: Goals for resuscitation of shock, *Crit Care Med* 21(suppl 2):S25, 1993.

Marion P: *The ICU book,* Philadelphia, 1991, Lea & Febiger.

Reed RL II: Oxygen consumption and delivery, *Current Opinions in Anaesthesia* 6:329, 1993.

Teich S, Chernow B: Specific cardiovascular drugs utilized in the critically ill, *Crit Care Clin* 1:491, 1985.

FLUIDS, ELECTROLYTES, AND ACID-BASE MANAGEMENT

Robert B. Noone

I. BODY FLUIDS

A. TOTAL BODY WATER
1. **60% of the total body weight in males**
2. **50% of body weight in females**
3. **75% to 80% of body weight in infants:** Decreases with age so that by 1 year of age, total body water approximately equals that of an adult; less water in fat than in muscle

B. COMPARTMENT DISTRIBUTION
1. **Intracellular fluid compartment:** 40% of body weight
2. **Extracellular fluid compartment:** 20% of body weight
   a. Interstitial fluid compartment: 15% of body weight
   b. Intravascular fluid compartment (plasma volume): 5% of body weight

C. REGULATION OF PLASMA VOLUME
Plasma volume is primarily a function of the total amount of sodium in the body; positive sodium balance will increase plasma volume. Plasma volume is most directly sensed by atrial receptors and is regulated by the renin-angiotensin-aldosterone axis.
1. **Volume deficit** is the most common volume disorder encountered in surgery. Typical causes include emesis, blood loss, and third space fluid losses resulting from an inflammatory process or tissue injury.
2. **The signs and symptoms** of acute volume loss include the following:
   a. CNS signs (lethargy and apathy progressing to stupor and coma) are the first to occur.
   b. Cardiovascular signs include orthostasis, tachycardia, and diminished pulses.
   c. Tissue signs (decreased turgor, soft tongue with longitudinal wrinkles) and muscle atony usually do not appear before 24 hours.
   d. Body temperature decreases.
3. **Acute volume overload is almost always iatrogenic.**
   a. Young patients can compensate for moderate to severe overload.
   b. The signs include distended veins, a bounding pulse, functional murmurs, edema, and basilar rales.

II. ELECTROLYTES

A. ELECTROLYTE COMPOSITION
1. **Intracellular**
   a. Principal intracellular anions: proteins and phosphates
   b. Principal intracellular cations: potassium and magnesium
2. **Extracellular**
   a. Principal extracellular anions: chloride and bicarbonate
   b. Principal extracellular cation: sodium

3. **Body fluids:** Table 3-1 shows usual electrolyte content of various body fluids.

B. **OSMOLARITY**

1. **Osmolarity refers to the number of osmotically active particles in solution.**

2. **Normal osmolarity is 290 to 310 mOsm/L.** Plasma osmolarity is calculated as follows:

$$P_{osm} = 2[Na] + \frac{glucose}{18} + \frac{BUN}{2.8}$$

3. **Nonpermeable plasma proteins** are responsible for the effective oncotic pressure between the plasma compartment and the interstitial fluid compartment (the colloid oncotic pressure).

4. **The effective oncotic pressure** between extracellular and intracellular compartments is regulated primarily by sodium, which does not freely cross the cell membrane.

5. **Because water diffuses freely between compartments, the effective oncotic pressures within the fluid compartments are equal.**

C. **REGULATION OF SERUM SODIUM**

Serum sodium concentration reflects the water balance of the body and is an index of how much sodium is diluted by water. Serum sodium concentration is a reliable index of serum osmolarity. Osmoreceptors in the brain are stimulated by a rise in serum osmolarity, stimulate the thirst mechanism to increase water intake, and release ADH, which increases free water resorption in the collecting duct of the kidney.

TABLE 3-1

ELECTROLYTE CONTENT OF BODY FLUIDS (mEq/L)

Fluid	Na$^+$	K$^+$	Cl$^-$	HCO$_3^-$	Volume (L/day)
Saliva	30	20	35	15	1.0-1.5
Gastric juice, pH < 4	60	10	90	—	2.5
Gastric juice, pH > 4	100	10	100	—	2
Bile	145	5	110	40	1.5
Duodenum	140	5	80	50	
Pancreas	140	5	75	90	0.7-1.0
Ileum	130	10	110	30	3.5
Cecum	80	20	50	20	
Colon	60	30	40	20	
Sweat	50	5	55	—	0-3
New ileostomy	130	20	110	30	0.5-2.0
Adapted ileostomy	50	5	30	25	0.4
Colostomy	50	10	40	20	0.3
Diarrhea fluid	25-50	35-60	20-40	30-45	

III. INTRAVENOUS FLUID THERAPY

Intravenous (IV) fluids are necessary when adequate oral intake is not possible. The fluids delivered should fulfill the maintenance requirements of the patient, replace previous losses, and replace ongoing losses.

A. ELECTROLYTE CONTENT OF IV FLUIDS (Table 3-2)

B. MAINTENANCE FLUID REQUIREMENT (Table 3-3)

1. Daily fluid requirements (per 24 hours)

a. 100 ml/kg for the first 10 kg

b. 50 ml/kg for the second 10 kg

c. 20 ml/kg for each kilogram thereafter

d. 30-35 ml/kg for adults

2. Daily maintenance requirements can usually be met with D_5W 1/2 NS plus 20 mEq KCl/L at the above rate for adults.

C. REPLACEMENT OF PREVIOUS FLUID LOSSES (Table 3-4)

1. If the patient is hemodynamically unstable, 2 L of lactated Ringer's solution should be given, but if the patient has evidence of metabolic alkalosis, normal saline should be given.

2. Dextrose should only be given with the replacement if there is hypoglycemia.

3. Risks of large infusions of crystalloid include the development of peripheral and pulmonary edema. Patients should receive colloids if (1) they have CHF, liver failure, and ascites, and; (2) if after CPB they

TABLE 3-2

ELECTROLYTE CONTENT OF INTRAVENOUS FLUIDS (mEq/L)

Fluid	Na^+	K^+	Ca^{++}	Cl^-	HCO_3^-
Lactated Ringer's	130	4	2.7	109	28
Normal saline (0.9%)	154	—	—	154	—
½ Normal saline (0.45%)	77	—	—	77	—
¼ Normal saline (0.21%)	34	—	—	34	—
Hypertonic saline (3%)	513	—	—	513	—

TABLE 3-3

DAILY FLUID AND ELECTROLYTE LOSSES

Losses	H_2O (ml/day)	Na^+ (mEq/day)	K^+ (mEq/day)
SENSIBLE LOSSES			
Urine	800-1500	10-150	50-80
Stool	0-250	0-20	Trace
Sweat	0-100	10-60	0-10
INSENSIBLE LOSSES			
Lungs	250-450	—	—
Skin	250-450	—	—
TOTAL OUTPUT	1300-2750	20-230	50-90

TABLE 3-4

**ESTIMATED FLUID AND BLOOD LOSSES IN ACUTE INJURY
(CLASSES OF SHOCK)**

	Class I	Class II	Class III	Class IV
Blood loss (% blood volume)	15%	15%-30%	30%-40%	>40%
Blood loss (ml) for a 70-kg man	750	750-1500	1500-2000	>2000
Pulse	<100	>100	>120	>140
Blood pressure	↔	↔	↓	↓
Pulse pressure	↔ or ↑	↓	↓	↓
Respiratory rate	14-20	20-30	30-40	>35
Urine output	>30	20-30	5-15	Minimal
Mental status	Slightly anxious	Mildly anxious	Anxious, confused	Confused, obtunded
Fluid replacement	Crystalloid	Crystalloid	Crystalloid and blood	Crystalloid and blood

already have evidence of peripheral edema but have low intravascular volumes from fluid losses.

4. **Patients should receive colloids after they receive the initial 2 L of crystalloid if hemodynamic stability is not attained.** Whereas 100 ml of 25% albumin increases plasma volume by 450 ml, 1000 ml of lactated Ringer's solution increases plasma volume by 200 ml.

5. **The primary risk of receiving colloids is pulmonary edema,** especially when coupled with any process that increases capillary permeability.

6. **After hemodynamic stability is achieved, replace half the remaining volume deficit (based on weight loss, history, and physical examination) within the first 8 hours.** The remainder can be replaced over a 16- to 24-hour period.

7. **Follow the patient's hemodynamics, urine output, electrolytes, and plasma osmolarity and adjust as indicated.**

D. **REPLACEMENT OF ONGOING FLUID LOSSES** (Table 3-5)

1. **Fever:** Add 2 to 2.5 ml/kg/day of insensible loss for each degree above 37°C.

2. **Third space losses:** Fluids of extracellular composition shift into a pathologic space that cannot be regulated (interstitium, retroperitoneum, and visceral parenchyma). Therefore this fluid is lost for the physiologic compartments. In adults, 1 L of fluid is lost to the third space for each quadrant of the abdomen explored, traumatized, or inflamed.

3. **Osmotic diuresis:** This is secondary to urea, mannitol, glucose, myoglobin, hemoglobin, or dextran. Urine output is high at the expense of intravascular volume.

4. **Tubes and drains:** Measure electrolyte composition and replace as needed. Specific body fluid losses can be estimated from Table 3-1.

TABLE 3-5

REPLACEMENT OF BODY FLUIDS

Fluid	Replacement Fluid
Sweat	D_5W ¼ NS + 5 mEq KCl/L
Gastric	D_5W ½ NS + 30-40 mEq KCl/L
Biliary or pancreatic	Lactated Ringer's
Small bowel	Lactated Ringer's
Colon	Lactated Ringer's
Third space losses	Lactated Ringer's

E. ASSESSMENT OF ADEQUACY OF INTRAVENOUS THERAPY

1. **History:** Thirst with minimal clinical signs indicates a 2% body weight water deficit. Marked thirst, dry mouth, oliguria, and previous poor oral intake indicates a 6% body weight water deficit. All of the above, in addition to weakness and changes in mental status, indicates a 7% to 14% body weight water deficit.
   a. Adults: Adequate urine output is 0.5 to 1.0 ml/kg/hr
   b. Children older than 1 year of age: Adequate urine output is 1.0 ml/kg/hr
   c. Children less than 1 year of age: Adequate urine output is 2.0 ml/kg/hr
2. **Examination includes the following considerations:**
   a. Signs of hypovolemia (see Table 3-4):
      (1) Vital signs: Tachycardia, orthostatic blood pressure, and hypotension
      (2) Flat neck veins when the patient is horizontal
      (3) Dry mucous membranes and skin tenting
      (4) Oliguria
   b. Signs of hypervolemia
      (1) Pitting edema
      (2) Rales on pulmonary auscultation
      (3) If the patient is over 40 years of age, a dull, low-pitched, early diastolic murmur heard most clearly at the apex with the patient in the left lateral decubitus position (S_3) may indicate hypervolemia and heart failure
3. **Laboratory assessment includes the following:**
   a. Serial serum electrolytes are important until stability is achieved.
   b. Urine electrolytes and osmolarity need to be drawn either before diuretics are given or no less than 12 hours after the last diuretic.
4. **Central venous monitoring:** This is especially helpful in patients with multisystem disease, elderly patients with limited cardiopulmonary reserve, and patients with a prior history of moderate to severe heart failure or COPD.

IV. ELECTROLYTE ABNORMALITIES

A. SODIUM

The daily requirements are 1 to 2 mEq/kg/day, and the normal serum sodium is 136 to 144 mEq/L.

3

FLUIDS, ELECTROLYTES, AND ACID-BASE MANAGEMENT

1. **Hyponatremia:** Obtain serum osmolality
   a. Hypertonic (osmotic) hyponatremia: Secondary to hyperglycemia or hypertonic infusions (glucose, mannitol, glycine). Na^+ decreases 1.6 mEq/L every 100 mg/dl increase in glucose or mannitol.
   b. Pseudohyponatremia: Excess plasma volume in nonaqueous phase resulting in false measurement of low sodium (e.g., hyperlipidemia; hyperproteinemia; or isotonic infusions of glucose, mannitol, or glycine). Current techniques using ion-selective electrodes measure only aqueous phase and do not result in this error.
   c. "True" (hypotonic) hyponatremia: Excess of free water relative to Na^+ (Table 3-6). Divide by clinical evaluation into hypovolemic (tachycardia, poor skin turgor, hypotension), isovolemic, and hypervolemic (edema).
      (1) Hyponatremia with hypervolemia: Often decreased *effective* volume stimulates ADH
         (a) Nephrotic syndrome
         (b) CHF
         (c) Cirrhosis
         (d) Iatrogenic overadministration of free water
      (2) Hyponatremia with isovolemia
         (a) SIADH
            (i) Tumors (especially small cell carcinoma of the lung)
            (ii) CNS disease (meningitis and encephalitis may affect the osmoreceptors that regulate ADH secretion)
            (iii) Pulmonary infections
            (iv) Drugs: clofibrate, cyclophosphamide, or chlorpropamide (increase ADH secretion or renal sensitivity to ADH)
         (b) Acute water intoxication
            (i) Psychogenic polydipsia
            (ii) Iatrogenic water administration
      (3) Hyponatremia with hypovolemia: Increase in ADH secretion because volume regulation takes priority over osmolarity regulation; have signs and symptoms of hypovolemia
         (a) Secretory diarrhea
         (b) Adrenal insufficiency
         (c) Salt-losing renal failure
      (4) CNS signs
         (a) Muscle twitching
         (b) Hyperactive tendon reflexes
         (c) Convulsions
         (d) Hypertension
   d. Acute hyponatremia—onset of symptoms occur when $Na^+ < 130$ mEq/L; gradual hyponatremia—symptoms occur when $Na^+ < 120$ mEq/L
   e. Evaluation
      (1) Serum and urine osmolarity
      (2) Urine sodium to see if renal loss (>20 mEq/L) or nonrenal loss (<10 mEq/L)

TABLE 3-6

HYPOTONIC HYPONATREMIA

	Hypovolemia		Isovolemia		Hypervolemia	
	U_{osm}	U_{Na}		U_{osm}	U_{Na}		U_{osm}	U_{Na}

Hypovolemia	U_{osm}	U_{Na}
GI losses	↑	↓
Third space losses	↑	↓
Diuretics	Iso	↑
Adrenal insufficiency	↑	↑

Isovolemia	U_{osm}	U_{Na}
H_2O intoxication	↓	↓
SIADH	↑	↑
Renal failure	Iso	↑
Postsurgical	↑	↑

Hypervolemia	U_{osm}	U_{Na}
CHF	↑	↓
Renal failure	Iso	↑
Cirrhosis	↑	↓
Nephrotic syndrome	↑	↓

3

FLUIDS, ELECTROLYTES, AND ACID-BASE MANAGEMENT

   f. Treatment
      (1) Treat the underlying cause of the hyponatremia.
      (2) Free water restriction is usually sufficient unless the cause is hypovo-
          lemic hyponatremia. In this case, treat volume deficits with isotonic
          fluids.
      (3) Use hypertonic sodium infusions only if the patient becomes acutely
          hyponatremic and is profoundly symptomatic. Serum sodium should
          (usually) only be corrected to 125 mEq/L.
      (4) Raise serum sodium 2 mEq/L/hr using a 3% NaCl at a rate of:

$$\frac{(2 \text{ mEq/L})(0.6 \times \text{body weight})}{513 \text{ mEq/L}} \times 1000 \text{ ml/hr}$$

      (5) Stop hypertonic saline when symptoms resolve because the risks of
          rapid correction of hyponatremia are permanent brain damage, sei-
          zures, and pontine myelinolysis.
      (6) Note that low serum sodium concentration can be an artifact of
          measurement. Hyperlipidemia and hyperproteinemia result in
          exclusion of sodium from a water-free space in the plasma
          sample.

 2. Hypernatremia
   a. Etiology: Table 3-7
      (1) Central diabetes insipidus: Renal water loss secondary to inadequate
          ADH secretion; causes include closed head injury, anoxic encepha-
          lopathy and meningitis
      (2) Nephrogenic diabetes insipidus: Insensitivity of renal collecting duct
          to ADH
      (3) Evaporation through the skin and from burn defects or profuse
          sweating from sepsis (sweat is hypotonic)
      (4) Evaporation through the lungs (e.g., inadequate vaporization of air in
          a ventilated patient)
   b. Symptoms: Restlessness, weakness, delirium, and maniacal behavior
   c. Signs
      (1) Dry, sticky mucous membranes
      (2) Decreased salivation
      (3) Decreased lacrimation
      (4) Red, swollen tongue
      (5) Elevated body temperature
   d. Evaluation and treatment
      (1) Hypernatremia is usually limited by thirst mechanism if there is
          access to free water.
      (2) Slowly replace the lost water after calculation of water deficit:

$$\text{Water deficit (L)} = (0.6 \times \text{body weight})\left[\frac{\text{current } P_{Na^+}}{140} - 1\right]$$

TABLE 3-7

HYPERNATREMIA

	Hypovolemia Water loss > Na$^+$ loss			Isovolemia Loss of water		Hypervolemia Na$^+$ gain > water gain	
	U$_{osm}$	U$_{Na}$		U$_{osm}$			
Diuretics	→	←	Central diabetes insipidus	<200	Adrenal hyperfunction		
Glycosuria (HNKC)	→	→	Nephrogenic diabetes insipidus	200-500	Iatrogenic hypertonic fluid administration		
Urea diuresis	→	←	Reset osmostat	variable			
Renal failure	→	←	Skin loss	↑			
Adrenal insufficiency	←	←					
GI, respiratory, skin water losses	←	→					

HNKC, Hyperosmolar nonketotic coma.

3

FLUIDS, ELECTROLYTES, AND ACID-BASE MANAGEMENT

(3) If an intracranial process is suspected, check urine and serum osmolarity. Diabetes insipidus results in dilute urine (<200 mOsm) despite a concentrated serum (>320 mOsm).

(4) If patient is alert and given access to water, desmopressin (1-deamino-8-arginine vasopressin; DDAVP) is an ADH analogue that can be given intranasally (10-40 μg qd or divided in 2-3 doses) as a long-term management to prevent complications of polyuria (bladder distention, hydroureter, and hydronephrosis).

(5) If patient is not alert or is unable to have free access to water because of other injuries, replace the lost free water slowly and begin DDAVP 1-2 μg SC/IV bid.

(6) If the cause is nephrogenic diabetes insipidus, give the patient thiazide diuretics and initiate salt restriction.

B. POTASSIUM

The daily requirements are 0.5 to 1.0 mEq/kg/day, and the normal serum potassium concentration is 3.5 to 5.0 mEq/L.

1. Hypokalemia
a. Etiology
  (1) Transcellular shift
    (a) β-Agonists
    (b) Metabolic alkalosis: Correction factor for potassium is 0.6 mEq/L K^+ per 0.1 pH unit
  (2) Potassium depletion
    (a) Renal loss
    (b) Diuretics
    (c) Osmotic diuresis (as in diabetic ketoacidosis)
    (d) Hyperaldosteronism
    (e) Renal tubular acidosis
    (f) Gastrointestinal loss (vomiting, diarrhea, fistula)
b. Symptoms: Weakness, ileus, tetany, vasoconstriction, and cardiac arrhythmias (especially with digoxin)
c. Treatment
  (1) Oral potassium if possible
  (2) Intravenous potassium at a maximum rate of 20 to 40 mEq/hr; replacement depends on total deficit:

Serum K^+ (mEq/L)	K^+ deficit (mEq)
3-4	100-200
2-3	200-400

2. Hyperkalemia
a. Etiology
  (1) Inadequate renal excretion of potassium: Renal failure, hypoaldosteronism, or diuretics that inhibit potassium secretion
  (2) Shift of potassium from the intracellular compartment (at the time of cell death)

b. Cardiac manifestations: ECG—changes progress from peaked T waves to prolonged PR interval, followed by decrease in P wave size; QRS complex widens, and T wave merges with QRS complex to form a "sine wave"; finally followed by ventricular fibrillation
c. CNS manifestations: Paralysis and confusion
d. Therapy: Depends on the severity of the hyperkalemia
   (1) If ECG changes are present:
      (a) Calcium gluconate: 10 ml of a 10% solution intravenously to stabilize the myocardial membrane and block the effect of potassium on the heart
      (b) Insulin and glucose: 10 to 15 U regular insulin (Humulin) in 50 to 100 ml of $D_{50}W$ intravenously to drive the potassium into cells until it is removed from the body
      (c) Potassium trapping resins: e.g., sodium polystyrene sulfonate (Kayexalate) (20 to 60 g in 100 to 150 g sorbitol), orally or as a retention enema
      (d) Dialysis: Necessary in refractory cases
   (2) If potassium is 5.0 to 6.5 mEq/L, without ECG changes:
      (a) Monitor ECG and stop all potassium administration
      (b) Treat underlying cause

C. CALCIUM

The daily intake is 800 to 1200 mg/day (2% of adult body weight is calcium), and the normal plasma calcium is 9.0 to 10.5 mg/dl. The normal ionized calcium level is 1.12 to 1.23 mmol/L.

1. Calcium metabolism

a. Calcium is nearly equally divided between the ionized (50%) and protein-bound phase (45%), with the remainder (5%) bound to lactate, bicarbonate, phosphate, sulfate, or citrate; 80% of protein-bound calcium is bound to albumin and the remainder to globulins. For every 1 g/dl decrease in albumin lower than 4.0 g/dl, subtract 0.8 mg/dl from the serum calcium.
b. The distribution of calcium is a function of body fluid pH and albumin concentration. One pH unit change results in a 1.7-unit change in ionized calcium (mg/dl).
c. Measurement of ionized calcium is a more accurate reflection of physiology.
d. The proximal small bowel is the site of active calcium absorption of most of the daily calcium intake. Passive calcium absorption occurs in the distal small bowel.
e. There is a regulated renal excretion of calcium of 100 to 400 mg/day.

2. Hypocalcemia

a. Etiology
   (1) Sepsis
   (2) Renal failure
   (3) Acute pancreatitis

       (4) Severe hypomagnesemia

       (5) Hypoparathyroidism

       (6) Vitamin D deficiency

  b. Symptoms: Tetany

       (1) Peripheral and perioral paresthesias

       (2) Carpal spasm

       (3) Seizures

       (4) Bronchospasm; laryngospasm

       (5) Chvostek's sign

       (6) Trousseau's sign

  c. Treatment

       (1) Acute management: Calcium gluconate IV (10 to 20 ml 10% solution) over 10 to 15 minutes, then titrate with IV drip (6 to 8 10-ml amps of 10% calcium gluconate in 1 L of D_5W). Calcium chloride (5 to 10 ml 10% solution) preferred for cardiac resuscitation but can cause soft tissue necrosis if extravasates.

       (2) Chronic management

          (a) Calcium carbonate: Initially 1 to 2 g PO tid, then 0.5 to 1 g PO tid

          (b) Vitamin D: Dihydroxy-vitamin D_3 (0.25 to 1 mg PO qd) or vitamin D_2 (50,000 to 100,000 U PO qd)

3. Hypercalcemia

  a. Etiology

       (1) Hyperparathyroidism

       (2) Malignancy (breast, lung, kidney, colon, thyroid, multiple myeloma)

       (3) Sarcoidosis

       (4) Vitamin D intoxication, vitamin A intoxication

       (5) Milk-alkali syndrome

       (6) Thyrotoxicosis

       (7) Adrenal insufficiency

       (8) Immobilization

       (9) Idiopathic hypercalcemia of infancy

      (10) Paget's disease

      (11) Thiazide diuretics

  b. Manifestations

       (1) Muscle weakness

       (2) Nausea and vomiting, resulting in hypovolemia

       (3) Weight loss

       (4) Fatigue, drowsiness

       (5) Confusion

  c. Acute therapy (basic management principles): Hypercalcuria causes osmotic diuresis and causes hypovolemia; focus on restoring intravascular volume and maximizing renal clearance of calcium with loop diuretics

       (1) If serum calcium < 12 mg/dl, hydrate with normal saline solution and give low-dose diuretic.

(2) If serum calcium > 15 mg/dl, rapidly volume load with 5 to 6 L of NS and administer high-dose diuretic. Place a central venous catheter and maintain a CVP at 10 cm H_2O while carefully monitoring for hypokalemia, hypomagnesemia, and pulmonary edema.

(3) If serum calcium = 12 to 15 mg/dl, clinical judgment should determine the appropriate management based on the above algorithm.

d. Chronic therapy

(1) Mithramycin: Administer 25 mg/kg IV qd for 3 to 4 days and then repeat at 1-week or more intervals. The effects are seen within 12 hours, and risks include thrombocytopenia, hepatocellular necrosis, and decreased clotting factors.

(2) Corticosteroids: Administer hydrocortisone 250 to 500 mg IV q8h or prednisone 40 to 100 mg PO. The effects are seen in several days.

(3) Calcitonin: Administer 4 IU/kg and increase to 8 IU/kg q6h. Use if rehydration, salt loading, and furosemide fail.

(4) Phosphate: Phosphate is reserved as the final therapeutic option. Oral Neutra-Phos 250 mg tid to qid or 100 ml Fleet retention enema can be used to elevate the serum phosphate level to reduce calcium mobilization from bone and decrease gut absorption of calcium. Oral supplementation is much safer than intravenous administration. IV supplementation (1500 mg over 6 to 8 hours) should be used only emergently and only to restore a normal phosphate level. The risks of IV phosphate are fatal hypocalcemia, renal cortical necrosis, metastatic calcification, and fatal shock. Never give IV phosphate if the patient is hyperphosphatemic.

D. MAGNESIUM

The daily requirements are 300 to 400 mg/day, and the normal serum magnesium is 1.3 to 2.1 mEq/L.

1. Hypomagnesemia: Very often unrecognized. Serum levels do not correlate well with body Mg^{++} stores. Have high index of suspicion and recognize clinical signs.

a. Etiology

(1) Diuretic and aminoglycoside use

(2) Alcoholism: hypomagnesemia can be severe in acute ETOH withdrawal

(3) Renal magnesium wasting resulting from systemic and intrinsic renal disease

(4) Extracellular fluid expansion caused by hyperaldosteronism and SIADH

(5) Osmotic diuresis resulting from glycosuria: Depletes magnesium body stores

b. Manifestations

(1) Other electrolyte abnormalities

(a) Refractory hypokalemia: must correct Mg^{++} before fixing hypokalemia

(b) Hypocalcemia, hyponatremia, hypophosphatemia

      (2) Arrhythmias: May potentiate digitalis toxicity; Mg^{++} administration can help control post-MI or other intractable arrhythmias

      (3) Weakness, including respiratory muscles

      (4) Muscle fasciculations

      (5) Tremors

      (6) Personality changes

      (7) Vertigo

      (8) Seizures

  c. Treatment

      (1) Acute management: For seizures or tetany, give 1 to 2 g of magnesium sulfate as 10% solution over 15 minutes, then 1 g IM q4-6h depending on clinical setting. If patellar reflexes are absent, stop replacement.

      (2) Moderate depletion: 6 g $MgSO_4$ over 3 hours, then follow up with 5 g over each 12 hours for 5 days.

      (3) Chronic management: Administer magnesium oxide 1200 mg PO qd.

2. Hypermagnesemia

a. Etiology: Poisoning after oral or rectal administration of antacids or cathartics in the setting of renal failure

b. Manifestations: Usually associated with magnesium >4.0 (magnesium >12 may be fatal)

    (1) Refractory hypotension

    (2) Flaccid paralysis

    (3) Decreased reflexes

    (4) Hypothermia

    (5) Coma

    (6) Respiratory failure

c. Treatment: 10 ml of 10% calcium gluconate repeated as necessary (calcium antagonizes magnesium's effect on nerves and muscle); hemodialysis in refractory cases

E. PHOSPHATE

The daily requirements are 800 to 1200 mg/day, and the normal serum phosphate is 2.5 to 4.3 mg/dl.

1. Phosphate homeostasis

a. Serum calcium and phosphate vary inversely.

b. Most of the body stores are in the teeth and bones.

c. Intestinal absorption of phosphate is 80% to 90% efficient.

2. Hypophosphatemia

a. Etiology

    (1) Respiratory alkalosis

    (2) Diabetic ketoacidosis

    (3) Dextrose infusions: in alcoholic or otherwise debilitated patients

    (4) Sepsis

    (5) Follows TPN administration if phosphate is not included initially

    (6) Phosphate loss in the urine from renal tubular insufficiency

    (7) Hepatic resection

b. Symptoms
   (1) Anorexia
   (2) Dizziness
   (3) Bone pain
   (4) Muscle weakness
   (5) Hyporeflexia
   (6) Paresthesias
   (7) Cardiac failure, respiratory failure
   (8) Seizures
   (9) Coma
c. Associated findings
   (1) Rhabdomyolysis
   (2) Decreased phagocytosis
   (3) Platelet dysfunction
   (4) Hemolysis
d. Treatment
   (1) If the patient has mild hypophosphatemia (1-2.5 mg/dl), treat the cause and consider giving Neutra-Phos 500 PO bid-tid.
   (2) If the patient has severe hypophosphatemia (<1 mg/dl), give IV sodium or potassium phosphate 2.5 to 5 mg/kg in 100 D_5W over 6 hours at 17 ml/hr via a central venous catheter. Repeat this procedure until the phosphate level is > 2.0 mg/dl. The risks of IV phosphate include hypocalcemia, metastatic calcification, and hypotension.

3. Hyperphosphatemia
a. Symptoms: No definite symptoms, although prolonged elevations lead to abnormal calcium phosphate deposits.
b. Treatment: Aluminum hydroxide antacids

V. ACID-BASE MANAGEMENT

Normal blood pH is maintained at 7.37 to 7.43 to allow optimal function of cellular enzymes, clotting factors, and contractile proteins. This regulation is possible because of intracellular buffers, extracellular buffers, and respiratory compensation. Normal values for arterial and venous blood are shown in Table 3-8.

A. INTRACELLULAR BUFFERS

1. Proteins, Hgb, bone, and organic phosphates serve as intracellular buffers.

2. Approximately 50% of the H^+ generated by nonvolatile acids diffuses within minutes to hours into cells where it is buffered by proteins, bone, and organic phosphates.

TABLE 3-8

NORMAL ACID-BASE VALUES

	pH	H^+	Pco_2 (mm Hg)	HCO_3^- (mEq/L)
Arterial	7.37-7.43	37-43	36-43	22-26
Venous	7.32-7.38	42-48	42-50	23-27

3. **H_2CO_3 is almost entirely buffered intracellularly by deoxygenated Hgb within red cells.**

B. **EXTRACELLULAR BUFFERS**

Bicarbonate-carbonic acid system

1. **In extracellular fluids,** acids (inorganic acids, such as hydrochloric, sulfuric, and phosphoric acids; and organic acids, such as lactic, pyruvic, and keto acids) combine with sodium bicarbonate to form the sodium salt of the acid and carbonic acid.

2. **Carbonic acid then dissociates into water and CO_2,** and CO_2 is excreted in the lungs. Because it is in equilibrium with CO_2, H_2CO_3 is called a volatile acid. The following equation represents this process:

$$CO_2 + H_2O \leftrightarrow H^+ + HCO_3^-$$

3. **The acid anion is excreted by the kidney with hydrogen or ammonium ions.** Extracellular fluid pH is determined by ratio of base bicarbonate to the amount of carbonic acid in the blood. At a pH of 7.4, this ratio is 20:1. Regardless of the absolute values, a ratio of 20:1 keeps the pH at 7.4. This process is defined by the Henderson-Hasselbalch equation:

$$pH = 6.1 + \log \frac{[HCO_3^-]}{Pco_2 \times 0.03}$$

4. **Changes in Pco_2 or HCO_3^- will change the ratio and alter pH.**

5. **Physiologic compensation for changes in pH serve to limit the extent of the acidemia or alkalemia** as calculated above. For example, a fall in $HCO_3^- \rightarrow$ fall in pH $\rightarrow$ stimulate increases respiration $\rightarrow$ fall in $Pco_2 \rightarrow$ increase ratio $\rightarrow$ increased pH. See Table 3-9.

6. **Figure 3-1** shows a nomogram useful for *simple* acid-base disorders. Note that this will not work for combined disorders.

7. **H_2SO_4 and H_3PO_4 are produced through protein catabolism and incomplete oxidation of fat and carbohydrates.** Because they are not in equilibrium with CO_2, they are called nonvolatile acids. H_2CO_3 that is generated by oxidative metabolism cannot be buffered by the bicarbonate—carbonic acid system because the addition of H^+ and HCO_3^- regenerates H_2CO_3.

VI. ABNORMALITIES IN ACID-BASE METABOLISM

A. **RESPIRATORY ACIDOSIS**

Increase in serum Pco_2 secondary to hypoventilation

1. **Mechanism:** Increased $Pco_2 \rightarrow$ increased $H_2CO_3 \rightarrow$ decreased ratio $\rightarrow$ decreased pH.

2. **Acute compensation:** Intracellular buffers $\rightarrow$ increase in HCO_3^- (1 mEq/L for each 10 mm Hg rise in CO_2). Any elevation of HCO_3^- above 30 mEq/L suggests a metabolic alkalosis as well.

3. **Chronic compensation:** Acid salts are excreted by the kidneys over the next 2 to 3 days in exchange for bicarbonate. This leads to an increased

TABLE 3-9

EXPECTED COMPENSATION FOR SIMPLE ACID-BASE DISORDERS

Primary Disorder	Initial Change	Compensatory Response	Expected Compensation
Metabolic acidosis	$\downarrow HCO_3^-$	$\downarrow Pco_2$	$Pco_2 = 1.5 [HCO_3^-] + 8 \pm 2$ Pco_2 = last 2 digits of pH
Metabolic alkalosis	$\uparrow HCO_3^-$	$\uparrow Pco_2$	$Pco_2 = 0.9 [HCO_3^-] + 9$ $Pco_2 \uparrow 0.6$ mm Hg each mEq/L $\uparrow HCO_3^-$
Respiratory acidosis	$\uparrow Pco_2$	$\uparrow HCO_3^-$	Acute: $\uparrow [HCO_3^-]$ 1 mEq/L every 10 mm Hg $\uparrow Pco_2$ Chronic: $\uparrow [HCO_3^-]$ 3.5 mEq/L every 10 mm Hg $\uparrow Pco_2$
Respiratory alkalosis	$\downarrow Pco_2$	$\downarrow HCO_3^-$	Acute: $\downarrow [HCO_3^-]$ 2 mEq/L every 10 mm Hg $\downarrow Pco_2$ Chronic: $\downarrow [HCO_3^-]$ 5 mEq/L every 10 mm Hg $\downarrow Pco_2$

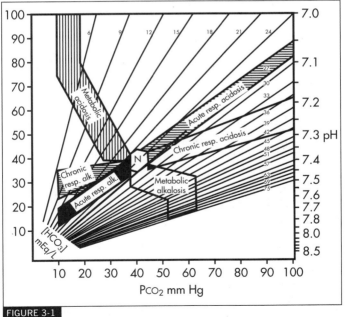

FIGURE 3-1

Nomogram for simple acid-base disorders.

ratio, which in turn leads to an increased pH. This process increases HCO_3^- by 3 to 4 mEq/L for each 10 mm Hg rise in Pco_2.

4. **Differential diagnosis includes the following:**
   a. Acute CNS suppression (drugs, stroke, sleep apnea, O_2 therapy in COPD)
   b. Chronic CNS suppression (tumor, obesity)
   c. Impaired respiratory muscle function
   d. Airway obstruction
   e. Impaired pulmonary gas exchange (pneumonia, ARDS, pneumothorax, COPD)
   f. Inadequate ventilator settings or ventilator dysfunction
5. **Treatment:** The decision to urgently intubate a patient should be based on physical examination and should not require evaluation of the blood gas. Time spent waiting on the laboratory values in a patient who is dyspneic, obtunded, and with obvious signs of increased work of breathing (i.e., accessory muscle use, diaphragmatic breathing, and intercostal muscle retractions) only jeopardizes the patient.

B. RESPIRATORY ALKALOSIS

Decrease in serum Pco_2 secondary to hyperventilation

1. **Mechanism:** Decreased $Pco_2 \rightarrow$ decreased $H_2CO_3 \rightarrow$ increased ratio $\rightarrow$ increased pH.
2. **Acute compensation:** Buffers (intracellular and extracellular) compensate, allowing HCO_3^- to decrease 1 to 2 mEq/L for each 10 mm Hg fall in Pco_2. This compensation will allow HCO_3^- to fall to as low as 18 mEq/L.
3. **Chronic compensation:** Acid salts are resorbed by the kidneys in exchange for bicarbonate, which is excreted. This leads to a decreased ratio, which in turn leads to a decreased pH. This allows HCO_3^- to decrease 4 to 5 mEq/L for each 10 mm Hg fall in Pco_2.
4. **Differential diagnosis includes the following:**
   a. Ventilator settings in excess
   b. Hypoxemia
   c. Sepsis
   d. Medications (salicylates, progesterone, catecholamines, theophylline)
   e. CNS process (CVA, infection, tumor, trauma)
   f. Cirrhosis
   g. Psychogenic hyperventilation
5. **Symptoms:** These include lightheadedness, cramps, circumoral numbness, acral paresthesias, and altered mental status.
6. **Treatment:** Assess ventilator settings and rule out hypoxemia. Consider the other diagnoses listed above, and address the underlying cause.

C. METABOLIC ACIDOSIS

Decrease in serum HCO_3^- resulting in retention or gain of acid or a loss of bicarbonate

1. **Mechanism:** Decreased $HCO_3^- \rightarrow$ decreased ratio $\rightarrow$ decreased pH.
2. **Acute compensation:** Increased alveolar ventilation $\rightarrow$ decreased $Pco_2 \rightarrow$ decreased $H_2CO_3 \rightarrow$ Restores ratio $\rightarrow$ increased pH. This compensation results in a 1 to 1.3 mm Hg fall in Pco_2 for each 1 mEq/L decline in HCO_3^-.

3. **Symptoms and signs:** These include lethargy, confusion, cool extremities, arrhythmias, hyperkalemia, and pulmonary hypertension.
4. **Evaluation:** Determine anion gap (anion gap = $[Na^+] - [Cl^-] - [HCO_3^-]$). Normal anion gap is 8 to 12 mmol/L.
5. **Differential diagnosis:** See Table 3-10.
6. **Causes of lactic acidosis:** See Box 3-1; normal lactate is 0.5 to 1.5 mEq/L.
7. **Treatment includes the following:**

a. Stabilize the intensive care patient while efforts to correct the underlying process proceed. Optimize the volume status, correct hypoxemia, and evaluate for sepsis, cardiac failure, and renal failure. Rule out diabetic ketoacidosis.
b. Administer sodium bicarbonate if pH < 7.2 after calculation of base deficit:

$$\text{Base deficit} = 0.4 \times \text{weight (kg)} \times [\text{desired } HCO_3^- - \text{measured } HCO_3^- \text{ (mEq/L)}].$$

c. Give half of the calculated deficit and then follow serial blood gases as you titrate the $NaHCO_3$ to raise pH > 7.2. Optimizing the volume status and oxygenation of the patient, as well as treating the underlying cause, will usually prevent the need for exclusive use of $NaHCO_3$ to completely correct the pH.
d. If $NaHCO_3$ is given too aggressively, the CO_2 produced (upon buffering H^+) can diffuse intracellularly and result in myocardial intracellular acidosis and cardiac dysfunction. This CO_2 production and shift can also cause cerebral suppression.

TABLE 3-10

DIFFERENTIAL DIAGNOSIS OF METABOLIC ACIDOSIS

Normal Anion Gap	Elevated Anion Gap
Inability to excrete acid	Ketoacidosis
Distal renal tubular acidosis	Diabetes
Addison's disease	Starvation
Hypoaldosteronism	
Excessive loss of HCO_3^-	
GI fistula (biliary/pancreatic)	Drugs or ingestions
Diarrhea	Methanol
Proximal renal tubular acidosis	Ethylene glycol
Ureterosigmoidostomy	Salicylates
Early renal failure	Paraldehyde
Carbonic anhydrase inhibitors	
Administration of acid	Uremia
Blood transfusions	
Ammonium chloride	
Arginine hydrochloride	
Hyperalimentation	Lactic acidosis (see Box 3-1)

FLUIDS, ELECTROLYTES, AND ACID-BASE MANAGEMENT

3

BOX 3-1

DIFFERENTIAL DIAGNOSIS OF LACTIC ACIDOSIS

I. Increased lactate production

A. Increased pyruvate production
   1. Enzymatic defects in glycogenolysis or gluconeogenesis
   2. Respiratory alkalosis

B. Impaired pyruvate utilization
   1. Decreased activity of pyruvate dehydrogenase or pyruvate decarboxylase
      a. Congenital
      b. ? role of diabetes mellitus, Reye's syndrome

C. Altered redox state favoring pyruvate conversion to lactate
   1. Enhanced metabolic rate
      a. Grand mal seizure
      b. Severe exercise
      c. Hypothermic shivering
   2. Decreased O_2 delivery
      a. Shock (cardiogenic, septic, hypovolemic)
      b. Asphyxia ($Pao_2 < 30$ mm Hg)
      c. CO poisoning
      d. Cardiac arrest
   3. Reduced O_2 utilization
      a. Cyanide intoxication (high-dose SNP)
      b. ? Phenformin
   4. D-Lactic acidosis (abnormal gut flora)

II. Primary decrease in lactate utilization

A. Liver disease

B. Alcoholism

C. Severe acidemia (pH < 7.1)

III. Mechanism uncertain

A. Diabetes mellitus

B. Malignancy

C. Hypoglycemia

D. Idiopathic

---

   e. Other side effects of $NaHCO_3$ administration include hypernatremia, hypokalemia, hyperosmolarity, and fluid overload. Monitor serum potassium after $NaHCO_3$ administration.

D. METABOLIC ALKALOSIS

Increase in serum HCO_3^- secondary to a loss of fixed acid or a gain of bicarbonate

1. **Mechanism:** Increased HCO_3^- → increased ratio → increased pH.
2. **Compensation (mainly renal):** Acid salts (such as chloride) are resorbed by the kidneys in exchange for bicarbonate, which is excreted. This leads to a decreased ratio, which in turn leads to a decreased pH.

3. **Respiratory compensation (occasionally):** Respiratory compensation → decreased alveolar ventilation → increased Pco_2 → increased H_2CO_3 → restores ratio → decreased pH. Appropriate compensation by hypoventilation leads to a 5 to 7 mm Hg rise for each 10 mEq/L elevation in HCO_3^-.

4. **Evaluation:** Determine the volume status of the patient by physical examination, urine output, and CVP monitoring. Hypovolemic patients typically have low urine chloride and will respond to saline therapy.

5. **Differential diagnosis includes the following:**
   a. Hypovolemic and low urine chloride (<10 mEq/L)
   b. Loss of gastric fluid (emesis or NG aspirate)
   c. Diuretic therapy, which mediates a contraction alkalosis
   d. Hypomagnesemia
   e. Relief of prolonged hypercapnia
   f. Bicarbonate therapy of organic acidosis
   g. Administration of bicarbonate-producing organic salts (citrate, lactate, acetate)
   h. Milk-alkali syndrome
   i. Severe hypokalemia
   j. Excess mineralocorticoid (exogenous steroids, Cushing's syndrome, ACTH-secreting tumors, hyperaldosteronism, renal artery stenosis)

6. **Treatment includes the following:**
   a. For all alkalotic states, hypokalemia must be avoided. Potassium is in competition with hydrogen ions for resorption of sodium at the level of the renal tubule. In alkalosis, preferential excretion of potassium in exchange for sodium allows conservation of hydrogen ions. If renal tubule potassium is insufficient because of low serum potassium, hydrogen ions cannot be resorbed and alkalosis will persist. In hypokalemic metabolic alkalosis (commonly seen after prolonged emesis) the renal tubule prioritizes sodium resorption to restore volume status. Consequently, potassium and hydrogen are excreted, which leads to "paradoxic aciduria" and further alkalosis. Volume and potassium replacement should be performed concurrently.
   b. If hypovolemia and low urine chloride are present, correct volume state with saline infusion and appropriate potassium supplementation to raise potassium to 4.5 to 5.0 mEq/L.
   c. Histamine antagonists can diminish hydrogen ion secretion in gastric contents.
   d. If isovolemia and high urine chloride are present, eliminate the excess mineralocorticoid and correct potassium to 4.5 to 5.0 mEq/L or magnesium to 2.0 mEq/L.
   e. If severe alkalosis is present, acetazolamide 250 to 500 mg IV can cause bicarbonate excretion.

f. As a final option in the setting of severe renal failure or life-threatening metabolic alkalosis (pH > 7.6, $HCO_3^- > 40$ mEq/L), give 0.1 N HCl via a central venous catheter after calculation of chloride deficit:

$$\text{Chloride deficit (mEq)} = (20\% \times \text{body weight}) \times (\text{normal plasma chloride} - \text{actual plasma chloride})$$

g. Infuse 100 mEq of HCl/L at a rate no faster than 125 ml or 2 mEq/kg/hr. Slower infusions are preferable and serial ABGs are vital in monitoring these patients. Complications include hemolysis and tissue necrosis.

SUGGESTED READINGS

Lyerly HK, Gaynor JW, editors: *Handbook of surgical intensive care: practices of the surgical residents of the Duke University Medical Center,* ed 3, St Louis, 1992, Mosby.

Marino PL: *The ICU book,* ed 2, Baltimore, 1998, Williams & Wilkins.

CARDIOPULMONARY RESUSCITATION

Alan P. Kypson

I. BASIC LIFE SUPPORT

The initiation of basic life support (BLS) begins with the assessment of the patient, determination of unresponsiveness, and activation of emergency medical services (EMS). The health care provider then follows the ABCs of BLS. The major objective is cardiopulmonary support to maintain tissue perfusion until personnel trained in advanced cardiac life support (ACLS) arrive.

A. AIRWAY

To determine if the patient is breathing, one must do the following:

1. Position patient supine on a firm, flat surface.

2. Open airway (tongue is most common cause of airway obstruction in unconscious patient).

a. Head tilt–chin lift

b. Jaw-thrust maneuver (safest approach in suspected neck injury)

B. BREATHING

1. Determine breathlessness—look, listen and feel: if the patient resumes breathing, roll to recovery (decubitus) position to maintain airway patency; if not, perform rescue breathing

2. Methods

a. Mouth-to-mouth: Simplest technique

b. Mouth-to-mask: The use of a barrier device to protect the health care provider from patient secretions

c. Bag-valve-mask: Optimal method of supporting ventilation in the hospital setting because 100% oxygen may be delivered to the patient

d. Cricoid pressure: Useful adjunct when an assistant is available to prevent gastric distention, regurgitation, and aspiration during cardiopulmonary resuscitation (CPR)

3. Goals of ventilation

a. Deliver two initial breaths to determine whether there is upper airway obstruction, followed by 10 to 12 breaths per minute. If attempts to ventilate are unsuccessful, reposition patient's head. If still unable to ventilate, proceed with airway obstruction management.

b. Approximate tidal volume is 800 to 1200 ml.

c. Allow 1.5 to 2 seconds for exhalation.

C. CIRCULATION

1. Determine pulselessness (carotid or femoral)

2. Chest compressions

a. Patient must be in a supine position.

b. Use a backboard when available for more efficient chest compressions.

c. Position your hands over the xiphoid process so that the heel of one hand rests on the sternum and the other hand is positioned over the first hand—fingers should be off the chest.

d. With elbows locked and shoulders positioned directly over the hands, compress the chest 1½ to 2 inches at a rate of 80 to 100 compressions per minute, using the hips as a fulcrum.

e. Adequacy of chest compressions is judged by the presence of a carotid or femoral pulse.

f. Chest compressions must be coupled with appropriate rescue breathing for successful resuscitation (15:2 ratio in one-rescuer CPR and 5:1 in two-rescuer CPR).

D. ONE-RESCUER CPR

See Figure 4-1.

E. TWO-RESCUER CPR

See Figure 4-2.

F. PEDIATRIC CONSIDERATIONS

1. **Epidemiology of cardiopulmonary arrest is different from adults;** trauma (motor vehicles, pedestrian injuries, bicycle injuries, drowning, and firearm injuries) and foreign-body airway obstruction are the leading causes of cardiopulmonary arrest in infants (<1 year) and children (1 to 8 years).

2. **Airway:** Assess and open as in the adult patient.

3. **Breathing**

a. If the victim is an infant, place mouth over infant's nose and mouth.

b. If the victim is a large infant or child, use mouth-to-mouth seal.

c. The correct volume for each breath is the volume that causes the chest to rise.

d. Rescue breathing is one breath every 4 seconds in children and every 3 seconds in infants.

4. **Circulation**

a. Palpation of the brachial artery is recommended in infants.

b. In children the carotid artery can be used for the pulse check.

5. **Chest compressions**

a. In infants the area of compression is the lower half of the sternum using the index and middle fingers. Depth of compressions should be about ½ to 1 inch at a rate of *at least* 100 times per minute.

b. In children the area of compression is the lower half of the sternum using the heel of the hand. Depth of compressions should be about 1 to 1½ inches at a rate of 100 times per minute.

II. ADVANCED CARDIAC LIFE SUPPORT

ACLS includes specific training of health care providers to continue BLS and stabilize the patient hemodynamically using appropriate pharmacologic and electrical therapy. Certification includes training and testing in the recognition and management of cardiac arrhythmias and use of airway adjuncts, defibrillator/cardioverter units, transcutaneous and transvenous pacemakers.

A. AIRWAY/BREATHING

1. **Oxygen:** Use as soon as possible; because oxygen content and delivery are compromised during distress, a system that provides 100% oxygen concentration should be used

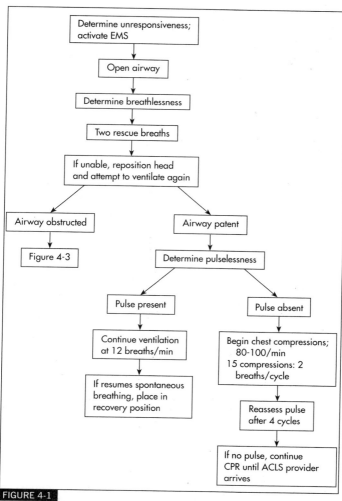

FIGURE 4-1

One-rescuer CPR.

2. Airway management/adjuncts

a. Head tilt–chin lift or jaw-thrust maneuver should be attempted before any airway adjunct is used.

b. Oropharyngeal airway: Can be used in patients who are not intubated to maintain airway patency. Holds the tongue away from the posterior wall

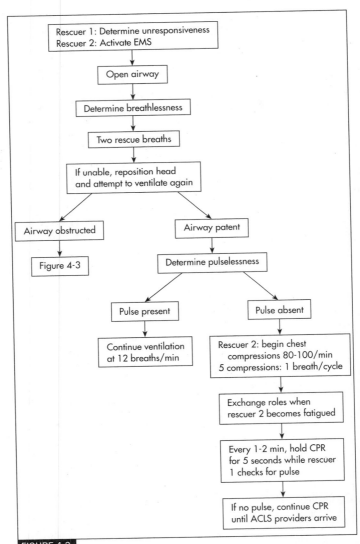

FIGURE 4-2

Two-rescuer CPR.

of the pharynx. Should only be used in the unconscious patient because it may stimulate vomiting or laryngospasm in the conscious or semiconscious patient.

c. Nasopharyngeal airway: Can be used when insertion of oropharyngeal airway is difficult or impossible. Can be used in the semiconscious patient.

d. Bag-valve-mask: Useful alternative to mouth-to-mouth breathing because oxygen may be easily added into the circuit and disease transmission is less likely between rescuer and patient. Must maintain airway patency and provide leakproof seal to the face to be most effective.

e. Endotracheal intubation: Should be performed as soon as possible by appropriately trained personnel to isolate the airway, keep it patent, reduce risk of aspiration, provide access for suctioning and drug delivery, and ensure delivery of high concentration of oxygen with selected tidal volume to maintain adequate lung inflation.

f. Cricothyrotomy: Acceptable emergency airway in the setting of severe facial trauma or when airway control is not possible by other methods.

3. Airway obstruction (Figure 4-3)

a. Foreign-body obstruction usually occurs during eating. In adults, meat is the most common cause of obstruction, whereas in children, small objects are the most frequent cause. In non–foreign-body obstruction, the tongue is the most common cause.

b. The patient is unable to ventilate and is clutching the neck (universal distress sign).

c. Symptoms include coughing, wheezing, and inability to phonate. If gas exchange worsens with increasing distress, stridor, and cyanosis, treat as a total airway obstruction.

d. Do not interfere with patient's efforts to expectorate the foreign body. If the patient is unsuccessful in clearing the foreign body, activate EMS.

e. The Heimlich maneuver is performed from behind the patient with the fist of one hand placed with the thumb against the abdominal wall. The other hand is placed on top of the fist, and a brisk upward abdominal thrust is delivered. If the patient is supine, the rescuer should straddle the victim and use the heel of one hand with the other hand on top to perform abdominal thrusts. Hands must be positioned in the midline above the umbilicus and below the xiphoid process to prevent potential complications.

f. Chest thrusts are reserved for gravid and markedly obese patients and are similar to performing chest compressions during CPR.

g. The use of the finger sweep (tongue-jaw lift and insertion of index finger to sweep the oropharynx) may remove the foreign body. Reserve this method for the unconscious victim only.

B. APPLICATION OF ACLS ALGORITHMS

1. It is essential to perform ACLS algorithms as soon as possible. Appropriate application of the monitor to the patient and arrhythmia recognition is central to ACLS.

4

CARDIOPULMONARY RESUSCITATION

2. **Defibrillation paddles should be positioned with one over the sternum and the other lateral to the left nipple at the midaxillary line.** Acceptable alternatives include the use of a back paddle placed posteriorly behind the heart and an anterior paddle placed over the precordium. A conductive gel must be applied to the paddles before defibrillation to decrease the resistance at the paddle-skin interface.

3. **Peripheral access is the first choice during CPR** and is usually a more-than-adequate route for administering necessary drugs. Central access,

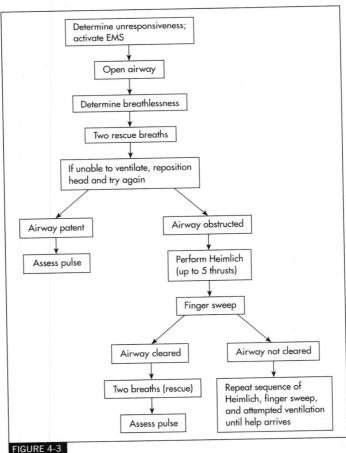

FIGURE 4-3
Foreign-body airway obstruction algorithm.

when available, provides faster drug delivery to the heart and peripheral circulation. In the temporary absence of IV access, use the endotracheal tube to deliver *a*tropine, *l*idocaine, *i*soproterenol, *e*pinephrine, and *n*aloxone (mnemonic ALIEN). Intraosseous access is also a valid, temporary route to administer fluids and medications, especially in children.

4. **Frequently used agents in ACLS:** See Table 4-1.
5. **Universal approach to the patient:** See Figure 4-4.
6. **Ventricular fibrillation/pulseless ventricular tachycardia:** See Figure 4-5.
7. **Pulseless electrical activity:** See Figure 4-6.
8. **Asystole:** See Figure 4-7.

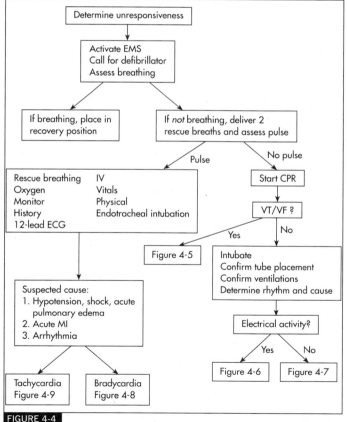

FIGURE 4-4

Universal approach for adult ACLS.

CARDIOPULMONARY RESUSCITATION

4

TABLE 4-1

FREQUENTLY USED AGENTS IN ACLS

Drug	Action	Indication	Dose (IV)
Adenosine	Depresses SA and AV nodes	PSVT	6 mg, then 12 mg 1-2 min later
Aminone	Phosphodiesterase inhibitor	Refractory CHF	0.75 mg/kg over 2-3 min; infusion 2-15 μg/kg/min
Atropine	Vagolytic	Bradyasystolic arrest, symptomatic bradycardia, first-degree AVB, Mobitz type II	0.5-1.0 mg every 3-5 min to 3 mg total
Bretylium	Sympatholytic	Refractory VT/VF	5 mg/kg, then 10 mg every 5-30 min to 35 mg/kg max; infusion of 2 mg/min
Calcium chloride	Direct inotrope	Hyperkalemia, hypocalcemia, Ca^+ channel blocker toxicity	2-4 mg/kg every 10 min
Diltiazem	Ca^{++} channel antagonist	PSVT, to slow ventricular response in atrial fibrillation/flutter	0.25 mg/kg, then 0.35 mg/kg 15 min later; infusion 5-15 mg/hr
Dobutamine	β-agonist	RV infarct, CHF	Infusion 2-20 μg/kg/min
Dopamine	Mixed α-, β-, DA-agonist	Hypotension	Infusion 2-20 μg/kg/min
Epinephrine	Mixed α-, β-agonist	VF, pulseless VT, PEA	1 mg every 3-5 min, then up to 0.1 mg/kg every 3-5 min; Infusion 2-10 μg/min

		...pulmonary significant tachycardia, brady-cardia in transplanted heart	2-10 µg/min
Lidocaine	Type Ib antiarrhythmic	VT, VF	1-1.5 mg/kg, then 0.5-1.5 mg/kg to 3 mg/kg max load; infusion 2-4 mg/min
Nitroglycerin	Direct vasodilator	CHF in patients with ischemic heart disease	12-25 µg: infusion 10-500 µg/min
Nitroprusside	Direct peripheral vasodilator	Hypertensive emergency, acute LVF	Infusion 0.1-8.0 µg/kg/min
Norepinephrine	Mixed α-, β-agonist	Refractory hypotension	Infusion 2-30 µg/min
Procainamide	Type Ia antiarrhythmic	Persistent arrest due to VF, PVC and VT not controlled with lidocaine, SVT	20-30 mg/min to a max dose of 17mg/kg; infusion 1-4 mg/min
Sodium bicarbonate	Corrects acidosis	Severe metabolic acidosis, hyperkalemia	1 mEq/kg, then 0.5 mEq/kg every 10 min
Verapamil	Ca++ channel antagonist	PSVT to slow ventricular response in atrial fibrillation/flutter	2.5-5 mg over 1-2 min, then 5-10 mg every 15-30 min to a max of 30 mg

SA, Sinoatrial; *AV*, atrioventricular; *PSVT*, paroxysmal supraventricular tachycardia; *CHF*, congestive heart failure; *AVB*, atrioventricular block; *VT*, ventricular tachycardia; *VF*, ventricular fibrillation; *RV*, right ventricle; *DA*, dopamine; *PEA*, pulseless electrical activity; *LVF*, left ventricular failure; *PVC*, premature ventricular contraction; *SVT*, supraventricular tachycardia.

CARDIOPULMONARY RESUSCITATION

4

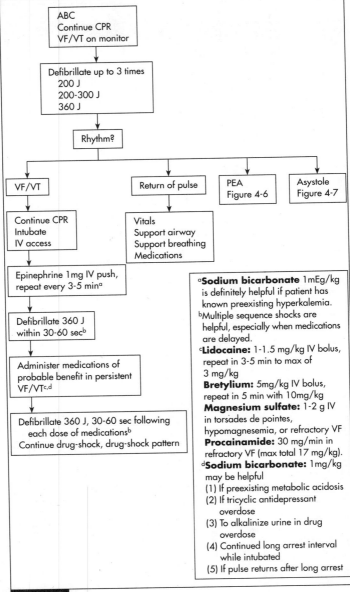

FIGURE 4-5

Ventricular fibrillation/pulseless ventricular tachycardia algorithm.

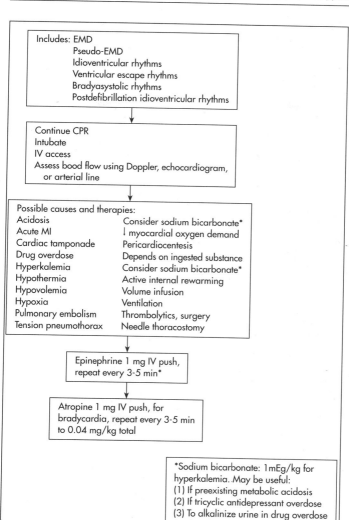

FIGURE 4-6

Pulseless electrical activity algorithm.

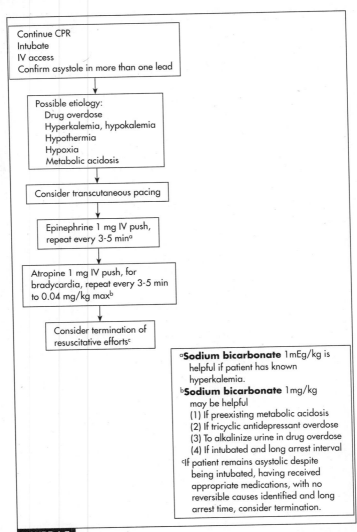

Continue CPR
Intubate
IV access
Confirm asystole in more than one lead

↓

Possible etiology:
  Drug overdose
  Hyperkalemia, hypokalemia
  Hypothermia
  Hypoxia
  Metabolic acidosis

↓

Consider transcutaneous pacing

↓

Epinephrine 1 mg IV push,
repeat every 3-5 min[a]

↓

Atropine 1 mg IV push, for
bradycardia, repeat every 3-5 min
to 0.04 mg/kg max[b]

↓

Consider termination of
resuscitative efforts[c]

[a]**Sodium bicarbonate** 1mEg/kg is
  helpful if patient has known
  hyperkalemia.
[b]**Sodium bicarbonate** 1mg/kg
  may be helpful
  (1) If preexisting metabolic acidosis
  (2) If tricyclic antidepressant overdose
  (3) To alkalinize urine in drug overdose
  (4) If intubated and long arrest interval
[c]If patient remains asystolic despite
  being intubated, having received
  appropriate medications, with no
  reversible causes identified and long
  arrest time, consider termination.

FIGURE 4-7
Asystole algorithm.

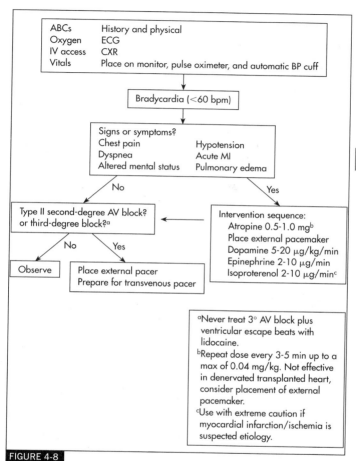

ABCs	History and physical
Oxygen	ECG
IV access	CXR
Vitals	Place on monitor, pulse oximeter, and automatic BP cuff

Bradycardia (<60 bpm)

Signs or symptoms?
Chest pain — Hypotension
Dyspnea — Acute MI
Altered mental status — Pulmonary edema

No → Yes →

Type II second-degree AV block?
or third-degree block?[a]

No → Observe

Yes → Place external pacer
Prepare for transvenous pacer

Intervention sequence:
Atropine 0.5-1.0 mg[b]
Place external pacemaker
Dopamine 5-20 μg/kg/min
Epinephrine 2-10 μg/min
Isoproterenol 2-10 μg/min[c]

[a]Never treat 3° AV block plus ventricular escape beats with lidocaine.
[b]Repeat dose every 3-5 min up to a max of 0.04 mg/kg. Not effective in denervated transplanted heart, consider placement of external pacemaker.
[c]Use with extreme caution if myocardial infarction/ischemia is suspected etiology.

FIGURE 4-8

Bradycardia algorithm.

9. Bradycardia: See Figure 4-8.
10. Tachycardia: See Figure 4-9.
C. PEDIATRIC ALGORITHMS
1. Frequently used agents in pediatric advanced life support (PALS): See Table 4-2.
2. Bradycardia: See Figure 4-10.
3. Asystole and pulseless arrest: See Figure 4-11.

4

CARDIOPULMONARY RESUSCITATION

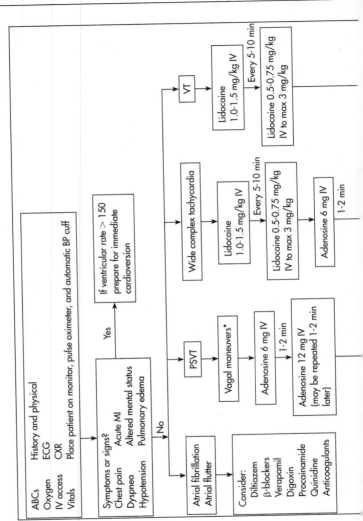

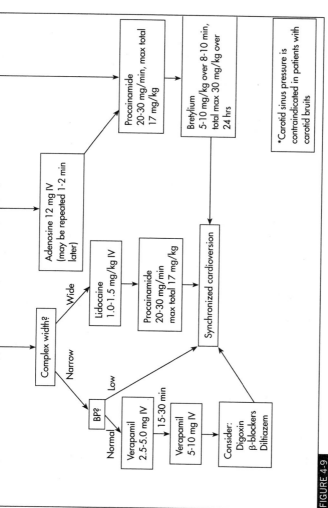

FIGURE 4-9
Tachycardia algorithm.

CARDIOPULMONARY RESUSCITATION

4

TABLE 4-2
FREQUENTLY USED AGENTS IN PALS

Drug	Action	Indication	Dose (IV)
Adenosine	Depresses SA and AV nodes	SVT	0.1-0.2 mg/kg, max single dose of 12 mg
Atropine*	Vagolytic	Symptomatic bradycardia	0.02 mg/kg, max dose of 0.5 mg in children and 1.0 mg in adolescents
Calcium chloride	Direct inotrope	Hypocalcemia, hyperkalemia	20 mg/kg
Dobutamine	β-agonist	CHF, especially in setting of ↑ SVR	2-20 μg/kg/min
Dopamine	Mixed α-, β-, DA-agonist	Hypotension	2-20 μg/kg/min
Epinephrine*	Mixed α-, β-agonist	Cardiac arrest, symptomatic bradycardia, hypotension not due to hypovolemia	0.01 mg/kg IV, IO; 0.1 mg/kg ET; repeat dose 0.1 mg/kg every 3-5 min; infusion of 0.1-1.0 μg/kg/min
Lidocaine*	Type Ib antiarrhythmic	Recurrent VT, VF, or symptomatic ventricular ectopy of unknown origin after resuscitation	1 mg/kg; infusion of 20-50 μg/kg/min
Naloxone*	Narcotic poisoning, respiratory depression, sedation, hypotension	Opiate antagonist	≤5 years old or ≤20 kg: 0.1 mg/kg; >5 years old or >20 kg: 2.0 mg
Sodium bicarbonate	Corrects acidosis	Severe acidosis due to prolonged resuscitation, hyperkalemia, tricyclic antidepressant overdose	1 mEq/kg/dose

*For endotracheal administration, dilute medication with NS to a volume of 3 to 5 ml.

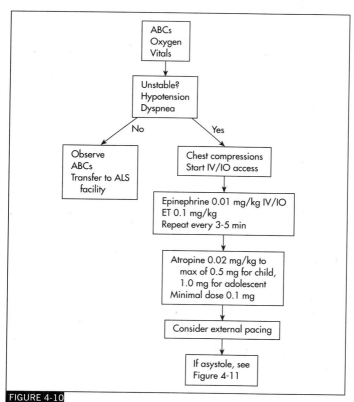

FIGURE 4-10

Pediatric bradycardia algorithm.

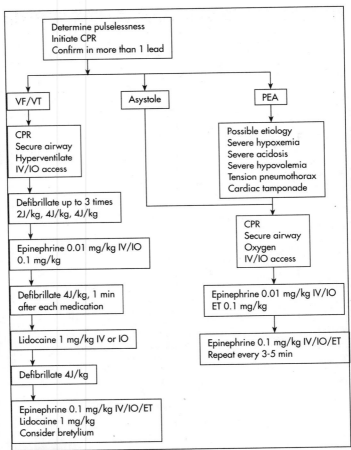

FIGURE 4-11
Pediatric asystole/pulseless arrest algorithm.

SUGGESTED READINGS

Chameides L, Hazinski MF, editors: *Pediatric advanced life support,* Dallas, 1997, American Heart Association.

Chandra NC, Hazinski MF, editors: *Basic life support for healthcare providers,* Dallas, 1997, American Heart Association.

Cummins RO, editor: *Advanced cardiac life support,* Dallas, 1997, American Heart Association.

Emergency Cardiac Care Committee and Subcommittees AHA: Guidelines for cardio-pulmonary resuscitation and emergency cardiac care. III: adult advanced cardiac life support, *JAMA* 268:2242-2250, 1992.

4

CARDIOPULMONARY RESUSCITATION

PROCEDURES

Lisa A. Clark

I. CONTROL OF THE AIRWAY

A. BAG-MASK VENTILATION

1. Indications: Immediate control of airway and ventilation

2. Equipment

a. Oxygen source

b. Ambu-bag, mask

c. Suction

3. Technique

a. Place patient in head-tilt or jaw-thrust position to open the airway.

b. Clear secretions.

c. Place mask over the mouth and nose, creating an air-tight seal.

d. Compress bag every 3 seconds.

e. Ensure that oxygen line is in place.

4. Complications and difficulties

a. Interference with spontaneous respiration

b. Emesis (cricoid pressure minimizes gastric air entry and emesis)

c. Failure of ventilation (auscultate, monitor oxygen saturation; proceed to endotracheal intubation as appropriate)

B. ENDOTRACHEAL INTUBATION

1. Indications

a. Unsuccessful bag-mask ventilation

b. Airway protection in an unresponsive patient

c. Respiratory insufficiency

d. Cardiopulmonary arrest

2. Equipment

a. Oxygen source

b. Bag and mask

c. Intravenous access, fluid, and medication for analgesia and sedation

d. Suction

e. Laryngoscope, several sizes of endotracheal tubes (generally 7.0 to 7.5 for women and 7.5 to 8.0 for men; children require a tube size according to the formula ([age + 4]/4) and malleable stylet

3. Technique—orotracheal approach

a. Place the patient supine, head tilted back.

b. Apply cricoid pressure.

c. Hyperventilate the patient with 100% oxygen using a bag and mask.

d. Ensure adequate analgesia and sedation.

e. Standing at the head of the patient, hold the laryngoscope in the left hand and open the patient's mouth, displace the tongue to the left, and advance the blade in the midline to the base of the tongue.

f. Visualize the vocal cords and the glottic opening, and place the endotracheal tube through the glottis opening, advancing the cuff 2 cm past the vocal cords into the trachea.

5

g. Inflate the cuff and secure the tube.

h. Auscultate breath sounds bilaterally, check end-tidal CO_2, and obtain a chest x-ray for positioning.

i. If intubation has not been achieved after 30 seconds, ventilate the patient again with 100% oxygen with the face mask before attempting again.

4. Technique—nasotracheal approach

a. It is necessary to have some respiratory effort to accomplish nasotracheal intubation.

b. Hyperventilate the patient with a bag and mask if necessary.

c. Anesthetize the largest naris with 4% aerosolized lidocaine solution.

d. Lubricate the endotracheal tube (½ to 1 size smaller than for orotracheal intubation) with K-Y Jelly or lidocaine jelly and slowly advance through the naris, following the breath sounds towards the trachea, advancing during each inspiration.

e. Inflate the balloon and auscultate.

5. Complications

a. Oropharyngeal and dental trauma

b. Tracheal laceration or rupture, vocal cord injury, avulsion of the arytenoid cartilage

c. Esophageal perforation, vomiting, and aspiration (risk is lessened with cricoid pressure)

d. Intubation of the right main stem bronchus (auscultate both axillae carefully after tube placement)

e. Intubation of the piriform sinus (nasal intubation is contraindicated in a patient with facial trauma)

C. EMERGENT CRICOTHYROIDOTOMY

1. Indications

a. Trauma to the oropharynx

b. Immediate airway management after unsuccessful endotracheal intubation

c. Upper airway obstruction

2. Equipment

a. Scalpel

b. Pediatric endotracheal tube or 14-gauge catheter-over-needle

c. Bag-valve unit with oxygen source

3. Technique—surgical cricothyroidotomy

a. Position the patient supine with the head extended but cervical spine protected in the trauma patient.

b. If time permits, prepare with antiseptic solution.

c. Palpate the cricothyroid membrane between the thyroid and cricoid cartilages.

d. Incise the skin and insert the knife through the cricothyroid membrane.

e. Insert the knife handle through the cricothyroidotomy and rotate 90 degrees.

f. Insert the pediatric endotracheal tube through the opening, inflate the cuff, and begin ventilation.

4. **Technique—needle cricothyroidotomy**
a. Puncture the cricothyroid membrane with a catheter-over-needle and remove the needle.
b. Mount the hub of the catheter with the barrel of a 12-ml syringe, which serves as a connector for oxygen, and begin ventilation.

5. **Complications**
a. Hemorrhage
b. Perforation of the esophagus
c. Inability to cannulate the trachea

D. NASAL PACKING FOR EPISTAXIS

1. **Indication:** Epistaxis unrelieved by 30 minutes of manual compression

2. **Equipment**
a. Ring forceps
b. Roll of 1- or 2-inch plain Nu-Gauze or Merocel pack

3. **Technique**
a. Obtain adequate IV access and give appropriate analgesia.
b. Correct any coagulation factor or platelet defects.
c. Use ringed forceps to tightly pack gauze into the naris or nares (be certain that one end of the gauze is accessible for later pack removal).
d. Remove 12 to 24 hours later with equipment available to repack, if needed.

4. **Complications**
a. Difficulty breathing and aspiration (intubation may be necessary, particularly when packing both nares)
b. Continued bleeding

II. ARTERIAL/VENOUS ACCESS

A. CENTRAL VENOUS CATHETERIZATION

1. **Indications**
a. Administration of fluids, vasoactive drugs, drugs that irritate veins, and total parenteral nutrition
b. Vascular access when peripheral access is poor
c. Hemodialysis and plasmapheresis
d. Central venous and pulmonary artery monitoring

2. **Equipment**
a. 18-gauge needle and guide wire (several centimeters longer than the catheter to be placed)
b. Catheter (single-, double-, or triple-lumen) or introducer-sheath combination
c. Antiseptic solution, cap, mask, sterile gloves, and sterile towels
d. Local anesthetic

3. **Technique—general**
a. Wear a cap, mask, and sterile gown and gloves, and prepare the skin with antiseptic solution.
b. Position supine and in Trendelenburg's position (15 degrees) for subclavian and jugular approaches.
c. Turn the patient's head away from the desired side of cannulation.

d. Determine the length for catheter placement (catheter tip in the superior vena cava) by measuring from the point of insertion to the angle of Louis (Figure 5-1).

e. Infiltrate the desired area with lidocaine.

f. Puncture the skin with the 18-gauge needle mounted on a 10-ml syringe, maintaining constant negative pressure, and advance slowly until blood appears, then disengage the syringe and cover the needle with a sterile gloved finger.

g. Insert the wire through the needle and advance slowly into the vein. (The wire should pass with minimal resistance over its entire length.)

h. Remove the needle over the guide wire and pass a dilator over the wire into the vein, retaining control of the guide wire.

i. Remove the dilator over the guide wire and thread the catheter over the guide wire, into the vein to the measured depth.

j. Remove the wire through the catheter and cap all ports.

k. To insert an introducer and sheath, enlarge the puncture site to 1 cm with a sterile blade before passing the introducer and sheath together over the wire.

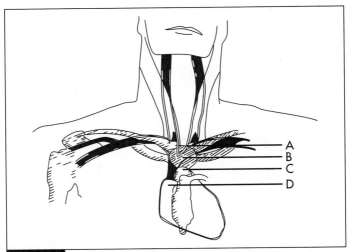

FIGURE 5-1

Superficial anatomic landmarks used to determine the depth of central venous catheters. **A,** Sternoclavicular joint subclavian vein. **B,** Manubrium brachiocephalic vein. **C,** Angle of Louis superior vena cava. **D,** Five centimeters inferior to Angle of Louis right atrium. *(From Kaye W: Intravenous techniques. In* Textbook of advanced cardiac life support, *Dallas, 1981, American Heart Association.)*

I. Aspirate and flush all ports of the catheter or sheath. Secure the catheter to the skin with a suture and dress with povidone-iodine ointment, sterile gauze, and clear polyurethane.

m. Verify the location of the catheter in the superior vena cava or cavoatrial junction with a chest x-ray.

4. Technique—internal jugular vein cannulation

a. Anatomy: As the internal jugular vein emerges at the base of the skull, it enters the carotid sheath posterior to the internal carotid artery and continues posterior and lateral to the common carotid artery until it crosses anterior to the common carotid artery near its termination. The internal jugular vein is medial to the sternocleidomastoid muscle superiorly, crossing deep to it and emerging at the triangle between the sternal and clavicular heads of the sternocleidomastoid. It continues behind the clavicular head, where it joins the subclavian vein (Figure 5-2).

b. Central approach:

   (1) Identify the triangle formed by the sternal and clavicular heads of the sternocleidomastoid muscle (Figure 5-3).

   (2) Insert the needle just lateral to the carotid pulse at the apex of the triangle of the sternocleidomastoid, directing the needle inferiorly and laterally along the medial aspect of the clavicular head toward the ipsilateral nipple.

5

PROCEDURES

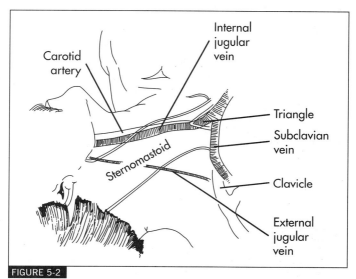

FIGURE 5-2

Anatomy of the internal jugular vein. *(From Kaye W: Intravenous techniques. In* Textbook of advanced cardiac life support, *Dallas, 1981, American Heart Association.)*

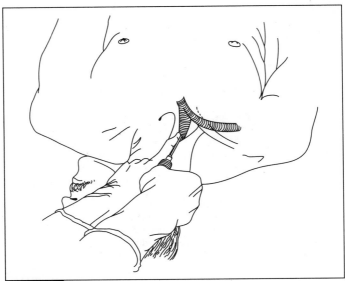

FIGURE 5-3

Anatomic landmarks for cannulation of the internal jugular vein using the central approach. *(From Kaye W: Intravenous techniques. In* Textbook of advanced cardiac life support, *Dallas, 1981, American Heart Association.)*

    (3) If the vein is not entered on the first pass (3 to 4 cm), maintain negative pressure in the syringe while slowly withdrawing the needle (in difficult cases a 22-gauge "seeker" needle may be useful in locating the jugular vein before inserting the 18-gauge needle).

    (4) When venous blood is encountered, remove the syringe and follow the Seldinger technique as described above.

  c. Posterior approach:

    (1) Introduce the needle deep to the lateral border of the sternocleidomastoid muscle, 5 cm superior to the clavicle, and just superior to the junction of the sternocleidomastoid and the external jugular vein (Figure 5-4).

    (2) Direct the needle inferiorly and anteriorly toward the suprasternal notch. If the vein is not entered on the first pass (5 cm), maintain negative pressure in the syringe while slowly withdrawing the needle. If venous blood is encountered, remove the syringe and follow the Seldinger technique as described previously. If venous blood is not encountered, reassess the landmarks and make a second pass. If arterial blood is encountered, immediately remove the needle and maintain pressure over the artery for 10 minutes before resuming.

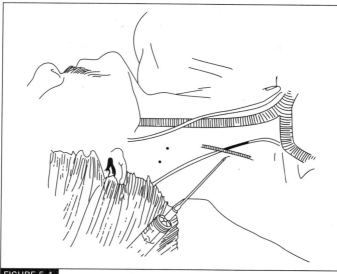

FIGURE 5-4

Anatomic landmarks for cannulation of the internal jugular vein using the posterior approach. *(From Kaye W: Intravenous techniques. In* Textbook of advanced cardiac life support, *Dallas, 1981, American Heart Association.)*

5. Technique—subclavian vein cannulation

a. Anatomy: The subclavian vein crosses over the first rib anterior to the anterior scalene muscle, which separates the subclavian vein and artery. The subclavian vein continues posterior to the medial third of the clavicle (to which it is attached) to join the internal jugular vein deep to the sternocostoclavicular joint (Figure 5-5).

b. Technique:

(1) Insert the needle 1 cm inferior to the junction of the middle and medial thirds of the clavicle. Direct the needle superiorly and medially, just deep to the clavicle and over the first rib, toward the suprasternal notch (Figure 5-6). If the vein is not entered on the first pass (5 cm), maintain negative pressure in the syringe while slowly withdrawing the needle.

(2) When venous blood is encountered, rotate the needle 90 degrees so that the bevel faces inferiorly. Remove the syringe and follow the Seldinger technique as described previously. If venous blood is not encountered, reassess the landmarks and make a second pass.

6. Technique—femoral vein access

a. Anatomy: The femoral vein lies immediately medial to the femoral artery

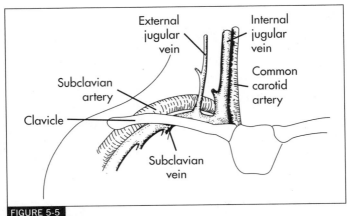

FIGURE 5-5

Anatomy of the subclavian vein. *(From Sladen A:* Invasive monitoring and its compli-cations in the intensive care unit, *St Louis, 1990, Mosby.)*

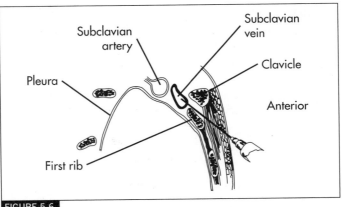

FIGURE 5-6

Sagittal section through the medial third of the clavicle. *(From Kaye W:* Intravenous techniques. In Textbook of advanced cardiac life support, *Dallas, 1981, American Heart Association.)*

  b. Technique:
    (1) Place two fingers of the nondominant hand on the pulse and after infil-tration of the area with 2 to 3 ml of local anesthetic, insert the needle approximately 2 cm medial to these fingers, several centimeters below the inguinal ligament at a 45-degree angle until blood returns easily.
    (2) Continue with the Seldinger technique, as described previously.

   c. Complications:
      (1) Pneumothorax
      (2) Arterial puncture (During needle insertion into the internal jugular or femoral vein, if arterial blood is encountered, immediately remove the needle and maintain pressure over the artery for 10 minutes before resuming. Compression is ineffective in the subclavian approach, thus it is important to ensure normal platelet count and coagulation parameters before attempting this procedure.)
      (3) Hematoma and hemothorax (remove the needle to the level of the skin before redirecting to avoid the laceration of blood vessels)
      (4) Air embolism (To treat suspected air embolism, place the patient in the left lateral decubitus position, administer 100% oxygen, attempt to aspirate the air through the catheter and consider hyperbaric oxygen [HBO] for a large, symptomatic embolus.)
      (5) Brachial plexus injury
      (6) Tracheal laceration
      (7) Subclavian vein thrombosis and sepsis (minimized by meticulous sterility of placement and care of lines)

B. INTRAOSSEOUS ACCESS

1. Indications: Impossible or insufficient IV access in a child less than 6 years of age

2. Equipment

a. Short, large-caliber bone-marrow aspiration needle or short 18-gauge spinal needle with stylet
b. Sterile gloves and antiseptic solution
c. Lidocaine

3. Technique

a. Position supine.
b. Pad an uninjured lower extremity to create a 30-degree angle at the knee.
c. Cleanse and infiltrate with local anesthesia 1 to 3 cm below the tibial tuberosity.
d. Insert the needle at this point at a 90-degree angle, with the bevel towards the foot.
e. Twist gently, advancing the needle through the bone cortex and into the bone marrow.
f. Remove the stylet and replace with a saline-filled syringe.
g. Draw back on the syringe to check for bone marrow. If no bone marrow returns, flush the needle gently with several milliliters of saline. If this flushes easily and without visible swelling, positioning is appropriate, and IV fluid may be started.
h. Cover with antibiotic ointment and a sterile dressing.
i. Remove as soon as the emergent resuscitation is complete and other access can be obtained.

4. Complications

a. Infection (use sterile technique and remove as soon as possible)
b. Hematoma (limit needle manipulation)

5

PROCEDURES

c. Physeal plate injury (insert the needle at least 1 to 2 cm from the tibial tuberosity)

C. GREATER SAPHENOUS VEIN CUTDOWN

1. **Indication:** Emergent need for medications and/or fluids and inadequate IV access

2. **Equipment**
   a. Sterile gloves, antiseptic solution
   b. Scalpel
   c. Hemostat
   d. 3.0 and 4.0 nonabsorbable suture
   e. 12- or 14-gauge IV catheter

3. **Technique**
   a. Locate the saphenous vein at the ankle, approximately 2 cm anterior and superior to the medial malleolus.
   b. Prepare the area with antiseptic solution and infiltrate with local anesthetic.
   c. Create a full-thickness skin incision, approximately 2.5 cm in length.
   d. Using a curved hemostat for blunt dissection, identify and isolate the vein, freeing it for a length of at least 2 cm.
   e. Ligate the distal vein with a 3.0 nonabsorbable suture, leaving the tie in place for gentle traction.
   f. Pass a tie around the proximal vein to hold in place while making a small transverse venotomy with a scalpel tip. Enlarge the venotomy slightly with the hemostats and slide the catheter into the vein.
   g. Ensure blood return and flush with saline.
   h. Secure with sutures proximal and distal on the vein.
   i. Close the skin around the site with interrupted 4.0 nonabsorbable sutures and cover with a sterile dressing.

4. **Complications**
   a. Infection (use sterile technique)
   b. Hematoma (minimize catheter manipulation)
   c. Damage to the nearby nerve and artery (avoided by knowledge of the anatomy and careful dissection)

D. PULMONARY ARTERY (PA) CATHETERIZATION

1. **Indications**
   a. Continuous hemodynamic monitoring in an unstable or potentially unstable patient
   b. To guide the fluid management in complicated patients, particularly those with right heart insufficiency
   c. Sampling of mixed venous (pulmonary arterial) blood for oxygen content
   d. Access to the right ventricle for cardiac pacing

2. **Equipment**
   a. Supplies for catheter sheath placement
   b. Pulmonary artery catheter
   c. Transducer, oscilloscope, and monitor (all calibrated)
   d. Cardiac defibrillator, lidocaine, and atropine (at bedside)

3. Technique

a. Ensure continuous ECG and IV access.

b. Sterile technique is used as previously described.

c. Cannulate the internal jugular vein or the subclavian vein using the Seldinger technique as described previously, and insert the catheter sheath.

d. After securing the sheath, thread the catheter through its sterile protective sleeve and ensure that the PA catheter has been properly flushed and that the balloon is functional.

e. With the balloon deflated, insert the catheter through the sheath to a depth of 20 ml.

f. Inflate the balloon and advance the catheter slowly while inspecting the ECG for arrhythmias and the pressure tracing for the succession of characteristic waveforms (Figure 5-7).

g. Once the proper position has been reached (pulmonary capillary wedge), the balloon is deflated. The tracing should return to that of the PA.

h. Draw the protective sleeve over the catheter and secure the connector. Verify the position. The disappearance of the characteristic PA waveform when the balloon is inflated and its prompt return when the balloon is deflated is mandatory. In addition, the oxygen saturation of blood samples drawn with the balloon inflated should be greater than that of systemic arterial blood.

i. Obtain a chest film to ascertain that the tip of the catheter is in a main branch of the PA and to rule out pneumothorax.

4. Complications

a. Cardiac arrhythmias (premature ventricular contractions, ventricular tachycardia, ventricular fibrillation, and right bundle branch block), readily treated by withdrawing the catheter and administering prepared antiarrhythmics or external cardiac pacing; a left bundle branch block is a relative contraindication to the use of a PA catheter because its passage may result in complete heart block; pulmonary hemorrhage and

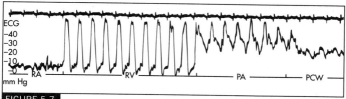

FIGURE 5-7

Succession of pressure waveforms observed during the advancement of pulmonary artery catheter through the right atrium (RA), right ventricle (RV), pulmonary artery (PA), and to the pulmonary capillary wedge (PCW) position. *(From Kaye W: Intravenous techniques. In* Textbook of advanced cardiac life support, *Dallas, 1981, American Heart Association.)*

5

PROCEDURES

pulmonary infarct (do not leave catheter in the "wedged" position, and ensure the catheter is not overwedged)

b. Catheter entanglement (follow tracings for advancement of catheter; if it becomes tangled, involve interventional cardiology or radiology; fluoroscopy may be useful for catheter placement in difficult cases)

c. Cardiac perforation or valvular damage (always deflate the balloon before withdrawing)

d. Endocarditis and sepsis (observe sterile technique in catheter placement and care)

E. ARTERIAL CATHETERIZATION

1. Indications

a. Continuous monitoring of arterial pressure

b. Access for frequent arterial blood samples

2. Equipment

a. Appropriately sized catheter-over-needle

b. Flexible guide wire

c. Antiseptic solution, sterile gloves, towels, razor, and surgical soap

d. Lidocaine (1% solution without epinephrine)

e. Pressure tubing, transducer, and monitor

3. Technique—arterial cannulation

a. Wearing sterile gloves, shave and prepare the area with antiseptic solution.

b. Infiltrate the region with local anesthetic.

c. Once the needle is successfully introduced into the artery, a Seldinger approach may be taken (as described previously) or the catheter may be advanced over the needle directly into the artery. If the artery cannot be cannulated in three attempts, discontinue the procedure and choose another site.

d. Remove the needle and attach the hub of the catheter to the pressure tubing. If arterial blood returns but cannulation is unsuccessful, withdraw the needle and maintain pressure for 5 to 10 minutes before resuming.

e. Secure the catheter to the skin with a suture or tape, apply antibiotic ointment, and cover with a sterile dressing.

4. Technique—radial artery cannulation

a. Perform Allen's test: Occlude the radial and ulnar arteries digitally until blanching of the hand is noted. Release the ulnar artery. Ulnar collateral circulation is considered inadequate if more than 5 seconds elapse before blushing of the hand occurs, in which case another site is selected.

b. Place the hand in dorsiflexion with a roll of gauze under the wrist and secure the palm and lower arm to the board.

c. Insert the 20-gauge needle-catheter over the radial pulse, just proximal to the head of the radius at a 30-degree angle to the skin with the bevel down. Advance the catheter and needle until blood appears at the hub of the needle, then proceed as above.

5. Technique—femoral artery cannulation

a. Anatomy: The femoral artery is found at the midpoint of a line between the anterior superior iliac spine and the symphysis pubis. Medial to the femoral artery is the femoral vein; lateral to the femoral artery is the femoral nerve.

b. Enter the skin several centimeters below the inguinal ligament at a 45-degree angle to a distance of 3 to 4 cm.

c. When arterial blood is encountered, proceed as described above.

6. Technique—dorsalis pedis artery cannulation

a. Anatomy: The dorsalis pedis artery, an extension of the anterior tibial artery, is found on the dorsum of the foot, parallel and lateral to the extensor hallucis longus. In 12% of the population, the dorsalis pedis artery is absent.

b. Demonstrate the presence of collateral flow by assessing the flow in the posterior tibial artery by palpation, or by using a Doppler flow meter.

c. Insert a 20-gauge needle-catheter over the palpable pulse at a 30-degree angle to the skin with the bevel down.

d. Advance the catheter and needle until blood appears at the hub of the needle, then proceed as described above.

7. Technique—axillary artery

a. Anatomy: The axillary artery is the continuation of the subclavian artery entering the axilla at the lateral border of the first rib; at the teres major muscle, it becomes the brachial artery. The axillary sheath contains the axillary artery, axillary vein, and the brachial plexus (Figure 5-8).

5

PROCEDURES

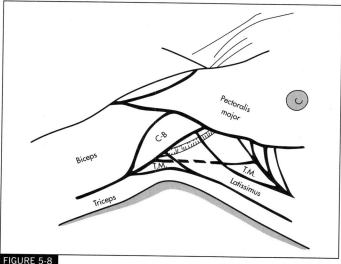

FIGURE 5-8

Anatomic landmarks for cannulation of the axillary artery. *C-B*, coracobrachialis muscle; *T.M.*, teres major muscle. *(From Sladen A:* Invasive monitoring and its complications in the intensive care unit, *St Louis, 1990, Mosby.)*

Interruption of flow in the axillary artery will not lead to ischemia in the arm because of extensive collateral flow from the thyrocervical trunk and the subscapular artery.

b. Hyperabduct, externally rotate, and immobilize the arm.

c. Enter the skin as high as possible in the axilla over the palpable pulse and proceed as above.

8. Complications

a. Thrombosis and thromboembolism

b. Distal ischemia (remove a catheter immediately when signs of distal ischemia appear; brachial artery cannulation is not recommended because of its inadequate collateral circulation and unacceptably high incidence of complications)

c. Hemorrhage and hematoma

d. Infection

e. Arteriovenous fistula

f. Neurologic complications (brachial plexus injury)

III. CARDIOTHORACIC PROCEDURES

A. PERICARDIOCENTESIS

1. Indications

a. Relief of cardiac tamponade emergently in patients with respiratory distress or progressive hypotension

b. To obtain fluid for diagnostic study

2. Equipment

a. Antiseptic solution, cap, mask, sterile gown, gloves, towels, and drapes

b. Lidocaine (1% solution without epinephrine)

c. 16-gauge (4-inch) needle, short-beveled attached to a 50-ml syringe

d. Sterile alligator connector (for ECG V-lead)

3. Technique

a. If the indication for pericardiocentesis is cardiac tamponade, the infusion of volume intravenously may improve cardiac performance until the pericardium can be drained.

b. Place the patient in the supine position.

c. Continuous ECG monitoring is mandatory.

d. Prepare the skin with antiseptic solution and create a sterile field with towels and drapes.

e. Connect the ECG V-lead to the needle with the sterile alligator clip. ST segment elevation during the procedure indicates ventricular contact with the needle, and PR segment elevation suggests atrial contact.

f. Infiltrate the skin and subcutaneous tissue to the left of the xiphoid process with lidocaine.

g. Insert the needle 1 cm to the left of the xiphoid at a 30-degree angle to the frontal plane while continuously aspirating the syringe. Advance the needle while observing the ECG. If grossly bloody fluid is obtained, assess it for coagulation. Clotting suggests intracardiac penetration, whereas pericardial fluid should not coagulate. If successfully entered, the pericardium should be completely drained. This may require the placement of a catheter, either through the needle or using a guide wire.

4. Complications

a. Cardiac arrhythmias

b. Cardiac puncture, myocardial or coronary artery laceration

c. Air embolism to a cardiac chamber or coronary artery

d. Pneumothorax

e. Hemorrhage

B. INTRAAORTIC BALLOON PUMP

1. Indications

a. Intractable cardiac failure after a cardiac surgical procedure

b. Refractory angina, despite maximal medical management

c. Perioperative treatment of the complications of myocardial infarction

d. Failed percutaneous coronary angioplasty and support during complex angioplasties

e. As a bridge to cardiac transplantation

The main contraindication to its use is severe aortic regurgitation.

Details regarding the indications and use of the intraaortic balloon pump are discussed in Chapter 16, and here only the placement of the device is presented.

2. Equipment

a. Long 18-gauge needle

b. 20-ml balloon catheter

c. 9-F sheath with guide wire

d. 3.0 nonabsorbable suture

3. Technique

a. The covered catheter is measured to the appropriate distance, from the insertion point at the groin to the sternal notch, and this distance is noted.

b. Prepare and drape the groin, and infiltrate local anesthetic over the femoral artery several centimeters distal to the inguinal ligament.

c. Insert the needle at this point, at a 45-degree angle into the femoral artery.

d. When pulsatile blood flow is returned, the syringe is removed, a guide wire is threaded to a point above the level of the iliac artery bifurcation, and the needle is withdrawn.

e. Enlarge the incision site to approximately 0.5 cm with a scalpel and insert the introducer sheath over a vessel dilator. If a dual-lumen IABP is used, it is threaded over the wire to the premeasured length. Single-lumen catheters require the removal of the guide wire before their insertion.

f. Withdraw the introducer sheath slightly to lessen the risk of iliac obstruction.

g. Position the sterile sleeve over the sheath and secure with 3.0 nonabsorbable suture. Cover with a sterile dressing.

h. Check a chest x-ray. The catheter should come to lie just distal to the origin of the subclavian artery.

4. Complications

a. Infection; use good sterile technique in catheter placement and care and remove as soon as possible.

b. Bleeding; minimize catheter manipulation, ensure that the femoral artery is punctured below the inguinal ligament, where direct pressure can stop any bleeding, and place the guide wire gently to avoid vessel wall penetration.

c. Ischemia of the ipsilateral limb can occur, at which point the stability of the patient must be assessed, weighing the risk of balloon pump removal against potential loss of the affected limb.

d. Thrombocytopenia may be induced by heparin or the pump itself.

e. Ischemia to the kidneys, spinal cord, or bowels may occur from balloon compression of end-organ blood flow and can be promptly treated by balloon repositioning, although the end-organ damage may be irreversible.

C. THORACENTESIS

1. Indications

a. To obtain a sample of pleural fluid for diagnosis

b. Drainage of a restricting pleural effusion and relieve respiratory compromise

2. Equipment

a. 18-gauge catheter-over-needle with a stopcock and 20-ml syringe

b. Extension tubing and collecting vessel

c. Antiseptic solution and sterile drapes

d. Lidocaine (1% solution without epinephrine)

3. Technique

a. Position the patient, if possible, in the sitting position, with the arms supported on a bedside table. (As an alternative, place the patient in the supine position, with the head of the bed elevated to 90 degrees.)

b. Locate the fluid level by percussion. Perform thoracentesis two interspaces below the percussed fluid level but not lower than the eighth intercostal space.

c. Prepare the skin with antiseptic solution and drape the field.

d. Infiltrate the skin with lidocaine using a 25-gauge needle. Anesthetize the deeper tissues with a 20-gauge needle, including the periosteum of the rib below the chosen intercostal space. While aspirating the syringe to avoid intravascular injection of lidocaine, enter the pleural cavity over the superior aspect of the rib, avoiding the intercostal neurovascular bundle. Administer lidocaine through the pleura; subsequent aspiration should confirm the presence of pleural fluid.

e. Remove the needle and reenter the pleural space with the catheter-over-needle attached to a syringe.

f. Remove the needle, covering the hub of the catheter to prevent pneumothorax. Mount the stopcock and the 20-ml syringe to the catheter.

g. For diagnostic purposes, aspirate fluid directly.

h. For drainage of a large effusion, connect the extension tubing to the stopcock, so the pleural fluid can be withdrawn into the syringe and ejected through the tubing into a collecting container. Upon completion of the procedure, place a small sterile dressing.

i. Obtain a chest film to document the removal of the pleural fluid and the absence of pneumothorax.

j. The pleural fluid is collected under sterile conditions and analyzed for differential cell count, Gram's stain and bacterial culture, fungal and mycobacterial culture, cytology, protein and glucose, amylase, LDH, and pH.

4. Complications

a. Pneumothorax (maintain constant negative pressure on the syringe throughout the procedure)

b. Hemothorax (never manipulate the needle while it is within the pleural cavity)

c. Puncture of the lung, liver, or spleen (never puncture lower than the eighth intercostal space)

d. Postexpansion pulmonary edema (limit removal to 1-1.2 L)

D. TUBE THORACOSTOMY

1. Indications

a. Pneumothorax (greater than 20% in magnitude)

b. Hemothorax, hydrothorax, or chylothorax

c. Prophylaxis for high-risk patients before positive-pressure ventilation or after penetrating thoracic injury

2. Equipment

a. Thoracostomy tube (24 to 28 F for pneumothorax; 32 to 36 F for hemothorax)

b. Antiseptic solution; cap, mask, sterile gown, gloves, towels, and drapes

c. Lidocaine (1% solution without epinephrine)

d. Sterile instruments (knife, scissors, Kelly clamp)

e. Collection-suction apparatus

3. Technique

a. Position the patient in the supine.

b. The preferred site for tube thoracostomy is the fifth intercostal space in the anterior axillary line.

c. Prepare the skin with antiseptic solution wearing cap, mask, sterile gown, and sterile gloves.

d. Create a sterile field with towels and drapes, and measure the chest tube from the desired insertion site to the apex, noting the distance.

e. Infiltrate the skin with lidocaine using a 25-gauge needle. Anesthetize the deeper tissues using a 20-gauge needle, including the periosteum of the ribs above and below the chosen intercostal space. While aspirating the syringe to avoid intravascular injection of lidocaine, enter the pleural cavity over the superior aspect of the rib, avoiding the intercostal neurovascular bundle. Administer lidocaine through the pleura, and subsequent aspiration should confirm the presence of pleural air or fluid.

f. Remove the needle and incise the skin one interspace below the desired site of insertion. Create a subcutaneous tunnel with blunt dissection using the Kelly clamp. Enter the pleural space with the tip of the clamp, just over the superior margin of the rib; open the clamp, spreading the pleura.

g. With a gloved finger, confirm penetration into the chest by palpating the lung, sweeping away pleural adhesions if present.

h. Grasp the tip of the thoracostomy tube with the Kelly clamp, and insert both into the pleural space. Direct the tube posteriorly and superiorly for drainage of hemothorax or hydrothorax or anteriorly for pneumothorax. Ensure that the last hole in the tube is within the thoracic cavity.

i. Secure the tube to the chest wall with a suture and cover with a sterile dressing of petroleum-soaked gauze and sponges.

j. Inspect the collecting system for an adequate water seal and measure the amount of drainage. Inspect and secure all connections.

k. Obtain a chest film to assess the position of the catheter and the evacuation of air or fluid from the thoracic cavity.

4. Complications

a. Hemorrhage (minimize manipulation of instruments and thoracostomy tube in the pleural cavity)

b. Laceration of the lung or heart (performing a finger sweep to assess for adhesions minimizes the risk)

c. Infection

d. Subcutaneous placement (use the nondominant hand to palpate the tube as it enters the pleural cavity)

e. Reexpansion pulmonary edema (limit removal to 1000 ml of fluid at one time)

f. Intraperitoneal placement (placement at the fifth intercostal space should eliminate this possibility)

IV. GASTROINTESTINAL PROCEDURES

A. NASOGASTRIC TUBE PLACEMENT

1. Indications

a. Gastrointestinal decompression in the case of intubation, gastroparesis, or intestinal obstruction

b. Feeding and medications in the patient unable to take nutrition or medication orally

2. Equipment

a. 18-F nasogastric tube

b. Lidocaine jelly and cotton-tipped swabs

c. 60-ml catheter tip syringe

3. Technique

a. Saturate the tips of several cotton-tipped swabs with lidocaine jelly and place in the posterior nasopharynx to anesthetize the region, then remove.

b. If possible, tilt the patient's head forward, which will make passage down the GI tract more direct.

c. Lubricate the end of the NG tube and pass straight back through the largest naris.

d. When the tube reaches the nasopharynx, ask the patient to swallow, which will facilitate the movement of the tube down the esophagus. Some discomfort and a gagging feeling is common, but if the gagging sensation progresses to the inability to speak, the catheter is likely in the airway and should be withdrawn until the patient is able to speak. Another attempt can then be made.

e. Once the tube reaches the stomach, a catheter tip syringe filled with air is connected to the tube, air injected and the abdomen auscultated to confirm placement. If there is any question of placement, obtain a KUB to confirm placement.

4. Complications

a. Bleeding from the nares is common in small amounts but may be profuse in the patient with a coagulopathy. Direct pressure is usually sufficient to stop the bleeding, but nasal packing may be required if pressure is ineffective.

b. Inadvertent placement into the lung. This is more common in the comatose patient. Tilting the head forward during placement will help avoid this, and it is imperative to check position by auscultation and KUB each time a tube is placed in a patient with a diminished level of consciousness.

B. NASODUODENAL TUBE

1. Indication: Inability to take oral feeds and the presence of gastroparesis and/or significant aspiration risk

2. Equipment

a. Nasoduodenal tube with a central, removable wire

b. Lubricating jelly

c. 10-ml syringe filled with air

3. Technique

a. The placement of this tube is identical to the nasogastric tube until the tube reaches the stomach, at which time the patient should be placed (when possible) in the right lateral position to facilitate movement of the tube through the pylorus.

b. Very slowly advance the tube, allowing normal gastric motility and pyloric opening to carry it into the duodenum. The position of the tip can be monitored by periodically injecting air and auscultating over the abdomen.

c. Once the tube has passed the pylorus, the loudest sounds will no longer be heard in the stomach but over the right upper quadrant.

d. At this point, an additional 10 cm of tubing should be advanced through the nose to encourage the tube as far into the duodenum as possible.

e. The position should then again be assessed by auscultation, and in any patient with altered mental status, a KUB should be obtained before the initiation of feeds.

f. After the KUB is checked, the inner wire is removed and feeding is begun.

4. Complications: Similar to those of NGT placement

5

PROCEDURES

C. SENGSTAKEN-BLAKEMORE TUBE

1. **Indication:** Compression of endoscopically proven variceal hemorrhage by tamponade of the gastroesophageal junction

2. **Equipment**
   a. Sengstaken-Blakemore tube
   b. Suction apparatus
   c. 50-ml syringe
   d. Pressure manometer
   e. Nasogastric and Ewald tubes
   f. Lubrication
   g. Supplies for endotracheal intubation

3. **Technique**
   a. Adequate fluid resuscitation should take precedence over attempts to treat upper gastrointestinal bleeding and placement may be performed in conjunction with other therapeutic modalities in the management of variceal hemorrhage.
   b. Most patients will require intubation, and this should be accomplished before tube placement.
   c. Place the patient in the left lateral decubitus position.
   d. Empty the stomach by passing a large orogastric or Ewald tube.
   e. Test the balloons of the Sengstaken-Blakemore tube carefully before insertion.
   f. Lubricate the tube well and pass nasally to the 50-cm mark.
   g. Fill the gastric balloon with 150 to 200 ml of air or a dilute radiocontrast solution and clamp the tube. Using gentle traction, withdraw the tube until resistance is encountered at the gastroesophageal junction. Secure the tube to the patient's face under minimal traction.
   h. Irrigate the distal tube with saline. In the absence of continued bleeding, leave the esophageal tube deflated. If bleeding has not ceased, inflate the esophageal balloon to 40 torr.
   i. Pass a nasogastric tube through the contralateral nostril until resistance is sensed at the level of the esophageal balloon. Continuously aspirate the blind esophageal segment to prevent regurgitation and aspiration of esophageal secretions.
   j. Obtain a chest film to confirm correct positioning.
   k. The esophageal tube may remain deflated in the absence of bleeding but should be inflated to 40 torr if bleeding ensues in the first 24 hours after placement. The balloon(s) of the Sengstaken-Blakemore tube remain inflated for 24 hours and are then deflated if no further bleeding has occurred. The tube may be removed after a second 24-hour period without bleeding.

4. **Complications**
   a. Esophageal rupture secondary to malposition of the gastric balloon
   b. Aspiration of blood, gastric secretion, or saliva
   c. Refractory variceal hemorrhage

D. PARACENTESIS
1. Indications
a. To evaluate for spontaneous bacterial peritonitis
b. Relief of severe ascites causing respiratory compromise
2. Equipment
a. 20-gauge catheter-over-needle with stopcock and 50-ml syringe
b. Extension tubing and collecting vessel
c. Antiseptic solution, sterile gloves, and drapes
d. Lidocaine (1% solution without epinephrine)
3. Technique
a. Place the patient supine.
b. Confirm the presence of fluid by percussion.
c. The preferred site for paracentesis is lateral to the rectus abdominis muscle in the lower abdomen.
d. Prepare the skin with antiseptic solution and drape the field. Infiltrate the skin with lidocaine using a 25-gauge needle. Anesthetize the deeper tissues with the 20-gauge needle, making the needle track discontinuous using the Z-track technique.
e. While aspirating the syringe, advance the needle through the fascia and into the peritoneum until ascitic fluid returns; remove the needle.
f. Insert the catheter-over-needle in the same manner; when ascitic fluid is encountered again, advance the catheter and remove the needle.
g. Attach a three-way stopcock and the 50-ml syringe. For diagnostic purposes, aspirate fluid directly. For drainage of massive ascites, connect extension tubing to the stopcock so that fluid may be withdrawn into the syringe and ejected through the tubing into a collecting container.
h. Remove the catheter and place a sterile dressing.
i. The ascitic fluid is collected under sterile conditions and may be analyzed for differential cell count, Gram's stain and bacterial culture, fungal and mycobacterial culture, cytology, protein and glucose, amylase, LDH, and pH.
4. Complications
a. Hemorrhage
b. Infection
c. Bowel or bladder perforation (ultrasound guidance can be helpful in a patient suspected to have adhesions; a Foley catheter will decrease the risk of bladder perforation)
d. Persistent ascitic leak
e. Hypotension (secondary to withdrawal of excessive volume; many advocate the administration of albumin during the procedure to avoid this)

E. TENCKOFF CATHETER INSERTION
1. Indications
a. Temporary management of acute renal insufficiency
b. Long-term management of end-stage renal disease with continuous ambulatory peritoneal dialysis

2. Equipment

a. Tenckhoff catheter and obturator; detachable trocar and obturator; priming trocar or priming catheter; Faller guide

b. Cap; mask; sterile gown, gloves, towels, and drapes; antiseptic solution

c. Lidocaine (1% solution without epinephrine)

d. Sterile instruments (knife, scissors, clamps, forceps)

e. Peritoneal dialysis fluid and administration tubing

3. Technique

a. Contraindications to the insertion of a peritoneal dialysis catheter at the bedside include extreme obesity and previous abdominal surgery.

b. Place the patient in the supine position. The preferred site for placement is in the midline, inferior to the umbilicus.

c. Wear a cap, mask, sterile gown, and sterile gloves, create a sterile field with towels and drapes, and prepare the skin with antiseptic solution.

d. Infiltrate the skin and subcutaneous tissue with lidocaine.

e. Make a 3-cm midline incision 2 cm inferior to the umbilicus. Using blunt dissection, identify the linea alba and provide upward traction with a suture or a clamp.

f. Enter the peritoneum with a catheter-over-needle or trocar. Connect the priming catheter or trocar to the administration tubing and instill approximately 2 L of dialysis solution.

g. Lubricate the Tenckhoff catheter, its obturator, and the Dacron cuffs with sterile saline; insert the obturator into the Tenckhoff catheter. Remove the priming catheter or trocar and insert the detachable trocar and obturator. After correct positioning within the peritoneum, remove the obturator from the trocar.

h. Insert the Tenckhoff catheter and its obturator through the trocar into the peritoneum, directing the catheter deeply into the pelvis. Remove the trocar over the catheter, and then detach it. Remove the obturator from the catheter, and position the inner Dacron cuff to rest at the fascial level.

i. Test the catheter for patency. Secure the catheter to the fascia. Create an exit site lateral and inferior to the entrance with a stab wound so that the subcutaneous cuff is 2 cm below the skin; this site should be just large enough for the catheter.

j. Create a subcutaneous tunnel with the Faller guide, and carefully pull the end of the catheter through the tunnel; insert the titanium connector.

k. Suture the insertion wound and apply sterile dressings.

4. Complications

a. Bleeding from the abdominal wall (recognized as bloody effluent, this occurs in 30% of the cases)

b. Dialysis solution leaks, inadequate drainage, or extraperitoneal extravasation (the most common cause of early catheter failure is omental entanglement resulting from placement anteriorly in the peritoneum rather than deeper in the pelvis; positioning the catheter deep in the pelvis and avoiding areas of intestinal adhesions lessen the risk)

c. Intestinal perforation and peritonitis (use an open technique for entering the abdomen)

F. DIAGNOSTIC PERITONEAL LAVAGE

1. Indications: Unexplained drop in hematocrit or hemodynamic instability in a patient with the potential for unexplained intraabdominal blood loss

2. Equipment

a. Mask, cap, sterile gown, gloves, and antiseptic solution
b. Lidocaine (1% with epinephrine)
c. Peritoneal dialysis catheter with trocar and tubing
d. 1000-ml bag of NS or lactated Ringer's solution with macrodrip extension tubing
e. Sterile instruments (tissue forceps, clamps, scalpel)
f. 3-0 suture

3. Technique

a. Place a Foley catheter to decompress the bladder (unless contraindicated).
b. Decompress the stomach with a nasogastric tube.
c. Prepare and drape the lower abdomen.
d. Anesthetize a region in the midline of the lower abdomen, one third of the distance from the umbilicus to the symphysis pubis.
e. Make a 2- to 3-cm vertical incision in the skin and subcutaneus tissue, down to the fascia.
f. Grasp the edges of the fascia and incise the peritoneum.
g. Insert the peritoneal dialysis catheter with trocar and direct deep into the pelvis.
h. Remove the trocar and place a purse-string suture around the catheter.
i. Withdraw fluid into a syringe. If it is grossly bloody, proceed to the operating room for exploration.
j. If the fluid is not grossly bloody, infuse 500 to 1000 ml of warmed fluid into the abdomen, agitate it, and then lower the IV bag to allow the fluid to return to it.
k. This fluid is considered positive for intraabdominal injury if there are more than 100,000 RBCs/mm^3, more than 500 WBCs/mm^3, or visible particulate matter.

4. Complications: Similar to those for Tenckhoff catheter insertion

V. UROLOGIC PROCEDURES

A. URETHRAL CATHETERIZATION

1. Indications

a. Monitoring urine output in the critically ill, immobile, or neurologically compromised patient
b. Tube placement is contraindicated in any trauma patient with an abnormal prostate, blood at the meatus, or other suspicion of urethral trauma

2. Equipment

a. Antiseptic solution
b. Lubricating jelly

5

PROCEDURES

   c. Foley catheter

   d. Urometer

   e. Water-filled 5- to 10-ml syringe

3. Technique in the male

   a. Test the balloon by injecting 5 ml of water into the balloon part.

   b. Grasp the penis and retract the foreskin, if present, with the nondominant hand, keeping the dominant hand sterile.

   c. Cleanse the tip of the penis with antiseptic solution, lubricate the tip of the catheter and insert into the urethra using gentle constant pressure while holding the penis at a 90-degree angle to the stretcher. If resistance is met, do not force the catheter because this may create urethral injury and a false passage. Should catheter placement be impossible, attempt again with a smaller or larger tube, and then proceed to suprapubic cystostomy if this is not successful.

   d. Place the catheter into the urethra all the way to the hub of the catheter, then inflate the balloon with 5 ml of water.

   e. Connect the catheter to the urometer, and tape the hub of the catheter loosely to the thigh so as to avoid traction injury to the bladder or penis.

   f. Replace the foreskin to avoid the formation of a phyma.

4. Technique in the female

   a. Place the legs in a frog position, if possible.

   b. Use the nondominant hand to spread the labia and the dominant hand to cleanse the urethral opening with antiseptic solution, then place the lubricated catheter tip into the urethral opening.

   c. With the catheter completely inserted, inflate the balloon with 5 ml of water and connect the catheter to the urometer.

5. Complications

   a. Urinary tract infection (use sterile technique when placing the catheter and remove as soon as possible)

   b. Urethral trauma (particularly possible in the male, who has a longer urethra, or patient with pelvic trauma, in whom a urethral injury must be suspected and ruled out before catheter placement)

B. SUPRAPUBIC CYSTOSTOMY

1. Indications: Close monitoring of urine output in a patient who cannot technically have a Foley catheter placed

2. Equipment

   a. Cap, mask, sterile gown, gloves, antiseptic solution

   b. Lidocaine

   c. Sterile instruments (scalpel, hemostat, tissue forceps)

   d. 3.0 suture

   e. Suprapubic tube with trocar

   f. Syringe with long 18-gauge needle

3. Technique

   a. Prepare and drape the suprapubic area and lower abdomen.

   b. Infiltrate local anesthetic into the area in the midline, directly over the symphysis pubis.

c. Insert a needle directly over this point, at a 90-degree angle, until urine returns, then remove the needle.

d. Make a small incision in the skin and subcutaneous tissues at this point, until the suprapubic tube with trocar can be easily passed into the bladder.

e. Inflate the balloon, withdraw the trocar, and ensure the flow of urine.

f. Suture the tube in place and cover with sterile dressing.

4. Complications and difficulties

a. Bleeding

b. Infection

c. Puncture of a structure other than the bladder (palpation and percussion reduce this risk, and ultrasound can be helpful in a patient who is obese or who has previous abdominal incisions)

VI. NEUROSURGICAL PROCEDURE: LUMBAR PUNCTURE

1. Indications

a. Symptoms of meningitis

b. Unexplainable altered mental status

c. Lumbar puncture is contraindicated in the patient with increased intracranial pressure

2. Equipment

a. Cap; mask; sterile gloves, gown, and towels; antiseptic solution

b. Spinal needle with stylet

c. Local anesthetic

d. Sterile tubes for CSF collection

3. Technique

a. Place the patient in the lateral position, knees bent, back rounded, and chin to the chest; palpate the vertebrae.

b. Locate the midline between spinous processes L3 and L4, at the level of the superior iliac crests. L4-L5 or L5-S1 should be used in children because of the lower position of the conus medullaris.

c. Infiltrate the skin with local anesthetic and insert the spinal needle parallel to the floor and bevel parallel to the longitudinal axis of the spine. With dural penetration, a distinct "give" will be felt.

d. Remove the stylet to confirm CSF flow. If there is no CSF, confirm landmarks and repeat the attempt.

e. Once in the arachnoid space, the bevel is turned up and attached to a manometer for pressure readings, at which time the patient's flexed position may be slightly relaxed.

f. CSF is then collected for determination of pH, glucose, protein, cell count, Gram's stain, culture, and cytology, if indicated.

4. Complications

a. Hemorrhage and hematoma (diminished by checking platelet count and coagulation profile before the procedure, detected by serial examinations, and treated with surgical clot evacuation)

b. Infection (prevented by the observance of meticulous sterile technique, diagnosed by surrounding erythema or change in neurologic examination, and may require surgical drainage if severe)

c. Spinal headache (this can be diminished by the use of a smaller needle and is treated with fluids, caffeine, the supine position, or epidural blood patch in severe cases)

SUGGESTED READINGS

American College of Surgeons: *Advanced trauma life support for doctors,* Chicago, 1997, The College.

Civetta JM, Taylor RW, Kirby RR, editors: *Critical care,* Philadelphia, 1992, JB Lippincott.

Daldec DL, Krome RL: Thoracostomy, *Emerg Med Clin North Am* 4:441, 1986.

Dauphinee K: Orotracheal intubation, *Emerg Med Clin North Am* 6:699, 1988.

Kaye W: Intravenous techniques. In *Textbook of advanced cardiac life support,* Dallas, 1981, American Heart Association.

Rippe JM, Irwin RS, Fink MP, et al: *Procedures and techniques in intensive care medicine,* Boston, 1995, Little, Brown.

Sabiston DC, Lyerly HK: *Textbook of surgery,* Philadelphia, 1997, WB Saunders.

Shoemaker WC, Ayres SM, Grenvik A, et al: *Textbook of critical care,* Philadelphia, 1995, WB Saunders.

Sladen A: *Invasive monitoring and its complications in the intensive care unit,* St Louis, 1990, Mosby.

Taylor RW, Civetta JM, Kirby RR, editors: *Techniques and procedures in critical care,* Philadelphia, 1990, JB Lippincott.

Walls RM: Cricothyroidotomy, *Emerg Med Clin North Am* 6:725, 1988.

PART II

Pathophysiology

THE CARDIAC SYSTEM

Carmelo A. Milano

I. NORMAL CARDIAC PHYSIOLOGY

A. CARDIAC CYCLE

1. **Electrical activation:** The normal cardiac impulse originates in the sinus node, which is located at the right atrium and superior vena cava juncture. Electrical conduction then proceeds rapidly via internodal pathways to the atrioventricular (AV) node (rate of conduction 1000 mm/sec). The AV node is located in the membranous septum just above the tricuspid valve orifice; conduction through the AV node is slow (200 mm/sec). The AV node fibers converge and give rise to the bundle of His, which branches into the right and left bundle branches, both of which terminate into Purkinje fiber systems. Conduction through the Purkinje fiber systems within the ventricular tissues is most rapid (4000 mm/sec). Nodal delay results in depolarization of the atria before ventricular depolarization and enables atrial contraction to contribute to ventricular filling before ventricular contraction.

2. **Valve function:** The AV valves (tricuspid and mitral) open passively during diastole, allowing the ventricles to fill; atrial contraction occurs during the final third of diastole, contributing further to ventricular filling. As ventricular contraction occurs, ventricular pressure rises and results in closure of the AV valves. Isovolumic contraction then takes place until ventricular pressure exceeds pressures in the great vessels, at which point the aortic and pulmonic valves open and ejection begins. Shortly after the ventricle begins to relax (diastole), the aortic and pulmonic valves close. Isovolumic relaxation occurs until ventricular pressure falls below atrial pressure, at which point the AV valves open again and ventricular filling begins. The components of the cardiac cycle can be divided into diastole, which includes isovolumic relaxation, rapid filling, slow filling, and atrial contraction, and systole, which includes isovolumic contraction and rapid and slow ejection.

B. COMPONENTS OF CARDIAC OUTPUT

Heart rate (HR) multiplied by stroke volume (SV) equals cardiac output (CO) (L/min). Stroke volume is determined by preload, afterload, and contractility.

1. **Heart rate:** Normal rate is 60 to 100 beats/min. At slower rates, increases in rate result in increased cardiac output. Heart rate between 90 and 100 provides optimal cardiac output. In general, rates above 120 beats/min do not allow for adequate ventricular filling, and cardiac output may decline.

2. **Preload:** Preload consists of the end-diastolic ventricular volume, which affects the degree of sarcomere stretch. Starling's law states that, within limits, end-diastolic sarcomere stretch relates directly to stroke volume. Therefore increases in end-diastolic volume (preload) result in greater stroke volume. Clinically, preload is often gauged from pulmonary artery

6

wedge pressure (PAWP), which estimates left ventricular end-diastolic pressure and volume.

3. **Afterload:** Afterload is the force against which the ventricle contracts; clinically, this consists of peripheral vascular resistance. As afterload increases, stroke volume decreases.

4. **Contractility:** Contractility can be thought of as pump efficiency independent of preload and afterload. Contractility is determined by the functional myocardial mass, which may be reduced by infarction, ischemia, cardiomyopathy, or hypoplasia. Contractility is also negatively affected by acidosis, hypothermia, hypocalcemia, and β-adrenergic blocking agents. Positive inotropic agents enhance contractility and include calcium, endogenous catecholamines, exogenous β-adrenergic receptor agonists, phosphodiesterase inhibitors, and thyroid hormone.

C. MYOCARDIAL BLOOD FLOW

During rest, normal blood flow is 60 to 90 ml/min per 100 g of myocardium. The majority of blood flow occurs during diastole because ventricular contraction increases coronary vascular resistance. Myocardial oxygen extraction is relatively high (75%) under resting conditions and increases little during exercise. However, during exercise, coronary arteriolar vasodilation occurs in response to increased CO_2 tension and decreased pH, and coronary vascular resistance can decrease fivefold to tenfold, resulting in markedly increased coronary blood flow and oxygen delivery.

II. CONGESTIVE HEART FAILURE/CARDIOGENIC SHOCK

Congestive heart failure refers to chronic ventricular dysfunction, resulting ultimately in pulmonary edema. Cardiogenic shock generally refers to an acute condition in which cardiac dysfunction results in systemic hypoperfusion. Etiologies for both conditions are similar and include myocardial infarction, cardiomyopathy, congenital lesions, and cardiac valve dysfunction. Cardiac tamponade and tension pneumothorax are conditions that may be confused with cardiogenic shock because they result in severely diminished cardiac output; in these conditions, however, ventricular function is normal and the primary problem is impaired ventricular filling. Massive pulmonary embolus may also be confused with cardiogenic shock; again, cardiac function is normal but left ventricular filling is impaired because of obstruction of the pulmonary circulation.

A. DIAGNOSIS

1. **Physical examination:** Hypotension, tachycardia, altered mental status, oliguria, respiratory distress, bibasilar crackles or wheezes, and peripheral edema. Chronically reduced cardiac output may result in cachexia.

2. **Laboratory tests:** Chest x-ray may reveal cardiomegaly, pleural effusions, or frank pulmonary edema. Other findings include elevated BUN and Cr secondary renal hypoperfusion, lactic acidosis, and elevated transaminases due to hepatic congestion.

3. **Swan-Ganz catheter:** Cardiac index (CI) less than 2.0 L/min/m^2. PAWP and CVP greater than 18. Mixed venous saturations less than 60%.

B. TREATMENT

1. **Correct specific causes:** Cardiac ischemia, valvular stenosis, etc.
2. **Place Swan-Ganz catheter and optimize components of cardiac output to achieve CI greater than 2.0.** Maintain effective cardiac rate and rhythm (ideally sinus rate of 90 to 100); in the absence of pulmonary edema, judicious increases in preload with colloid boluses may improve output. A PAWP of 15 to 18 mm Hg generally indicates adequate filling. However, if the LV is chronically scarred or hypertrophied, pressures greater than 18 mm Hg may be required to achieve optimal LV preload. Mechanical ventilation with positive pressure may also falsely elevate PAWP and again higher pressures may be required to achieve adequate filling. Afterload reduction to achieve mean arterial BP of 70 mm Hg; acutely, sodium nitroprusside, nitroglycerin, or milrinone infusions may be used, and chronically, ACE inhibitors are effective. After HR, preload, and afterload have been optimized, if the patient remains in cardiogenic shock, parenteral inotropic agents should be started (Table 6-1).
3. **Intraaortic balloon pumps are indicated for acute cardiogenic shock unresponsive to medical treatments.** The device is usually inserted from the femoral artery using a Seldinger technique. Proper position is the descending thoracic aorta just distal to the left subclavian. Balloon inflation is timed to diastole, thereby augmenting coronary perfusion, and deflation occurs just before systole, providing reduced afterload. Generally, systemic anticoagulation with heparin is required. Specific contraindications include severe aortic insufficiency, extensive atherosclerosis, and aneurysmal disease of the descending aorta.
4. **Pulmonary edema:** Supplemental oxygen to achieve arterial saturation greater than 88% to 90%. Intubation and mechanical ventilation for progressive respiratory distress, hypoxia (oxygen saturation less than 80%), or hypercapnia ($Pco_2 > 50$). Furosemide (Lasix) 40 mg IV. Further diuretic management depends on initial response; if no response, repeat furosemide 80 mg IV, bumetanide (Bumex) 4 mg IV, or ethacrynic acid (Edecrin) 50 mg IV.
5. **Isolated right ventricular failure:** May result from RV infarct or chronic pulmonary hypertension. Treatment includes volume loading to provide a CVP greater than 20 mm Hg, pacing to achieve HR greater than 90; specific pulmonary vasodilators include nitric oxide 20 ppm (if patient is intubated), milrinone, and prostaglandins.

III. ISCHEMIC HEART DISEASE

A. PREOPERATIVE EVALUATION

1. **History and physical examination:** Previous history of MI, cardiac surgery, or arrhythmia should be elicited. Symptoms that may represent myocardial ischemia include classic angina, left arm pain (ulnar distribution), dyspnea at rest or with exertion, back pain, epigastric pain, decreased exercise tolerance, palpitations, and syncope. Diabetic patients

TABLE 6-1

VASOACTIVE DRUGS

Drug	Dose (μg/kg/min)	AR Activation*			Physiologic Response				
		α1	β1	β2	SVR	MAP	CO	HR	PAWP
Dopamine	<5	−	++	−	↕	↑	↑	↑	↕
	>5	++	++	−	⇈	⇈	↑	↑	↑
Dobutamine	2-20	−	++	+	↓	↑	↑	↑	↓
Epinephrine	<0.05	−	++	+	↓	↑	↑	↑	↑
	>0.05	++	++	+	⇈	⇈	↑	↑	↑
Norepinephrine	0.03-1.0	++	+	−	⇈	⇈	↕	↕	↕
Phenylephrine	0.6-2.0	++	−	−	⇈	⇈	↓	⇇	↑
Isoproterenol	0.03-0.15	−	++	++	↓	↕	↑	↕	↓
Milrinone	0.3-1.5	PDEI†	PDEI†		→	↕	↑	↕	↓
Amrinone	5-20	PDEI†	PDEI†		→	↕	↑	↕	↓

*AR, Adrenergic receptor activation; α1, peripheral vasculature; β1, myocardium; β2, peripheral vasculature and myocardium.
†Amrinone and milrinone are common phosphodiesterase inhibitors (PDEI).

may have myocardial ischemia without significant symptoms. Physical examination may identify a cardiac murmur, S_3 or S_4, or evidence of pulmonary edema, but patients with severe coronary artery disease often have a normal examination. ECG should be inspected for abnormal rhythm, ST or T wave changes, Q waves, and conduction disorders. Chest x-ray should be performed to identify cardiomegaly.

2. **Preoperative predictors of cardiac complications during noncardiac surgery:** These were first described by Goldman et al and are listed in Table 6-2.

3. **Stress test:** When significant risk factors are present, patients should be evaluated with a functional study to rule out myocardial ischemia (exercise treadmill stress study, dobutamine or adenosine chemical stress study). If the functional studies reveal ischemia or if the history is strongly positive, coronary angiography should be performed and significant coronary stenosis addressed before any major elective surgery.

B. PERIOPERATIVE MANAGEMENT

Patients with known ischemic heart disease who undergo emergent or urgent surgical procedures are at increased risk for MI. Specific recommendations are as follows: all antianginal medications must be continued and converted to parenteral forms if necessary. Specifically, β-blockers should be continued; intermittent intravenous metoprolol may substitute for longer-acting oral β-blockers. Intravenous nitroglycerin should be titrated to mean arterial BP of 70. Continue aspirin. Avoid significant hypotension or hypertension, and maintain euvolemia, which may require Swan-Ganz catheter monitoring or intraoperative transesophageal echocardiography. Maintain Hct greater than 30%. Avoid hypoxia and respiratory distress; use supplemental oxygen.

C. POSTOPERATIVE MYOCARDIAL INFARCTION

1. **Diagnosis:** Frequently atypical presentation, including pulmonary edema, arrhythmia, or hypotension without classic angina. Ruled out by serial ECG and CPK MB isoform measurements (q8h × 3). CPK MB is elevated as early as 4 to 6 hours after an MI, peaks at 24 hours, and

---

TABLE 6-2

PREDICTORS OF CARDIAC RISK DURING NONCARDIAC SURGERY

Factor	Definition
Ischemic heart disease	MI within 6 months, class III or IV angina
Congestive heart failure	Pulmonary edema, presence of S_3 gallop or jugular venous distention
Cardiac arrhythmias	Rhythm other than sinus, >5 PVCs/min
Valvular heart disease	Evidence for significant aortic stenosis
General medical status	Elevated serum creatinine, hypoxia, hepatic insufficiency
Age	Greater than 70
Type of surgery	Intraperitoneal or intrathoracic procedures

Modified from Mangano DT, Goldman L: *N Engl J Med* 333:1750, 1995.

returns to normal in approximately 72 hours. Troponin T and troponin I are proteins released from injured myocardium: newer assays allow rapid serial measurements that probably are more sensitive and specific for myocardial injury relative to CPK MB measurements. Patients who are being ruled out for MI should also have continuous cardiac monitoring. Transesophageal or transthoracic echocardiography may also be performed; new LV wall motion dysfunction further suggests myocardial infarction or severe ischemia.

2. Treatment

a. Medical management: β-adrenergic blockade to reduce myocardial work and oxygen demands (metoprolol [Lopressor] 5 mg IV initially followed by 25 to 50 mg PO q6h); goal HR 60 to 70. Aspirin and, if possible, intravenous heparin should be initiated. Intravenous nitroglycerin should be initiated with a goal mean arterial BP of 60 to 70. Thrombolytics are generally contraindicated in the early postoperative period. Hemodynamic instability or persistent ischemia despite these measures is an indication for intraaortic balloon pump placement.

b. Revascularization: Diagnostic catheterization should be performed, and significant coronary stenoses require angioplasty, coronary stenting, or coronary artery bypass surgery. The type of revascularization is dictated by the anatomy of the coronary artery disease. The timing of cardiac catheterization and revascularization in the setting of postoperative MI is controversial and should be individualized. However, the postoperative patient with ongoing ischemia despite medical treatment should be approached aggressively with early revascularization.

IV. VALVULAR HEART DISEASE

A. AORTIC STENOSIS

Most harmful valvular condition for patients undergoing noncardiac surgery. Represents important predictor of cardiac complication (see Table 6-2).

1. Etiology: Congenital bicuspid, degenerative (senile) calcific, and rheumatic.

2. Differential diagnosis: Includes congenital supravalvular lesions, subvalvular stenosis, and dynamic hypertrophic subaortic stenosis.

3. Diagnosis: Symptoms include angina, syncope, and congestive heart failure. Physical examination reveals a systolic murmur radiating into the neck; peripheral pulses have a retarded upstroke. Echocardiography confirms the diagnosis, and aortic valve area can be calculated from flow velocity. Cardiac catheterization allows measurement of the pressure gradient between the LV and aorta from which valve area is calculated. Severe aortic stenosis is defined as a valve area less than 1 cm^2 and is almost always symptomatic. Critical aortic stenosis is defined by an aortic valve area less than 0.75 cm^2 or 0.40 cm^2/m^2. A peak systolic pressure gradient of greater than 50 mm Hg is often used to define severe or critical aortic stenosis. However, the pressure gradient is dependent on cardiac output and is less accurate than valve area for quantifying stenosis; for example, a patient with severe stenosis may have a mild gradient under low output conditions.

4. **Treatment:** Asymptomatic aortic stenosis generally does not require treatment; hypovolemia must be avoided and invasive monitoring, including a Swan-Ganz catheter, is recommended. Severe aortic stenosis requires valve replacement before elective noncardiac procedures.

B. AORTIC INSUFFICIENCY

1. **Etiology:** Annuloaortic ectasia (aortic insufficiency with dilation of the annulus and aortic root), endocarditis, and aortic dissection.

2. **Diagnosis:** The chronic form is generally well tolerated and may be present for years before symptoms develop. Typical symptoms include dyspnea on exertion, orthopnea, and paroxysmal nocturnal dyspnea. Syncope and angina are rare. Endocarditis and aortic dissection can cause acute valvular insufficiency, which may present as pulmonary edema or cardiogenic shock. Physical examination reveals water-hammer pulses, widened pulse pressure, and a diastolic murmur. Chest x-ray reveals LV dilation. Echocardiography confirms the diagnosis and grades the insufficiency.

3. **Treatment:** Patients with mild, moderate, or asymptomatic aortic insufficiency usually tolerate noncardiac surgical procedures well; fluid balance should be carefully checked and may necessitate PA catheter placement to avoid pulmonary edema. Patients with severe and symptomatic aortic insufficiency require valve replacement.

C. MITRAL STENOSIS

1. **Etiology:** Rheumatic heart disease.

2. **Diagnosis:** Classic presenting symptom is dyspnea on exertion. Pulmonary edema, atrial fibrillation, and embolic complications are later features of the disease process. Physical examination reveals an opening click and a diastolic murmur. Chest x-ray demonstrates normal LV size, LA enlargement, and mitral calcification. Echocardiography and cardiac catheterization confirm the diagnosis. Moderate mitral stenosis is defined by a mitral valve area less than 1.5 cm^2, a point at which symptoms generally begin. Severe mitral stenosis is defined by a mitral valve area less than 1.0 cm^2 or by an LA/LV gradient of greater than 10 mm Hg.

3. **Treatment:** Medical treatments include diuretics for pulmonary edema and antiarrhythmics, including procainamide, amiodarone, or sotalol for maintaining sinus rhythm. Tachycardia reduces diastolic filling times and further increases LA/LV gradient. In patients with atrial fibrillation, warfarin (Coumadin) anticoagulation is warranted. The onset of symptoms generally indicates need for invasive treatments: percutaneous balloon valvuloplasty is indicated for noncalcified valves without left atrial thrombus or significant regurgitation. For more calcified valves or after balloon valvuloplasty failures, mitral valve replacement is warranted.

D. MITRAL INSUFFICIENCY

1. **Etiology:** Includes ischemic, rheumatic, and infective endocarditis; myxomatous degeneration; and mitral valve prolapse.

2. **Diagnosis:** Physical examination reveals a systolic murmur that is loudest at the apex and radiates to the left axilla. Pulmonary edema may develop, and V waves may be present on the pulmonary artery wedge tracing. Associated frequently with atrial fibrillation and left atrial enlargement. Diagnosis can be confirmed on echocardiography or ventriculography.

3. **Treatment:** Mild and even moderate mitral regurgitation usually can be managed medically. Afterload reduction with ACE inhibitors improves cardiac output and reduces regurgitant flow into the left atrium; mean arterial pressures of 60 to 70 should be the goal. Diuretics and antiarrhythmics can be added to avoid pulmonary edema and atrial fibrillation. Severe mitral insufficiency usually requires mitral valve repair or replacement and coronary revascularization for ischemic forms. For acute severe mitral regurgitation secondary to MI and papillary muscle rupture, intraaortic balloon pumping may help stabilize patients before surgery.

E. **ENDOCARDITIS**

1. **Etiology:** Bacterial seeding of morphologically abnormal valve or valve prosthesis, most common organisms in native valve endocarditis are *Streptococcus viridans, Staphylococcus aureus,* and *Enterococcus.* Most common organism in prosthetic valve endocarditis is *Staphylococcus epidermidis.*

2. **Diagnosis:** Most common symptom is fever (>75%); common signs include heart murmur, fever, and manifestations of emboli. Blood culture positivity approaches 100% when three sets are properly obtained before initiation of antibiotic therapy. Transthoracic and transesophageal echocardiography should also be obtained to confirm presence of vegetations and rule out annular abscess.

3. **Treatment:** Specific IV antibiotic therapy for 6 weeks. Indications for surgery include resistant heart failure, recurrent or severe embolic events, persistent bacteremia, valve abscess, complete heart block, valve dehiscence, or severe obstruction.

4. **Prophylaxis:** All patients with significant murmur, abnormal valve morphology, congenital cardiac lesions, or prosthetic valves should be treated with antibiotic prophylaxis before any procedure that may induce bacteremia (Table 6-3).

F. **PROSTHETIC VALVES**

1. **Bioprosthetic valves:** Usually bovine pericardial or porcine valvular tissue. Examples include Hancock, Carpentier-Edwards, and Ionescu-Shiley. Do not require chronic anticoagulation. Generally not as durable as mechanical prostheses.

2. **Mechanical prosthetic valves:** Includes St. Jude Medical, Medtronic-Hall, Carbomedics, Björk-Shiley, and Starr-Edwards. In any position, these require chronic anticoagulation with warfarin (INR 2.5 to 3.5). Surgical procedures should be performed through a heparin window with complete reversal of warfarin. For major bleeding complications,

TABLE 6-3

ADULT ENDOCARDITIS PROPHYLACTIC REGIMENS

Procedure/Patient	Dosing Regimen
DENTAL, ORAL, UPPER RESPIRATORY	
Standard regimen	Amoxicillin 3 g PO 1 hr before and 1.5 g 6 hr after initial dose
Penicillin allergy	Erythromycin stearate 1 g PO 2 hr before and 500 mg PO 6 hr after initial dose
	or
	Clindamycin 300 mg PO 1 hr before and 150 mg PO 6 hr after initial dose
GENITOURINARY/GASTROINTESTINAL	
Standard regimen	Ampicillin 2 g IV and gentamicin 80 mg IV 30 min before procedure and repeat 8 hr after initial dose
Penicillin allergy	Vancomycin 1 g IV and gentamicin 80 mg IV 1 hr before and repeat 8 hr after initial dose

Modified from Dajani AS, Bisno AL, Chung KJ, et al: *JAMA* 264:2919, 1990.

anticoagulation should be stopped and reversed with fresh frozen plasma (FFP) until bleeding is controlled; anticoagulation can then be gradually restarted with aspirin and low-dose heparin while monitoring for bleeding.

V. CARDIAC TAMPONADE

Typically develops as blood or other fluid accumulates in the pericardial sac and subsequently impairs diastolic filling.

A. ETIOLOGY

Malignancy, uremia, idiopathic or viral, acute infarct, trauma, cardiac surgery, bacterial infection, tuberculosis, radiation, myxedema, aortic dissection, postpericardiotomy syndrome, and systemic lupus erythematosus. Differential diagnosis includes primary ventricular dysfunction, superior vena cava syndrome, constrictive pericarditis, and tension pneumothorax.

B. DIAGNOSIS

Physical examination reveals hypotension, tachycardia, muffled cardiac tones, and distended neck veins. Pulsus paradoxus is a classic finding that is defined as a fall in the systolic BP greater than 10 mm Hg with inspiration. Invasive monitoring shows increased and equalized CVP and PAWP, and cardiac output is decreased. Echocardiography reveals pericardial effusion and impaired diastolic filling (RA and RV compression during diastole).

C. TREATMENT

Fluid boluses and inotropes may transiently improve hemodynamics in the setting of tamponade, but definitive treatment consists of pericardial drainage. Subxiphoid pericardial aspiration and drain placement is acutely effective for tamponade. Echocardiography is useful to guide aspiration and drain placement and avoid injury to the epicardial vessels. Bloody fluid that is aspirated should be kept; if the blood clots after several minutes, this suggests that the ventricle was aspirated. In the setting of trauma or after cardiac surgery, formal sternotomy or thoracotomy is required for drainage and control of the bleeding.

VI. ARRHYTHMIAS

A. SUPRAVENTRICULAR ARRHYTHMIAS

Generally narrow QRS (<0.12 sec) rhythms, with a ventricular rate dependent on the efficiency of AV nodal conduction. Atrial fibrillation and atrial flutter are the most common. Supraventricular arrhythmias often are caused by treatable conditions, such as thyrotoxicosis, myocardial ischemia, hypokalemia, hypoxia, or acidosis.

1. **Atrial flutter:** Regular rhythm with an atrial rate of approximately 300, and ventricular response rate is usually 150, reflecting 2:1 AV nodal conduction.

2. **Atrial fibrillation:** No organized atrial activity, and irregularly irregular ventricular response.
   Treatment for atrial flutter and atrial fibrillation are similar.

a. If hemodynamically unstable, immediate synchronous electrical cardioversion is indicated, initially with 100 J, then 200 J and 300 J.

b. For hemodynamically stable patients, rate control should be the first goal, and regimens include digoxin 0.5 mg IV followed by 0.25 mg twice at 4-hour intervals for a total load of 1 mg. Alternatively, diltiazem 10 mg IV over 5 minutes followed by an infusion of 10 to 20 mg/hr, or β-blockers such as metoprolol 5 mg IV over 5 minutes or esmolol. These agents can be combined to enhance rate control, but there is increased risk of bradycardias and heart block. Calcium channel blockers and β-blockers are also negative inotropes and may cause hypotension; serial BP measurements should be taken during administration.

c. After rate is controlled, a variety of agents are effective for chemical cardioversion and for maintaining a sinus rhythm. These include procainamide, quinidine, sotalol, and amiodarone (Table 6-4). Amiodarone is most effective, although it does have serious toxicities.

3. **Paroxysmal supraventricular tachycardia (PSVT):** Characterized by repeated episodes of a regular tachycardia with an abrupt onset lasting minutes to hours. Common rate is 180 beats/min. Mechanism often involves reentry patterns at the level of the AV node. Treatment includes synchronous electrical cardioversion if there is hemodynamic instability; in stable patients, calcium channel blockers (diltiazem and verapamil) are effective for cardioversion. Adenosine 6 or 12 mg IV push is also effective for cardioversion.

B. VENTRICULAR ARRHYTHMIAS

Includes ventricular tachycardia (VT) and ventricular fibrillation (VF). VT is defined as 3 or more beats of ventricular origin in succession at a rate of greater than 100. Frequently patients with good ventricular function are able to sustain some cardiac output during sustained VT. During ventricular fibrillation there is no organized ventricular depolarization and no cardiac

TABLE 6-4
ANTIARRHYTHMIC MEDICATIONS

Drug	Dose	Indications	Side Effects
Adenosine	6-12 mg IV push	PSVT	Flushing, dyspnea
Amiodarone	150 mg IV push over 30 min, then 1 mg/min for 6 hr, then 0.5 mg/min IV for 1-2 days, then continue 200-1000 mg PO qid	SVT, VT/VF	Pulmonary fibrosis
Bretylium	5-10 mg/kg IV over 20 min, then 1-2 mg/min IV	VT/VF	Hypotension
Diltiazem	0.25 mg/kg IV bolus over 5 min, then 5-15 mg/hr IV	PSVT, SVT	Heart block, hypotension
Lidocaine	1 mg/kg IV, then 1-4 mg/min IV	VT/VF	Mental status changes, seizures
Magnesium	1-2 g magnesium sulfate IV over 2 min, repeat as needed or based on serum level	VT/VF (particularly torsades de pointes)	Flushing, bradycardias
Procainamide	10-15 mg/kg IV load over 45 min followed by 2-4 mg/min IV	SVT, VT/VF	Skin rash, agranulocytosis
Quinidine	Sulfate form: 600 mg PO load followed by 300-600 mg PO tid; Gluconate form: 648 mg PO load followed by 324 mg PO tid	SVT, VT/VF	GI upset, mental status changes
Sotalol	40-80 mg PO q12h	SVT, VT/VF	Proarrhythmic

output. The terms *coarse* and *fine* have been used to define the amplitude of waveforms in VF.

1. **Etiology:** Most important is myocardial ischemia; others include hypokalemia, hypomagnesemia, hypoxia, acidosis, proarrhythmic effect of antiarrhythmic medications, V pacing, intracardiac catheters, and β-adrenergic agonists.
2. **Differential diagnosis:** Includes aberrantly conducted supraventricular tachycardias (e.g., atrial flutter with a bundle branch block). VT generally has a wider QRS (>0.14 sec) and more left axis deviation relative to aberrantly conducted supraventricular arrhythmias. VT may also display capture and fusion beats and AV dissociation. If the diagnosis of a wide, complex tachycardia is unclear, it should be treated as VT until proven otherwise.

3. **Treatment:** Sustained VT requires immediate synchronous electrical cardioversion; VF requires asynchronous electrical cardioversion. Lidocaine 1 to 2 mg/kg IV bolus followed by 2 mg/min IV infusion should be started. Specific causes should be considered and corrected. Other agents that are effective include procainamide, magnesium sulfate, bretylium, amiodarone, and sotalol (see Table 6-3). Recurrent ventricular arrhythmias require formal electrical physiology testing, and some patients benefit from internal defibrillators.

C. BRADYCARDIAS

1. **Types:** Includes sinus bradycardia, sinus arrest with a slow escape rhythm, and heart block.

2. **Classification of heart block:** First-degree heart block is prolongation of the PR interval greater than 0.2 sec with a normal P-to-QRS relationship. Second-degree heart block is intermittent failure of atrial activity to conduct to the ventricles (a P wave without an associated QRS complex). Second-degree is further divided into type I, in which there is successive prolongation of the PR interval before complete block, and type II, in which complete block is sporadically interspersed with normal conduction. Third-degree, or complete, heart block refers to complete dissociation between atrial and ventricular activity.

3. **Etiology:** Increased vagal tone may transiently cause bradycardias that usually are not clinically relevant. Sustained heart block and other bradycardia may result from medications: β-blockers, calcium channel blockers, and digoxin should be eliminated. First- or second-degree heart block is seen frequently after inferior MI and often resolves spontaneously. Anterior MI may result in persistent advanced second-degree or complete heart block. Valvular surgery and endocarditis may also result in transient or permanent heart block.

D. ACUTE THERAPY

Acute therapy for all forms of sustained symptomatic bradycardia should include intravenous atropine; an initial dose of 0.5 mg should be repeated every few minutes to a total dose of several milligrams as indicated. Transcutaneous pacing can be quickly established; many defibrillator units serve dual function as external pacers. For transvenous pacing, an introducer catheter is sterilely placed into the right internal jugular vein, through which a pacing wire is fluoroscopically guided into the apical portion of the right ventricle. Intravenous infusions of dopamine or isoproterenol can also be given to increase heart rate, although in the setting of myocardial ischemia, these agents may induce ventricular arrhythmias.

E. INDICATIONS FOR PERMANENT PACEMAKER

Complete heart block with or without symptoms, persistent type II second-degree heart block, symptomatic sick sinus syndrome, and symptomatic tachycardia-bradycardia syndromes.

F. PACEMAKER THREE-LETTER IDENTIFICATION CODE

1. **First position:** Denotes the chamber paced: A = atrium, V = ventricle, and D = dual.

2. **Second position:** Denotes the chamber sensed: O = none, A = atrium, V = ventricle, and D = dual.
3. **Third position:** Denotes response to sensing: O = none, T = triggered, I = inhibited, and D = dual (T + I).
4. **Newer code:** A newer code includes fourth position for denoting programmability and fifth position for antitachycardia function.

SUGGESTED READINGS

Dajani AS, Bisno AL, Chung KJ, et al: Prevention of bacterial endocarditis: recommendation of the American Heart Association, *JAMA* 264:2919, 1990.

Mangano DT, Goldman L: Preoperative assessment of the patient with known or suspected coronary disease, *N Engl J Med* 333:1750, 1995.

Cummins RO, editor: *Advanced cardiac life support,* Dallas, 1997, American Heart Association.

6

THE CARDIAC SYSTEM

THE PULMONARY SYSTEM

Lynne A. Skaryak

I. NORMAL LUNG ANATOMY AND FUNCTION

A. ANATOMY

1. Conducting airways

a. Includes trachea with branching to level of terminal bronchioles

b. Anatomic dead space without contribution to gas exchange

2. Respiratory zone

a. Respiratory bronchioles and alveolar ducts and sacs

b. Consists of 300 million alveoli; surface area for gas exchange is 50 to 100 m^2

c. Alveolar cells

    (1) Type I pneumocytes: involved in gas exchange

    (2) Type II pneumocytes: surfactant secretion (reduce surface tension, increase compliance, decrease respiratory work)

3. Circulation

a. Pulmonary arteries: Supply respiratory bronchioles and alveoli.

b. Bronchial arteries: Supply trachea to level of terminal bronchioles; abundant collaterals with pulmonary arteries that are important after pulmonary transplantation and sleeve resection, which result in interruption of bronchial circulation.

B. LUNG VOLUMES (Figure 7-1)

Measured with spirometry (direct) and washout techniques (indirect)

1. Tidal volume: TV is the volume of normal inspiration and normal expiration.

2. Inspiratory reserve volume: IRV is the difference between maximal inspiration and normal inspiration.

3. Expiratory reserve volume: ERV is the difference between maximal expiration and normal expiration.

4. Residual volume: RV is the volume remaining in the lung after maximal expiration.

5. Total lung capacity: TLC is the volume in the lung after maximal inspiration.

6. Vital capacity: VC is the volume expired between maximal inspiration and maximal expiration.

7. Inspiratory capacity: IC is the volume inspired between normal expiration and maximal inspiration.

8. Functional residual capacity: FRC is the volume in the lung at the end of normal expiration.

9. Forced expiratory volume: FEV_1 is the volume forcibly exhaled within 1 second from TLC.

C. RESPIRATORY VOLUMES

For predictors of postoperative morbidity and mortality, see Table 7-1.

1. Minute ventilation: V_E = TV × breaths per minute (bpm); the volume of air inspired per minute.

101

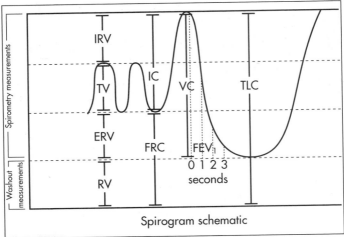

FIGURE 7-1

Lung volume spirogram.

TABLE 7-1

PREDICTORS OF POSTOPERATIVE MORBIDITY AND MORTALITY

Pulmonary Function Test	Increased Morbidity	Contraindication to Major Surgery
FEV_1	<30% predicted	<0.6 L
FVC	<50% predicted	<1.0 L
FEV_1/FVC	<60% predicted	<50%
$Paco_2$	50-55	>55
Pao_2	50-60	<50

2. **Alveolar ventilation:** V_A = fraction of V_E that reaches alveoli and is available for gas exchange.
3. **Dead space:** V_d = fraction of V_E not available for gas exchange.
D. **VENTILATION**
1. **Pulmonary compliance**
a. Defined as the change in lung volume per change in pressure.
b. The lung is elastic and tends to collapse; the chest wall is expansile and tends to expand the lung.
c. FRC is the point of equilibrium between the two opposing forces; decreased compliance is almost always associated with a decrease in FRC.
2. **Airway resistance**
a. Airway resistance (R_{AW}) = pressure difference between the mouth and the alveoli divided by the flow rate.

b. Resistance is proportional to the length of the airway and inversely proportional to square radius of the airway.

E. PERFUSION

1. **Pulmonary vascular bed:** Accommodates the entire cardiac output at a low perfusion pressure (15 mm Hg); normal pulmonary vascular resistance is approximately one fifth of systemic vascular resistance

2. **Alveolar hypoxia and hypercapnia (acidosis):** Induce pulmonary vasoconstriction, increase pulmonary vascular resistance, and redistribute pulmonary blood flow

3. **Fluid balance**

a. Fluid distribution across the capillary/alveolar membrane is determined mainly by capillary hydrostatic pressure, which forces fluid out of the capillary, and by capillary oncotic pressure, which draws fluid back into the capillary.

b. Normally there is a net flux of fluid out of the capillary into the interstitium, which is drained by pulmonary lymphatics. Pulmonary edema occurs when the net flux of fluid out of the capillary (e.g., with increased capillary hydrostatic pressure) exceeds the capacity of pulmonary lymphatics to remove fluid.

F. VENTILATION AND PERFUSION MATCHING

In the normal state, the distribution of ventilation parallels perfusion; ventilation/perfusion (V/Q) mismatch is the most common cause of hypoxemia. The following scenarios are possible:

1. **V/Q = 0:** Alveoli are perfused but not ventilated; this constitutes physiologic shunt (see below). Concentration of O_2 and CO_2 in the alveoli are equal to the concentration in mixed venous blood ($Po_2 = 40$ mm Hg; $Pco_2 = 45$ mm Hg).

2. **V/Q < 1:** Ventilation is less than perfusion, but gas exchange does occur; concentrations of O_2 and CO_2 in alveoli are between those of mixed venous blood and normal arterial blood ($Po_2 = 40$-100 mm Hg; $Pco_2 = 40$-45 mm Hg).

3. **V/Q = 1:** Ventilation matched by perfusion and normal gas exchange occurs; alveolar and arterial $Po_2 = 100$ mm Hg and $Pco_2 = 40$ mm Hg.

4. **V/Q > 1:** Ventilation exceeds perfusion and only a fraction of the ventilated lung takes part in gas exchange; concentrations of alveolar O_2 and CO_2 are between those of normal arterial blood and inspired gas ($Po_2 = 100$-150 mm Hg; $Pco_2 = 0$-40 mm Hg). The fraction of ventilation that does not take part in gas exchange contributes to the physiologic dead space.

G. SHUNT

A shunt is defined as mixed venous gas that does not participate in gas exchange. Shunts cause decrease in arterial O_2 concentration with minimal effect on CO_2. Administration of 100% Fio_2 does not completely correct shunt hypoxemia. An anatomic shunt refers to blood that does not pass through the pulmonary circuit (e.g., an intracardiac shunt). Physiologic shunting refers to blood that passes through pulmonary circulation without undergoing gas exchange (V/Q = 0). This is seen with consolidation. Shunt fraction is the ratio of blood flow through the shunt to total cardiac output. The normal shunt fraction is 1% to 2% and not clinically relevant.

H. WORK OF BREATHING

1. **Definition:** The product of volume and pressure.
2. **Requires oxygen consumption:** May also constitute up to 20% of the overall oxygen consumption in critically ill patients.
3. **Components of work.**
   a. Elastic recoil of lung and chest wall
   b. Frictional resistance of airway
   c. Frictional resistance of endotracheal tube and mechanical ventilator
4. **Respiratory muscle fatigue:** Occurs in processes disturbing the balance between energy supply and work requirement. Decreased respiratory muscle and energy supply may occur, for example with malnutrition or hypophosphatemia or during low cardiac output states. Increased work requirements are seen during sepsis, after multiple trauma, or when compliance decreases. During respiratory failure, rapid shallow breathing and increased use of accessory muscles precedes respiratory arrest.

II. CAUSES OF RESPIRATORY FAILURE

A. HYPERCAPNIC RESPIRATORY FAILURE

1. **Primary hypoventilation, respiratory acidosis, and secondary hypoxia**
2. **Etiology**
   a. Disorders of neural system, which controls ventilation: CVA, sedatives, sleep apnea, spinal cord injury, Parkinson's disease, multiple sclerosis, amyotrophic lateral sclerosis (ALS), and diabetic neuropathy
   b. Primary disorders of respiratory muscle (e.g., myasthenia gravis)
3. **Management:** If possible, treat underlying cause; supplemental oxygen, CPAP, and mechanical ventilation

B. ASTHMA

1. **Pathophysiology**
   a. Reversible bronchospasm with airway obstruction
   b. Inflammation: Eosinophils, T lymphocytes, macrophages, and mast cells
   c. Hyperresponsiveness of airway tone to a variety of stimuli
   d. Increased airway resistance, hyperinflation, and air trapping
   e. Increased work of breathing
   f. Increased FRC, RV, TLC
   g. Increased V/Q mismatch
   h. Increased dead space
2. **Management**
   a. Recognize high-risk patients: steroid use, need for intubation, or hospitalization history
   b. Oxygen: 25% to 40% to optimize oxygenation without exacerbating V/Q mismatch
   c. High-dose inhaled β-adrenergic agonists (albuterol, terbutaline, salbutamol, metaproterenol); repeat treatments every 20 minutes until effect seen

d. Systemic steroids: methylprednisolone (Solu-Medrol) 60 to 120 mg IV, followed by oral prednisone taper over 1 week

e. Inhaled anticholinergics (ipratropium bromide): decrease vagal tone and increase bronchial smooth muscle relaxation

g. Mechanical ventilation for progressive respiratory distress, depressed mental status, or CO_2 retention

h. Careful fluid management; avoid overhydration

C. CHRONIC OBSTRUCTIVE PULMONARY DISEASE

1. **Definition:** Irreversible changes in lung characterized by airflow obstruction; includes chronic bronchitis, emphysema, and chronic obstructive airway disease

2. **Etiology**
   a. Cigarette smoking
   b. Environmental pollution
   c. Recurrent respiratory infections
   d. α_1-Protease inhibitor deficiency

3. **Pathophysiology**
   a. Airway narrowing, obstruction, secretions, edema, and hyperreactivity
   b. Expiratory airflow limitation
   c. Hyperinflation: autoPEEP, increased dead space
   d. V/Q mismatch, secondary hypoxia
   e. Respiratory muscle fatigue
   f. Pulmonary artery hypertension
   g. Cor pulmonale
   h. Central respiratory drive abnormalities, secondary hypercapnia

4. **Management**
   a. Arterial blood gas to assess severity
   b. Inhaled β-adrenergic agonists
   c. Steroids: high dose followed by slow taper
   d. Antibiotics: low threshold to start in these patients with increased risk for postoperative infections
   e. Bronchoscopy is useful to obtain cultures and for pulmonary toilet; however, use caution in nonintubated patients because this can act as stimulant for further bronchoconstriction
   f. Correct hypoxemia: avoid respiratory depression/hypercarbia while using low levels O_2 to maintain Pao_2 of 55 to 60 mm Hg
   g. Reduce lung water with diuretics
   h. CPAP
   i. Intubation/mechanical ventilation: use minimal PEEP, low tidal volumes, limit peak inspiratory pressure, allow longer expiratory time, and beware of autoPEEP

D. ADULT RESPIRATORY DISTRESS SYNDROME

1. **Mechanism:** Capillary/alveolar membrane injury with resultant noncardiogenic pulmonary edema; causes include aspiration, pneumonia, inhalation of toxic fumes, sepsis, massive transfusions, long bone injuries, pulmonary contusions, radiation injury, and pancreatitis

2. Diagnosis

a. Precipitating condition or presence of risk factors
b. Acute onset
c. New bilateral fluffy infiltrates on CXR
d. No evidence of cardiac failure, fluid overload (PCWP less than 18 mm Hg), or previous lung disease
e. Pao_2/Fio_2 ratio < 150
f. Shunt fraction $> 20\%$

3. Features

a. Pulmonary edema
b. Decreased pulmonary compliance
c. Hypoxemia, dyspnea, and tachypnea
d. Increased airway resistance
e. Increased shunting and dead space

4. Management

a. Treat underlying cause
b. Rule out sepsis
   (1) Panculture
   (2) Bronchoalveolar lavage (BAL)
   (3) Abdominal CT
   (4) Sinus films
   (5) Thoracentesis if pleural effusions are present
   (6) Antibiotics: initially broad spectrum, then guided by culture results
c. Pulmonary artery catheter is useful to guide diuretic therapy, follow hemodynamics during increased PEEP or to evaluate effects of nitric oxide (NO) therapy
d. Supplemental oxygen
e. Mechanical ventilation should try to recruit alveoli while minimizing barotrauma
   (1) Tidal volumes of 10 ml/kg are generally sufficient.
   (2) PEEP should be titrated to reduce Fio_2 to less than 60% and to increase Pao_2/Fio_2 to > 200.
   (3) Pressure control ventilation induces less barotrauma than volume ventilation.
   (4) Inverse I:E ratio may be required, but patients should be sedated and paralyzed.
f. Corticosteroids (controversial): 1 to 2 mg/kg methylprednisolone q6h × 5 days in later stages to lessen interstitial fibroproliferation
g. Prone positioning to redistribute and mobilize lung edema and to recruit new alveoli
h. Nitric oxide to reduce pulmonary vascular resistance and improve V/Q mismatch

E. PNEUMONIA

1. Etiology

a. Primary pneumonia usually due to gram-positive organisms or *Haemophilus influenzae.*

b. Nosocomial pneumonia—most common infection in ICU setting. Causative organisms include gram-negative rods (GNR) 60% to 75%, gram-positive cocci 25% to 35%, anaerobes 2%, and *Candida albicans* 10%. Risk factors include:
    (1) Previous antibiotic therapy
    (2) Surgery
    (3) Prolonged hospitalization
    (4) Mechanical ventilation
    (5) Aspiration risk
    (6) COPD

2. Diagnosis
a. Physical examination: rhonchi and diminished breath sounds
b. New-onset purulent sputum or change in sputum quality
c. Positive sputum and blood cultures
d. CXR demonstrates new infiltrate, consolidation, cavitation, and pleural effusion

3. Differential diagnosis
a. ARDS
b. Pulmonary edema
c. Pulmonary embolism/infarct
d. Pulmonary hemorrhage

4. Treatment: IV antibiotic therapy based on organism sensitivities. Duration of therapy at least 10 days and based on clinical course. Virulent gram-negative organisms generally require two agents (e.g., a third-generation cephalosporin and an aminoglycoside). Bronchoscopy is indicated for diagnosis and to facilitate clearance of secretions. Tracheostomy is indicated to facilitate weaning from mechanical ventilation and to facilitate clearance of secretion.

F. AIRWAY HEMORRHAGE
1. Definitions
a. Massive hemoptysis: more than 600 ml in 24 hours
b. Exsanguinating hemoptysis: 150 ml/hr with total blood loss greater than 1000 ml, seldom responsive to medical treatments

2. Etiology
a. Bronchial artery bleeding
    (1) Bronchiectasis
    (2) Tuberculosis
    (3) Lung abscess
    (4) Malignancy
    (5) Necrotizing pneumonia
    (6) Bronchitis
    (7) Cystic fibrosis
b. Pulmonary arterial bleeding
    (1) Tuberculosis
    (2) Suppurative pulmonary disease
    (3) Pulmonary arteriovenous fistula

(4) Malignancy
(5) PA rupture from Swan-Ganz catheter
c. Innominate artery bleeding
(1) Tracheoinnominate fistula
(2) Tracheal resection
d. Rarely bleeding from aorta
(1) Aortic dissection
(2) Traumatic aortic transection

3. Management
a. Prevent asphyxiation
b. Establish airway and administer humidified O_2
c. Decubitus positioning with bleeding side down if site of bleeding is known
d. Resuscitate: large-bore IVs, type and cross 6 U blood, and assess/correct coagulopathies (PT/PTT, hematocrit, platelets, fibrinogen)
e. Bronchoscopy is the primary diagnostic and therapeutic procedure; it allows for removal of clot and restoration of ventilation, and it localizes bleeding and may establish etiology; bronchoscopy also allows for bronchial tamponade of bleeding site, and selective main stem intubation/ventilation of nonbleeding side
f. Arteriography/embolization: success rate is 75% to 85%, recurrence rate is 20%
g. Pulmonary resection

G. PULMONARY EMBOLUS
1. Risk factors
a. Congestive heart failure
b. Atrial fibrillation
c. Orthopedic procedure
d. Immobility longer than 72 hours
e. Malignancy
f. Obesity
g. Multisystem trauma
h. Prior history of PE or DVT
i. Pregnancy

2. Clinical presentation
a. Symptoms
(1) Dyspnea
(2) Pleuritic chest pain
(3) Hemoptysis
b. Signs
(1) Tachycardia
(2) Tachypnea
(3) Fever
(4) Hypotension
(5) Collapse
(6) Evidence of DVT

3. Diagnosis
a. CXR: Most often normal with PE, but other causes of hypoxia are ruled out (e.g., pneumothorax, ARDS, and pulmonary edema).
b. ABG: Significant hypoxia is almost always present: if PaO_2 on room air is greater than 80 mm Hg, PE is very unlikely.
c. ECG should be obtained to rule out myocardial infarction.
d. V/Q scan:
   (1) Negative scan excludes PE.
   (2) Intermediate- or low-probability scans are generally not diagnostic. Pulmonary angiography is required or lower-extremity Doppler ultrasound (if positive anticoagulation is initiated and angiogram can be avoided).
   (3) High-probability scan is diagnostic for PE.
e. Pulmonary angiography remains the gold standard.
f. Spiral chest CT scan with pulmonary embolus protocol

4. Treatment
a. Stabilize hemodynamics with fluid bolus and inotropes
b. Supplemental oxygen and mechanical ventilation for progressive hypoxia and respiratory failure
c. Anticoagulation alone is usually sufficient for most PEs without severe hemodynamic or respiratory compromise
   (1) Heparin IV bolus (80 U/kg) followed by continuous infusion (18 U/kg/hr) to keep PTT 2 to 3 times control
   (2) Oral anticoagulation concomitantly with heparin; discontinue heparin when international normalized ratio (INR) is 2.0 to 3.0 after minimum of 4 days' overlap
   (3) Contraindications: cranial surgery, head trauma, and hemorrhagic stroke
d. Thrombolytic therapy
   (1) Indicated for PEs with hemodynamic instability or severe hypoxia, unresponsive to conservative measures
   (2) Urokinase/tissue plasminogen activator given via pulmonary angiogram catheter embedded in clot for 24 hours
   (3) Major bleeding complication (10% to 20%)
   (4) Recurrence of PE (7%)
   (5) Contraindications: active or recent bleeding, hemorrhagic stroke, intracranial neoplasm, recent cranial surgery or trauma, bleeding diathesis, CPR, nonhemorrhagic stroke, surgery within 10 days, and uncontrolled hypertension
e. Surgical embolectomy
   (1) Indicated acutely with massive PE and shock or with chronic PE and persistent hypoxia and pulmonary hypertension
   (2) Stabilize patient with volume and vasoactive agents (norepinephrine) while waiting for OR
   (3) Most successful if performed within 30 minutes of massive PE

f. Suction catheter embolectomy
   (1) Performed in radiology or angio-operating room
   (2) Femoral or jugular vein cutdown
   (3) 5-F steerable catheter with suction cup for clot extraction

III. BRONCHOSCOPY

Indications:

1. Diagnosis

a. Airway obstruction
b. Biopsy of masses
c. Localization of hemorrhage
d. Obtaining accurate cultures
e. Assess traumatic airway injury
f. Evaluate suspected inhalation or caustic burn injury
g. Evaluate integrity of airway anastomosis

2. Therapy

a. Relief of airway obstruction
b. Removal of foreign bodies
c. Perform difficult intubations
d. Injection of epinephrine/tamponade for bleeding
e. Dilation of stenoses
f. Pulmonary toilet for lobar collapse, atelectasis, and thick secretions

3. Technique

a. Supplemental oxygen
b. Nebulized lidocaine
c. Topical anesthetic: nares, pharynx, trachea, and carina
d. Pulse oximetry/cardiac monitoring
e. IV access
f. Sputum trap and sterile saline available for lavage

4. Potential complications

a. Bronchospasm
b. Hypoxia
c. Arrhythmias
d. Aspiration
e. Pneumothorax
f. Hemorrhage
g. Vocal cord damage

IV. LUNG TRANSPLANTATION

A. POSTOPERATIVE DAY 0

1. Pulmonary

a. Ventilation: Pressure control mode initially to minimize barotrauma, followed by pressure support mode (maintain TV 7 to 10 ml/kg) for weaning
b. Many patients can be weaned to extubate within the first 24 hours
c. Monitor postoperative chest tube drainage and aggressively correct coagulopathy and hypothermia in bleeding patients

d. Bronchoscopy should be performed before extubation for inspection of the anastomotic site, pulmonary toilet, and BAL for cultures

e. Portable isotope perfusion scan is performed within first 2 to 3 hours of transplantation to evaluate perfusion homogeneity of transplanted lung and rule out major anastomotic problem

f. Special considerations

    (1) Decubitus position with transplant side up in single-lung patients

    (2) Reperfusion injury may occur during the first 24 to 48 hours and manifests as an infiltrate on CXR and progressive hypoxia; treatment involves:

        (a) Diuresis

        (b) Plasmapheresis

        (c) Nitric oxide

    (3) Nebulized colistin, amphotericin B, and tobramycin for known pre-operative recipient infections with GNR or fungus

2. Pain management: Best accomplished with an epidural catheter infusion of local anesthetic, this avoids high systemic levels of narcotics, which may inhibit respiratory drive

3. Laboratory/physiologic monitoring

a. Daily laboratory tests: CXR, electrolytes, BUN, creatinine, CBC, cyclosporine levels, ABG

b. Swan-Ganz catheter: cardiac output, pulmonary artery pressure, PCWP

B. POSTOPERATIVE DAYS 1 TO 3

1. Ambulation

2. Discontinuation of Foley, Swan-Ganz catheter, and chest tubes (if there is no air leak present)

3. Advance diet

4. Transition from IV to oral immunosuppression

5. Transition from epidural to oral agents

6. Daily spirometry: FEV_1 and FVC (10% decrease may signal rejection, but measurements are effort dependent)

7. Chest PT

C. SINGLE-LUNG TRANSPLANTATION CONSIDERATIONS

1. Hyperinflation/air trapping within native lung may result in compression atelectasis of transplanted lung. Treatment includes:

a. Bronchodilator therapy

b. Positioning patient with allograft side up

c. Split lung ventilation

d. Volume reduction procedure on the native lung

2. Barotrauma of emphysematous native lung.

a. Usually occurs with mechanical ventilation; volume ventilation can lead to higher airway pressures and greater injury; pressure-cycled ventilation helps reduce mean and peak airway pressure.

b. Prolonged chest tube may be required for air leaks and pneumothorax.

D. PHRENIC NERVE INJURY

Most are unilateral and transient; bilateral injuries need tracheostomy and prolonged ventilator wean.

E. CARDIOVASCULAR

1. **Diuresis helps reduce lung water and improves compliance, but severe hypovolemia must be avoided**
2. **ECMO for severe cardiopulmonary failure** (e.g., severe reperfusion injury with elevated pulmonary vascular resistance)
3. **Septic shock may present without classic fever or leukocytosis;** common etiology is bacterial from infected donor or recipient lung
4. **Arterial stenosis/pulmonary venous occlusion may require surgical revision**
5. **Pulmonary embolism**
6. **Myocardial infarction**
7. **Pulmonary hypertension:** sedation, pulmonary artery catheter monitoring, NO
8. **Arrhythmias:** Supraventricular tachycardia (SVT), atrial fibrillation

F. INFECTIOUS DISEASE

1. **Check donor cultures** and treat accordingly.
2. **Continue to treat pretransplant recipient cultures with customized antibiotics.**
3. **Panculture for temperatures greater than 38° C;** bronchoscopy should be performed to obtain reliable pulmonary sputum specimens, and then early empiric antibiotic coverage while cultures pending.
4. **Limit propofol use to 24 hours:** This increases risk of fungal infections in transplant population.

G. GASTROINTESTINAL COMPLICATIONS (AS HIGH AS 40%)

1. **Gastroparesis:** May result from vagus nerve injury; usually this resolves with time. Promotility agents, such as metoclopramide (Reglan) or cisapride, may help improve emptying.
2. **Malabsorption:** Commonly seen in cystic fibrosis patients; enzyme supplements must be continued.
3. **Pneumatosis intestinalis:** May be seen with CMV enteritis.
4. **Ulcer/gastritis prophylaxis.**

H. RENAL

1. **Acute tubular necrosis:** May occur secondary to intraoperative hypotension, hypovolemia from overaggressive diuresis, or from nephrotoxic drugs (cyclosporine, antibiotics).
2. **Adjust medications based on creatinine clearance.**
3. **Treatment:** Includes maintaining adequate renal perfusion with colloid infusions and renal dose dopamine.

I. NEUROPSYCHOLOGY

1. **Seizures:** Secondary to cyclosporine, electrolyte abnormalities, and CNS infections.
2. **Delirium:** Frequently caused by steroids, but may be manifestation of sepsis.

J. ACUTE REJECTION

1. **Decrease in FEV_1 or FVC**
2. **CXR:** Perihilar opacities, pleural effusions

3. **New or worsening dyspnea**
4. **Nonproductive cough, low-grade fever, malaise**
5. **Bronchoscopy:** BAL for cultures to rule out infection and transbronchial biopsy for histologic confirmation
6. **Therapy:** Pulse IV methylprednisolone 500 to 1000 mg/day × 3 days, may initiate before biopsy results if clinical suspicion is high

SUGGESTED READINGS

Miller A, editor: *Pulmonary function tests: a guide for the student and house officer,* Orlando, Fla, 1987, Grune & Stratton.

Simpson KP, Garrity ER: Perioperative management in lung transplantation, *Clin Chest Med* 18:277-284, 1997.

7

THE PULMONARY SYSTEM

THE RENAL SYSTEM

G. Chad Hughes

I. INTRODUCTION

A. NORMAL KIDNEY FUNCTIONS
1. **Regulation of water and electrolyte balance**
2. **Excretion of metabolic wastes and foreign chemicals**
3. **Assists in acid-base balance**
4. **Regulation of arterial BP**
5. **Regulation of erythrocyte production via erythropoietin secretion**
6. **Regulation of vitamin D activity:** conversion of vitamin D to active form (1,25-dihydroxyvitamin D_3) occurs in kidney

B. BASIC RENAL PROCESSES
1. **Kidneys lie on either side of the vertebral column** in the retroperitoneal space opposite the L1-L2 vertebral bodies, with the right kidney being approximately 1 cm lower than the left.
2. **Kidneys are 11.5 to 12.5 cm in length,** with no greater than 1 cm difference in length between the two; weight is 150 g each.
3. **The functional unit of the kidney is the nephron.** There are approximately 1 million nephrons per kidney. The nephron consists of the glomerulus and renal tubular system.
4. **Renal blood flow**
   a. Renal blood flow is determined by cardiac output and renal vascular resistance.
   b. Renal vascular resistance is primarily controlled at the arteriolar level. If renal perfusion pressure (RPP) decreases, the efferent arterioles constrict to maintain the glomerular filtration rate (GFR). If systolic BP falls to less than 70 mm Hg, this mechanism fails and the afferent arterioles constrict with a subsequent decrease in GFR and urine output.
   c. RPP depends upon several factors, including systemic mean arterial pressure (MAP), renal vascular resistance, and renal venous pressure.
   d. When RPP falls, renin secretion by the juxtaglomerular apparatus is increased, leading to increased production of angiotensin I, which is subsequently converted to angiotensin II. Efferent arteriole constriction in the face of reduced RPP is due to angiotensin II. This efferent arteriole constriction helps maintain GFR despite reduced RPP. Angiotensin II is a powerful vasoconstrictor that also directly leads to an increase in MAP and RPP via increasing peripheral vascular resistance.
   e. ACE inhibitors can lead to acute renal failure (ARF) in patients with a GFR dependent on high levels of angiotensin II (e.g., bilateral renal artery stenosis, severe congestive heart failure) via efferent arteriole dilation with consequent diminished GFR.
   f. Adequate blood flow largely controls GFR and is essential for normal renal function. Autoregulation maintains GFR between MAP of 60 and 200 mm Hg.

TABLE 8-1
DAILY RENAL SOLUTE EXCHANGE

	Filtered	Reabsorbed	Secreted	Urine
Sodium (mEq)	25,200	25,050	—	150 (100 mEq/L)
Potassium (mEq)	720	720	100	100 (67 mEq/L)
Chloride (mEq)	18,000	17,870	—	130 (87 mEq/L)
Bicarbonate (mEq)	4000	4000	—	0
Urea (mM)	900	500	—	400 (267 mM)
Creatinine (mM)	15	—	—	15 (10 mM)
Glucose (mM)	900	900	—	0
Total solutes (mOsm)	49,735	49,040	140	910 (607 mOsm/L)
Water (ml)	180,000	178,500	—	1500

5. **Glomerular filtration**
   a. GFR is the amount of ultrafiltrate generated by the glomerulus per unit time.
   b. GFR is approximately 125 ml/min or 180 L/day in a 70-kg male (10% of renal blood flow). GFR decreases with age.
   c. Glomerular capillary hydrostatic pressure is the most significant determinant of GFR and is directly proportional to RPP.
   d. The GFR is not easily measured and is usually estimated clinically by calculation of the endogenous creatinine clearance (see section II, C).
   e. Composition of ultrafiltrate: protein-free crystalloid solution with an electrolyte concentration nearly identical to that of circulating plasma.
6. **Tubular reabsorption:** Many of the filtered plasma solutes are either completely absent from the urine or present in substantially smaller quantities than in the initial ultrafiltrate (Table 8-1). The reabsorption capabilities of the renal tubules are demonstrated by the fact that 99% of the 180 L/day of ultrafiltrate is reabsorbed. Reabsorption of fluid and solutes in the tubule is accomplished via simple diffusion (concentration gradient), facilitated diffusion, active transport, or endocytosis.
7. **Tubular secretion:** Tubular secretion begins with simple diffusion of a substance out of the peritubular capillaries into the interstitium. Transport into the tubule may be active or passive, depending on the gradients of the particular solute. Tubular secretion plays a major role in hydrogen and potassium ion excretion.

II. CLINICAL ASSESSMENT OF RENAL FUNCTION
A. **HISTORY AND PHYSICAL**
1. **A history of azotemia, uremia, hypertension, hematuria, or proteinuria and review of all medications should be obtained.**
2. **Signs suggestive of renal insufficiency** include hypertension, alopecia, peripheral neuropathy, conjunctival calcification, band keratopathy, gynecomastia and/or testicular atrophy in males, peripheral edema, pericardial rub, and CHF.

B. URINALYSIS

1. Urine output

a. Under conditions of normal hydration, urine output should be within the range of 0.5 to 1.0 ml/kg/hr.

b. High urine output (polyuria) may indicate water diuresis ($U_{osm} <$ 250 mOsm/L) or solute diuresis ($U_{osm} >$ 250 mOsm/L). Water diuresis may be appropriate in the setting of primary polydipsia or intravenous infusion of dilute solutions; inappropriate causes include central and nephrogenic diabetes insipidus. Likewise, solute diuresis may be appropriate in the setting of saline loading or postobstructive diuresis and inappropriate in the setting of hyperglycemia or high-protein tube feeding.

c. Low urine output is described as either oliguria (<400 ml/day in an adult) or anuria (<100 ml/day).

2. Urine pH

a. Normal urine pH is 5.0 to 6.0 (range 4.5 to 8.0).

b. Urine pH normally varies with systemic acid-base balance.

c. In patients with metabolic acidosis, the urine pH should generally be less than 5.0. Urine pH greater than 5.3 in this setting indicates abnormal urinary acidification and the presence of renal tubular acidosis.

d. In patients with metabolic alkalosis resulting from volume contraction (saline responsive), a persistently low urine pH indicates inadequate volume repletion.

e. Diagnostic use of the urine pH requires that the urine be sterile as infection with any of the urease-producing pathogens results in pH elevation.

3. Urine specific gravity

a. Specific gravity ranges between 1.003 and 1.030 and is a measure of the density of urine.

b. Failure to reabsorb water is a sign of renal tubular dysfunction. This may be manifest as hyposthenuria (low urine osmolarity or specific gravity) in the face of plasma hyperosmolarity. The urine specific gravity correlates with urine osmolarity (U_{osm}) but can be influenced by many factors, including glycosuria and proteinuria, and is less accurate than U_{osm}. Consequently, specific gravity is an unreliable indicator of volume status or renal function in the presence of glycosuria, after use of intravenous radiographic contrast agents, or in patients receiving diuretics.

4. Urine dipstick

a. Glucose: Glucose is normally absent from urine. The normal renal threshold is approximately 180 mg/dl serum glucose level (range 165 to 200). Above this level, enough glucose is filtered to exceed maximal tubular reabsorption.

b. Protein
   (1) Chemical dipsticks used to detect protein react with albumin only.
   (2) Only positively charged proteins of low molecular weight usually cross the glomerular capillary membrane and appear in the urine (<200 mg/day excreted).

(3) With glomerular disease, the capillary membrane is disrupted and protein (albumin) becomes detected in the urine; massive proteinuria (>3.5 g/day) is diagnostic of glomerular disease.

(4) Proteinuria, if detected by dipstick, should be quantified in a 24-hour urine collection before elective operation. Excretion greater than 200 mg in 24 hours is indicative of significant renal parenchymal disease and warrants a more detailed evaluation before elective procedures.

c. Ketones

(1) Ketones are normally absent from urine.

(2) Ketonuria is seen with conditions of ketone body overproduction, including diabetic ketoacidosis, starvation, alcoholism, and pregnancy.

d. Leukocyte esterase and nitrite

(1) Leukocyte esterase detects abnormal numbers of WBCs in the urine and is 80% to 90% sensitive in detecting urinary tract infections (UTIs). However, leukocyte esterase will not differentiate urinary tract WBCs from WBCs from contamination (e.g., vaginal secretions) during specimen collection.

(2) Many bacteria produce the enzyme reductase that reduces urinary nitrates to nitrites, which are detectable by dipstick. Sensitivity of the nitrite test for UTI is about 50%.

(3) The combination of leukocyte esterase and nitrite further improve the sensitivity for UTI.

e. Bilirubin and urobilinogen

(1) Conjugated bilirubin is normally absent from urine but can be seen with elevated serum levels of bilirubin. Unconjugated bilirubin cannot pass the glomerular filter and does not appear in the urine. Consequently, patients with jaundice resulting from hemolytic anemia will have not have bilirubin detected in the urine.

(2) Urobilinogen is produced from both unconjugated and conjugated bilirubin by metabolic activity of bacteria in the duodenum and is subsequently absorbed into the bloodstream. Some of this reabsorbed urobilinogen is filtered by the kidneys and excreted in the urine. Thus increased levels of urobilinogen may be seen with elevated serum levels of direct and indirect bilirubin. Patients with complete biliary obstruction have no bile reaching the duodenum and consequently no urobilinogen formation. The test must be performed within 30 minutes of collection as urobilinogen rapidly oxidizes in air to nondetectable urobilin.

f. Hemoglobin

(1) A positive urine dipstick for hemoglobin is seen in most patients with at least 2 RBCs/hpf on microscopic examination.

(2) The dipstick also reacts with myoglobin.

5. Microscopic analysis of urinary sediment

a. Examination should be done within 1 hour of collection to avoid cell lysis.

b. RBCs (see section III, D): Gross urinary bleeding is usually seen with stones, acute glomerulonephritis, tumor, and trauma. Conditions associated with significant microscopic hematuria and occasionally gross bleeding include clotting disorders, blood dyscrasias, renal infarction, malignant hypertension, subacute bacterial endocarditis (SBE), collagen vascular disease, and UTI.

c. WBCs

(1) WBCs may originate from anywhere in the urinary tract.

(2) Pyuria of renal origin is usually accompanied by significant proteinuria. WBC casts are definite evidence that urinary WBCs originate in the kidney.

(3) UTI is usually accompanied by bacteruria.

d. Epithelial cells: The presence of more than 10 squamous epithelial cells per low-power field is an indicator of possible contamination. Urinary sample contamination rates may be as high as 30% in females.

6. **Urine electrolytes and fractional excretion of sodium (FE$_{Na}$)**

a. Normal urine electrolytes are listed in Table 8-1.

b. Urine sodium (U$_{Na}$) is generally an excellent indicator of tubular reabsorptive capacity. With volume contraction, renal tubular sodium reabsorption should increase, whereas U$_{Na}$ should decrease (<20 mEq/L). Therefore, in a patient with volume contraction, a high U$_{Na}$ (>20 mEq/L) likely indicates tubular dysfunction.

c. FE$_{Na}$ is the fraction of the sodium filtered that is ultimately excreted. As tubular reabsorption of sodium increases, FE$_{Na}$ falls. FE$_{Na}$ is an even more reliable indicator of volume status than U$_{Na}$ and is calculated by the formula:

$$FE_{Na} (\%) = (U_{Na}/P_{Na})/(U_{Cr}/P_{Cr}) \times 100$$

where   FE$_{Na}$ = fractional excretion of sodium
    (U$_{Na}$/P$_{Na}$) = ratio of urine and plasma sodium concentrations
    (U$_{Cr}$/P$_{Cr}$) = ratio of urine and plasma creatinine concentrations

(1) In the presence of hypovolemia and hypoperfusion the renin-angiotensin system is activated, and the subsequent release of aldosterone will induce the kidney to reabsorb sodium. Therefore an FE$_{Na}$ less than 1% is indicative of a prerenal etiology of ARF.

(2) FE$_{Na}$ greater than 3% is consistent with tubular injury or obstruction.

(3) FE$_{Na}$ between 1% and 3% is nonspecific and may be seen with mixed prerenal and renal parenchymal causes of ARF.

d. Assessment of renal function or volume status by urine electrolytes is unreliable in the presence of a preexisting prerenal state (e.g., CHF, cirrhosis), with diuretic therapy, or after the use of contrast dye.

C. **PLASMA CREATININE (P$_{Cr}$) AND CREATININE CLEARANCE (C$_{Cr}$)**

1. **Creatinine,** produced via conversion of muscle creatine in the liver, is removed from the plasma mainly by glomerular filtration (80%) with only minor secretion (20%) by the proximal tubule. Because the renal

excretion (clearance) of creatinine is approximately equal to its production, the plasma creatinine remains relatively constant. An increase of 1 mg/dl over baseline generally indicates a 50% decrease in GFR. An increase of more than 2 mg/dl/day suggests a rapid rate of protein breakdown, as might occur in the setting of rhabdomyolysis or resolving hematoma.

2. **As renal failure progresses, P_{Cr} is a less reliable indicator of GFR** because of increasing tubular secretion of creatinine.

3. **A gradual rise in plasma creatinine does not necessarily reflect continuing renal injury.** A steady state level will take several days to develop and the creatinine will rise continually until a new plateau is reached.

4. **In patients with decreased muscle mass,** P_{Cr} can remain within normal limits despite significantly impaired renal function.

5. **Certain drugs** (e.g., trimethoprim and cimetidine) may compete for tubular creatinine secretion and spuriously elevate P_{Cr} levels. Likewise, other substances may be measured as creatinine by the chemical assay. Examples of the latter include cefoxitin and acetone.

6. **C_{Cr} is a better estimate of GFR than P_{Cr}.**

a. C_{Cr} can be determined by measuring creatinine in a 24-hour urine collection and obtaining a simultaneous plasma creatinine. At Duke University Medical Center, we serially measure 2-hour creatinine clearance in the ICU to detect early changes in renal function not yet reflected in P_{Cr}. Studies have shown the 2-hour test to correlate highly with results obtained over longer collection periods.

b. Formula for determining actual creatinine clearance after a timed urine collection:

$$C_{Cr} \text{ (ml/min)} = U_{Cr} \times U_{vol}/P_{Cr}$$

where U_{Cr} = urinary creatinine (mg/dl)
   U_{vol} = urine volume (ml/minutes collected)
   P_{Cr} = plasma creatinine (mg/dl)

c. A diurnal variation in creatinine clearance exists with higher values generally obtained in the afternoon. This variation may be as much as ±25%. Because of this variation, creatinine clearance should be measured at the same time each day.

d. Incomplete urine collections lead to errors in calculating C_{Cr}. This can be checked by confirming that the daily urinary creatinine excretion (mg/24 hr) approximates the daily creatinine production (15 to 20 mg/kg/day in females; 20 to 25 mg/kg/day in males). Failure to achieve these levels of U_{Cr} invalidates the C_{Cr}, regardless of the degree of renal functional impairment.

e. C_{Cr} may also be estimated using the age (years), body weight (kg), plasma creatinine (P_{Cr} in mg/dl), and the formula:

$$C_{Cr} \text{ (ml/min)} = [(140 - \text{age}) \times \text{weight}/72 \times P_{Cr}] \, (\times 0.85 \text{ for females})$$

D. BLOOD UREA NITROGEN

1. **BUN** is the end-product of protein degradation via the urea cycle. It is freely filterable, but approximately 50% of filtered urea is reabsorbed. This reabsorption occurs passively and is dependent on water reabsorption to establish the diffusion gradient for urea. Therefore BUN reflects both the renal function and volume status of a patient.

2. Because urea generation is directly dependent on protein intake and degradation, **BUN may an unreliable indicator** of renal dysfunction in malnourished patients.

E. URINE OSMOLARITY (U_{osm}) AND PLASMA OSMOLARITY (P_{osm})

1. **Healthy kidneys excrete an osmolar load while retaining free water.** If damage to the renal tubules occurs, this ability to excrete hyperosmolar urine becomes impaired and urine and plasma osmolarity will approach equal values.

2. **U_{osm}** (40 to 700 mOsm/L) indicates the amount of solute in a given volume of urine. A U_{osm} less than 300 mOsm/L in the face of a P_{osm} greater than 290 mOsm/L is consistent with inappropriate water loss or diabetes insipidus.

3. **Maximal urine concentration** by the normal kidney is approximately 1400 mOsm/L.

4. **Normal P_{osm}** is 285 +15 mOsm/L.

5. **P_{osm} may be falsely elevated** because of osmotically active molecules, for example, glucose, urea, or ethanol, present in excess amounts. In the presence of hyperglycemia or elevated BUN, P_{osm} may be corrected by the formula:

$$P_{osm} = 2 \times [Na^+] + BUN\ (mg/dl)/2.8 + glucose\ (mg/dl)/18$$

F. RADIOLOGIC EVALUATION OF THE GENITOURINARY TRACT

1. **Table 8-2** lists the more commonly used techniques for imaging the genitourinary system, as well as their relative usefulness for assessing renal structure and function.

2. Because of its accuracy in evaluating kidney size and excluding obstruction, **renal ultrasonography is often the initial screening test for the evaluation of azotemia.**

III. PERIOPERATIVE MANAGEMENT OF THE RENAL SYSTEM

A. ESTABLISHED (CHRONIC) RENAL FAILURE

1. **Chronic renal failure** (CRF) is a syndrome that results from the irreversible impairment or destruction of nephrons, regardless of cause, and is assigned when renal insufficiency persists for more than 3 months. Conditions encountered with this syndrome include impaired fluid and electrolyte regulation, coagulopathy, suppressed erythropoiesis and immune function, atherosclerosis, hypertension, pericarditis, encephalitis, and peripheral neuropathy.

2. **Preexisting renal insufficiency** increases the risk of complications in the perioperative period. This risk increases with the severity of renal failure.

TABLE 8-2			
RADIOLOGIC EVALUATION OF THE KIDNEYS			
Study	Anatomy	Function	Utility
KUB	*	—	Nephrolithiasis, intraurinary air
Intravenous pyelogram	***	***	Nephrolithiasis, obstruction, pyelonephritis, tumors
Retrograde pyelogram	****	*	Obstruction, filling defects
Cystogram	***	**	Bladder and lower urinary tract anatomy and function
Ultrasound	***	—	Renal size, hydronephrosis, tumor, nephrolithiasis
CT	****	**	Renal, retroperitoneal, and adrenal anatomy
Technetium scan	*	***	Renal blood flow and glomerular filtration
Arteriogram	****	****	Renal vasculature, upper and lower urinary tracts

If GFR is greater than 50 ml/min, surgery is usually well tolerated and no specific precautions are needed. If GFR is less than 20 ml/min, perioperative complications are more likely to occur unless specific preventive steps are taken.

3. **Perioperative considerations** for patients with chronic renal failure.

a. Preoperative

   (1) Obtain a baseline weight preoperatively to help assess changes in volume status during the perioperative period.

   (2) For elective procedures in patients with end-stage renal disease, dialyze preoperatively and postoperatively. However, routine hemodialysis performed less than 6 hours before surgery or in the first 24 hours thereafter increases the risk of perioperative bleeding. If dialysis is absolutely necessary during these periods, it may be performed without heparin. Typically, patients should receive their last hemodialysis between 6 and 30 hours before surgery. If performed more than 30 hours before surgery, the risk of intraoperative hyperkalemia increases.

   (3) In patients on chronic peritoneal dialysis, the abdomen should be drained before induction of general anesthesia to reduce intraabdominal pressure, facilitate intraoperative mechanical ventilation, and decrease the risk of aspiration.

   (4) Because of suppressed immune function, prophylactic antibiotics and careful wound management are essential. Antibiotic dosing should be adjusted for the degree of renal impairment. To minimize the chance of vascular access infection, all patients on hemodialysis should receive antibiotic prophylaxis before any procedure that might cause bacteremia. The American Heart Association guidelines for endocarditis prophylaxis are applicable to patients on hemodialysis.

b. Intraoperative

(1) Muscle relaxants should be carefully chosen. Succinylcholine is generally well tolerated, although it produces a rise in the serum potassium level in both normal patients and those with CRF. This increase may be deleterious in CRF patients with an already elevated potassium level. The half-lives of D-tubocurarine and pancuronium are prolonged in patients with CRF. Vecuronium and atracurium are probably the muscle relaxants of choice in these patients, although cumulative effects of vecuronium may be seen with repeated doses. Atracurium is not affected by either renal or hepatic dysfunction and is thus ideal.

(2) General anesthesia of any type causes a reduction in renal blood flow that is proportional to the depth of anesthesia. Spinal anesthesia causes only minimal alterations in renal hemodynamics, although hypotension resulting from sympathetic blockade is to be avoided. Overall, the requirements of the procedure rather than the presence of CRF should dictate the choice of anesthesia.

c. Postoperative

(1) Initial postoperative assessment should begin with careful review of intraoperative fluid balance (urine output, blood loss, and fluid replacement) and hemodynamic course.

(2) Vital signs and urine output should be monitored immediately and throughout the postoperative period. Intravascular volume status must be assessed and consideration given to invasive monitoring of CVP, PCWP, and cardiac output for patients at risk for ARF. Daily weights are also essential.

(3) Patients with CRF are very sensitive to narcotic analgesics, and morphine metabolism may be diminished in renal failure. Consequently, morphine doses in these patients must be reduced to avoid respiratory depression. Meperidine (Demerol) should be avoided, especially in repeated doses, because accumulation of its primary metabolite, normeperidine, may accumulate and lead to seizures. Codeine doses may need to be reduced, as well.

(4) In non–end-stage renal disease patients, hourly urine output should be at least 0.5 ml/kg/hr.

(5) Nutrition: Patients with CRF are frequently malnourished, which may contribute to postoperative morbidity. Enteral and parenteral nutritional support have been shown to improve survival in patients with CRF undergoing surgery and should be considered early in the postoperative period.

(6) Aggressive application of renal replacement therapy (usually hemodialysis or peritoneal dialysis) is essential to minimize complications of CRF in the perioperative setting. Low-dose heparin hemodialysis techniques are typically used for the first postoperative week to decrease bleeding complications.

(7) Attention must be paid to preserving the vascular access of patients already on hemodialysis during the perioperative period. This

includes avoiding pressure on the limb where the access is located and minimizing hypotension during and after the procedure. No needle sticks should be performed in the extremity with the access.

4. **Potential perioperative complications of decreased renal function.**
   a. Fluid overload: The administration of large quantities of intravenous fluids can lead to extracellular fluid overload, particularly when GFR is less than 10 ml/min. However, maximum sodium excretion is decreased even in patients with moderate renal insufficiency, and large sodium loads given quickly may cause significant volume expansion.
   b. Acidosis: Chronic metabolic acidosis is usually present in patients with CRF. This acidosis is usually well compensated by respiratory hyperventilation, and blood pH is only slightly below normal. However, these patients may rapidly develop a severe acidosis in the perioperative period; consequently, the serum bicarbonate concentration should be 18 mEq/L or higher before surgery.
   c. Hyperkalemia: Although patients with moderate renal insufficiency can usually maintain a normal steady-state serum potassium concentration, they do not tolerate sudden shifts of potassium ions into the extracellular fluid. Consequently, hyperkalemia is a common complication of surgery in these patients. Because the risk of perioperative hyperkalemia correlates with the preoperative serum potassium level, this level should be below 5 mEq/L before surgery.
   d. Disorders of calcium and phosphate homeostasis: Marked hypocalcemia increases the cardiovascular risk of general anesthesia. Treatment of severe hypocalcemia should begin with control of the serum phosphate level. If phosphate is greater than 6 mg/dl in a patient with severe hypocalcemia, oral phosphate binders or dialysis should be used to lower it. Decreasing the serum phosphate to less than 5.5 mg/dl may lead to a slight increase in the serum calcium level and allow safe administration of calcium. Hypocalcemia can then be treated with oral calcium supplements ($\geq$1 g/day elemental calcium) and the vitamin D derivative 1,25-dihyroxycholecalciferol (0.5 to 0.75 μg/day). Intravenous calcium may be given if more rapid therapy is needed. Symptomatic hypocalcemia may develop in the postoperative period after release of intracellular phosphate. Serum phosphate levels should be controlled before direct efforts to increase serum calcium concentrations are made. Intravenous calcium should be considered only if definite signs of hypocalcemia are present.
   e. Bleeding: Patients with chronic renal failure have an increased bleeding tendency because of multifactorial defects in platelet aggregation. The bleeding time is the only test that correlates with clinical bleeding in uremic patients and should be obtained preoperatively in patients with CRF and a history of excessive bleeding. More intensive dialysis preoperatively may shorten the bleeding time. In addition, intravenous desmopressin (DDAVP) (0.4 μg/kg) may be given immediately before the procedure and is effective for 6 to 8 hours. Additional doses should

not be given in less than 24 hours because of the development of tachyphylaxis. Oral or intravenous estrogens may be given, as well. Their onset of action is slower, but the therapeutic effect lasts longer than that of DDAVP. Raising the hematocrit to at least 30% also decreases the bleeding time by improving platelet adhesion. Cryoprecipitate and platelet transfusions also decrease the bleeding time and reduce bleeding complications.

B. PREVENTION OF ACUTE RENAL FAILURE

1. **The preservation of renal function** in patients with CRF who have not yet progressed to end-stage renal disease is paramount in the perioperative period. Preexisting renal insufficiency is a major risk factor for the development of postoperative ARF.

2. **Maintenance of renal perfusion** by aggressive management of hypovolemia, hypoxemia, and low cardiac output are goals in the prevention of ARF.

3. **Contrast agents and nephrotoxic drugs** (NSAIDs, aminoglycoside antibiotics) should be used only when the benefits outweigh the risk of renal failure. When contrast studies are unavoidable in patients with CRF, an infusion of ½ normal saline should be started 1 to 2 hours before the study and continued for 4 to 6 hours thereafter.

4. **Diuretics confer no long-term benefit** in the treatment of ARF. Attempts to convert oliguric to nonoliguric renal failure by administering diuretics have shown no benefit; diuretic response merely identifies those patients with less severe degrees of renal dysfunction.

5. **Renal-dose dopamine (1 to 3 μg/kg/min) has no demonstrated efficacy** in the prevention of ARF.

C. URINARY OBSTRUCTION

1. **Most urinary obstruction** in the perioperative period consists of urinary retention. This may be due to interference with the autonomic nervous system by anesthesia or other drugs. This combined with bladder atonicity resulting from overdistention can lead to acute urinary retention.

2. **Bladder overdistention should be prevented** by having the patient void on call to the OR for short procedures or by placing a Foley catheter for prolonged operations.

3. **If a patient is unable to void in the postoperative period,** initial measures should include ambulation and placing a warm bag of saline over the suprapubic region. If this fails, bethanechol (5 mg SQ) may be administered in young patients with no contraindications to the drug (e.g., asthma, COPD, bowel obstruction, recent GI surgery, bladder outlet obstruction, cardiac disease). If bethanechol fails, or in patients with contraindications to its use, bladder catheterization should be performed. If the patient's urinary retention is caused by bladder outlet obstruction (e.g., benign prostatic hypertrophy in older men), the catheter should be left in place until the patient is fully ambulatory.

4. **Larger catheters (18 to 22 F) with Coude tips** are generally more effective if obstruction is at prostatic level. Smaller catheters (12 to 14 F) are more effective in urethral stricture disease.

5. **Before manipulation of the infected lower urinary tract,** broad-spectrum antibiotics should be administered, and the patient should be observed closely after manipulation for signs of sepsis.

6. **Watch closely for postobstructive diuresis** in the postrenally azotemic patient who has undergone relief of lower urinary tract (or bilateral upper tract) obstruction. Urine output should be replaced 0.5 ml/ml with D_5 ½ NS while monitoring serum electrolytes until resolution of the diuresis.

D. HEMATURIA

1. **Defined as greater than 1 RBC/hpf in males, greater than 3 RBC/hpf in females.**

2. **Bleeding** may arise from the urethra, prostate, bladder, ureter, or kidney. Hematuria in the first part of the stream is usually from the urethra, whereas terminal hematuria suggests a bladder neck or prostate source. Hematuria throughout the urinary stream suggests a bladder, ureteral, or renal source.

3. **A positive dipstick or even "gross" hematuria** must be confirmed by microscopic examination of the urinary sediment. False-positive dipsticks can result from hemoglobinuria, myoglobinuria, or ascorbic acid.

4. **Presence of RBC casts or dysmorphic RBCs** along with proteinuria (≥ 3 g) is consistent with glomerular disease.

5. **Presence of pyuria, dysuria, bacteruria, and WBC casts** are consistent with urinary tract infection (e.g., urethritis, cystitis, or pyelonephritis).

6. **If hematuria fails to clear after adequate treatment for UTI,** or in patients with no microscopic evidence for glomerular disease or UTI, cystoscopy and intravenous pyelography (IVP) are indicated to rule out urologic tumor.

7. **Posttraumatic hematuria**

   a. Hematuria in the trauma setting is defined as greater than 5 RBCs/hpf.

   b. Physical examination findings suggestive of potential renal injury include fractured lower ribs, flank ecchymoses or abrasions, and penetrating lower thorax or upper abdominal wounds. Pelvic fractures should raise concern for both urethral and bladder injuries (15% incidence with pelvic fracture). Blood at the meatus, high-riding prostate on rectal examination, and hematoma of the penis, scrotum, or perineum all suggest possible urethral injury.

   c. All patients with suspected urethral injury must undergo urethrography before catheterization. If the diagnosis of urethral injury is made, suprapubic cystostomy is the preferred method of draining the bladder.

   d. Blunt trauma.

      (1) The degree of hematuria does not necessarily correlate with injury severity. However, in blunt trauma victims (excluding rapid-deceleration injury) with microscopic hematuria alone and no evidence of shock, the incidence of significant urologic injury is less than 1%. These patients usually have a low-grade renal injury that can be managed conservatively, and no further evaluation is necessary.

(2) The incidence of significant urologic injury (usually renal) is increased in blunt trauma victims with microscopic hematuria and shock, and CT with IV contrast should be performed if the patient can be stabilized. One-shot IVP should be done in the OR for patients requiring immediate operative intervention.

(3) Trauma patients with gross hematuria require urgent renal imaging, usually with CT. Likewise, bladder rupture must be ruled out in this setting and may be done via CT cystogram.

(4) Although hematuria will be seen with most significant traumatic renal injuries, both renal pedicle avulsion and acute renal artery thrombosis may present without hematuria. These injuries do not normally occur as an isolated event and are commonly associated with closed head, abdominal, thoracic, and extremity injuries. The usual injury mechanism is rapid deceleration, as with motor vehicle crashes or falls from great heights. All patients with rapid-deceleration injury need urgent renal imaging. This can usually be performed in conjunction with imaging required for associated injuries.

e. Penetrating trauma.

(1) Any victim of penetrating trauma with either microscopic or gross hematuria requires further urologic evaluation. However, hematuria may be absent in patients with penetrating ureteral injury, so a high index of suspicion is needed in patients with penetrating injuries in the vicinity of the anatomic course of the ureters.

(2) Some 80% or more of patients with penetrating renal injuries will have associated abdominal injuries.

(3) CT is the study of choice in stable patients to evaluate potential renal or ureteral injury. Cystography (conventional or CT) will best define bladder injuries.

(4) Renal venous injuries are difficult to detect on CT or IVP and usually require selective venography.

(5) For penetrating trauma victims who remain hemodynamically unstable and require operative intervention, intraoperative one-shot IVP will provide information on the presence and function of both kidneys and may detail parenchymal and ureteral injuries.

IV. MANAGEMENT OF ACUTE RENAL FAILURE

A. GENERAL CONSIDERATIONS

1. **ARF** by definition is an abrupt decrease in kidney function that results in accumulation of nitrogenous solutes (azotemia). Clinically, this usually presents as a decrease in urine output (<0.5 ml/kg/hr in an adult) or a significant rise in serum creatinine. Most renal failure encountered in surgical patients is not single-organ failure and occurs in the context of simultaneous dysfunction of several organ systems (multisystem organ failure [MSOF]).

2. **Urine output in ARF may be oliguric (<400 ml/day) or nonoliguric,** in which urine output is normal or increased while solute clearance is

THE RENAL SYSTEM

8

markedly impaired. Mortality from nonoliguric ARF is significantly less than from oliguric renal failure, although many cases progress to oliguria with its accompanying poor outcome.

3. **Regardless of urine output, the sequelae of ARF are due to retention of metabolic wastes.** Hypervolemia and electrolyte imbalances further complicate management of oliguric ARF.

B. ETIOLOGY/EVALUATION (Figure 8-1)

1. **The pathogenesis of ARF** is commonly classified as postrenal, prerenal, or renal parenchymal disease. In some patients, more than one cause of

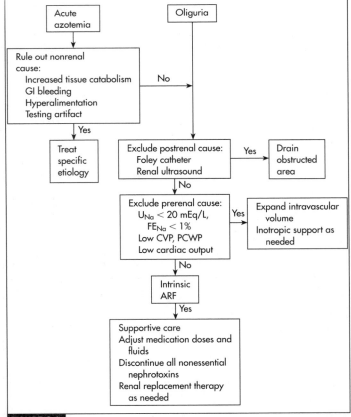

FIGURE 8-1

Management algorithm for acute renal failure.

renal dysfunction may be present, so all potential mechanisms should be considered.

2. Postrenal ARF (1% to 15% of cases).

a. Obstructive uropathy must always be ruled out in the oliguric patient.

b. Evaluation of a potential postrenal etiology of ARF includes the following:

(1) History: Patients may complain of flank pain resulting from acute distention of the renal capsule or suprapubic discomfort caused by bladder distention. It may be due to prostatic enlargement or a plugged Foley catheter.

(2) Physical examination: Examine for bladder distention and, if a Foley catheter is already in place, flush to make sure it is properly functioning.

(3) Diagnosis may be made by placing a Foley catheter and observing large output of urine after relief of bladder neck obstruction. In addition, renal ultrasonography is a quick and simple procedure to evaluate both the upper and lower urinary tracts for obstruction.

c. ARF is unlikely to result from unilateral upper urinary tract obstruction without pathology in the contralateral kidney.

3. Prerenal ARF (50% to 90% of cases).

a. ARF caused by renal hypoperfusion is classified as prerenal. This is the most common cause of an acute decrease in urine output in surgical patients and is usually the result of decreased intravascular volume. Other causes include primary myocardial dysfunction and decreased renal perfusion resulting from abdominal compartment syndrome.

b. Surgical patients are at risk for hypovolemia and hypoperfusion; therefore any patient with oliguria should be assumed to be hypovolemic until proven otherwise. Typical circumstances that precipitate prerenal ARF in surgical patients are listed in Box 8-1.

c. Evaluation of a potential prerenal etiology of ARF includes the following:

(1) History: Review fluid balance over the past several hours and days. Fluid output significantly greater than input suggests a prerenal

THE RENAL SYSTEM

BOX 8-1
CAUSES OF PRERENAL ARF IN SURGICAL PATIENTS
VOLUME CHANGES
Dehydration
Blood loss
Third space sequestration
HEMODYNAMIC CHANGES
Septic shock
Cardiogenic shock
Neurogenic hypotension
VASCULAR CHANGES
Renal artery stenosis
Renal vein thrombosis
Operative vessel occlusion

cause of oliguria. Likewise, review any changes in weight over the past few days. Weight loss in the acute setting is most likely secondary to fluid loss. Potential causes of fluid loss include the gastrointestinal tract (bowel obstruction with sequestration of large volumes of fluid in the intestine, nasogastric suction, vomiting, diarrhea), blood loss, and insensitive losses via the respiratory tract and skin, including burns and open wounds. It is important to realize, however, that patients with systemic infection, burns, major trauma, or other causes of the systemic inflammatory response syndrome (SIRS) may have liters of excess body fluid, as evidenced by peripheral edema and increased body weight, yet may still have intravascular volume depletion. If the patient has risk factors or a known history of cardiac disease, primary myocardial dysfunction should be considered. Other potential causes include renal vascular obstruction and intrarenal shunting resulting from the hepatorenal syndrome.

(2) Physical examination: Evaluate for flat neck veins, tachycardia, cool extremities, delayed capillary refill, and other signs of hypovolemia or decreased perfusion. Patients with primary myocardial dysfunction may have distended neck veins, however. If the abdomen is extremely firm, abdominal pressure may be measured by filling the bladder with sterile saline and transducing bladder pressure via the Foley catheter. If the pressure is greater than 40 cm H_2O, decompression should be considered.

(3) Urinalysis (Table 8-3): Urine should be checked for sodium, osmolarity, and specific gravity. A urine sodium less than 20 mEq/L along with an elevated urine osmolarity (>400 mOsm/L) and specific gravity (>1.024) demonstrate preserved concentrating function and suggest a prerenal cause.

TABLE 8-3

DIAGNOSTIC URINE CHEMISTRY

Test	Prerenal	Intrinsic (ATN)
GLOMERULAR FILTRATION		
Creatinine clearance (ml/min)	>40	<20
Urine/plasma creatinine	>40	<20
WATER REABSORPTION		
Specific gravity	>1.024	<1.015
Urine osmolarity (mOsm/L)	>400	<350
Urine/plasma osmolarity ratio	>1.5	<1
SODIUM REABSORPTION		
Urine sodium (mEq/L)	<20	>40
Fe_{Na} (%)	<1	>3
UREA		
Urine/plasma urea	>8	<3
BUN/creat$_{serum}$	>20	<15

(4) Fractional excretion of sodium (FE_{Na}) (see section II, B): In the presence of hypovolemia and hypoperfusion, the renin-angiotensin system is activated and the subsequent release of aldosterone promotes renal sodium reabsorption. Therefore an FE_{Na} less than 1% is indicative of a prerenal cause.

(5) FE_{Na} and urine sodium are the most reliable means of differentiating prerenal from other causes of ARF.

(6) Caution must be taken in interpreting any of these parameters in the presence of a preexisting prerenal state (e.g., CHF, cirrhosis), diuretics, or after the use of contrast dye.

(7) If the cause of ARF is still unclear after the above evaluation or if the patient does not respond appropriately to therapy, consider the use of a pulmonary arterial catheter to measure CVP, PCWP, and cardiac output to assist both diagnosis and further therapy. Also, consider the use of echocardiography to evaluate cardiac function in patients in whom the above tests suggest a prerenal cause yet intravascular volume status is adequate.

4. **Renal Parenchymal ARF (10% to 30% of cases).**

a. Renal parenchymal ARF is usually diagnosed by excluding prerenal and postrenal causes. Evaluation of a potential intrinsic renal cause of ARF should include the same work-up as outlined above for prerenal ARF. Findings suggestive of renal parenchymal ARF include normal volume status, normal perfusion, specific gravity less than 1.015, urine osmolarity less than 350 mOsm/L, urine sodium greater than 40 mEq/L, and FE_{Na} greater than 3%.

b. Potential causes include ATN resulting from ischemia or nephrotoxic agents, including pigment nephropathy and, rarely, drug-induced allergic interstitial nephritis. Other causes of parenchymal renal disease, such as acute glomerulonephritis and vasculitis, are not typically responsible for ARF in the surgical patient.

c. Acute tubular necrosis

(1) ATN accounts for the majority (80%) of intrinsic renal parenchymal failure.

(2) The major causes of ATN include ischemic and toxic insults. In general, the ischemic causes have a higher incidence of oliguria and a more prolonged clinical course.

(3) Severe hemorrhage, hypotension, and shock are typical examples of ischemic insults. Ischemia may also result from ACE inhibitor−induced efferent arteriole dilation (see section I, B) in patients with bilateral renal artery stenosis or severe CHF. Likewise, NSAIDs may compromise renal blood flow via inhibition of prostaglandin-induced vasodilatation in patients with cirrhosis, CHF, or volume depletion. Prolonged prerenal azotemia can also lead to ATN.

(4) Nephrotoxic agents include aminoglycoside antibiotics, various chemotherapeutic agents, radiographic contrast agents, and various

8

THE RENAL SYSTEM

heavy metals and solvents. In addition, hemoglobin and myoglobin may cause renal tubular damage.

(a) Nephrotoxic drugs: Drug-induced ARF is responsible for approximately 5% of all cases of ARF. The site of damage of several well-documented nephrotoxic drugs is listed in Box 8-2.

(b) Contrast media: Iodinated radiographic contrast agents are a common nephrotoxin. The incidence of contrast nephropathy is approximately 1% to 10% and may be predicted according to a number of risk factors. These include contrast load, age, preexisting renal insufficiency, and diabetes. The incidence in patients with normal renal function is significantly lower at 1% to 2%. Contrast nephropathy is usually experienced as an asymptomatic, transient rise in P_{Cr} but may progress to oliguric renal failure requiring hemodialysis. Induced diuresis with fluids

BOX 8-2
NEPHROTOXIC DRUGS
GLOMERULUS
Heroin
Hydralazine
Penicillamine
Probenecid
Procainamide
RENAL ARTERIOLES
Allopurinol
Penicillin G
Propothiouracil
Sulfonamides
Thiazides
PROXIMAL TUBULE
Aminoglycosides
Amphotericin B
Cephaloridine
Polymyxin B
DISTAL TUBULES
Amphotericin B
Lithium
Vitamin D intoxication
INTERSTITIAL
Acetaminophen
Aspirin
Methicillin
Penicillin G
Phenacetin

and diuretics before contrast injection may decrease the incidence and severity of ARF in high-risk patients.

(c) Pigment nephropathy (myoglobinuria and hemoglobinuria) may result from hemolysis or rhabdomyolysis and is a common cause of ARF after trauma, burns, transfusion reactions, CPB, seizures, alcohol or drug intoxication, prolonged muscle ischemia, or extended coma. Although myoglobin is not a direct nephrotoxin, in the presence of aciduria it is converted to ferrihemate, which is toxic to renal cells. Diagnosis can be made by finding elevated serum CPK, hemoglobin, or myoglobin, and urine sediment microscopy demonstrating prominent heme pigment without RBCs. Hyperkalemia and elevated P_{Cr} are also consistent with injury to muscle masses.

(d) Prevention of myoglobin-induced ARF includes generous hydration, use of osmotic agents, and alkalinization of the urine to a pH greater than 6. However, the most important factor is to maintain a urine output of at least 100 ml/hr until myoglobin is no longer detectable in the urine.

d. Interstitial nephritis

(1) Drug-induced allergic interstitial nephritis accounts for 90% of cases of acute interstitial nephritis and about 10% of cases of intrinsic renal failure. Numerous agents may produce the syndrome, including antibiotics (e.g., penicillins, cephalosporins, sulfonamides), NSAIDs, and various diuretics, among others.

(2) The time to onset is variable, usually days to weeks after the patient begins antibiotics, although the condition may develop weeks to months after starting therapy with NSAIDs. Most cases are idiosyncratic and not dose-related.

(3) Patients may have fever, skin rash, or eosinophilia. Arthralgias are also common. Eosinophiluria is present in most cases of antibiotic-related disease.

(4) The syndrome should resolve with discontinuation of the offending agent. Steroids may accelerate recovery.

e. SIADH

(1) SIADH does not represent true renal failure, although the condition may present with oliguria. Serum creatinine is normal.

(2) Potential causes include ectopic ADH production (e.g., carcinoma, lymphoma), CNS disorders (e.g., closed head injury [CHI], tumor, intracranial hemorrhage, infection), and pulmonary disorders (e.g., viral or bacterial pneumonia, TB, positive-pressure ventilation). All causes are characterized by the continuous, nonsuppressible secretion of ADH.

(3) Diagnosis based on finding high urine sodium (>30 mEq/L); normal to low serum sodium; high urine osmolarity (usually >400 mOsm/L) in the face of low serum osmolarity; and normal thyroid, adrenal, and renal function.

8

THE RENAL SYSTEM

(4) This disorder is treated by fluid restriction and loop diuretics, if needed. Hypertonic saline is used only if the patient is symptomatic from hyponatremia. SIADH usually resolves spontaneously with no adverse effects on the kidneys.

C. MANAGEMENT OF ACUTE RENAL FAILURE (see Figure 8-1)

1. Nonoliguric ARF

a. Rule out nonrenal causes of acute azotemia. Increased BUN may result from protein breakdown from tissue catabolism, corticosteroids, gastrointestinal bleeding, or hyperalimentation. Increased P_{Cr} may be seen with rhabdomyolysis and administration of certain drugs (see section II, C).

b. Treatment for nonoliguric ARF patients may differ only slightly from treatment required for identical patients with normal renal function. Unlike patients with oliguric renal failure, a fluid challenge should not be used in these patients.

c. All medications should be reviewed and any nonessential nephrotoxic agents discontinued. In addition, all medications should be dose-adjusted for the degree of renal dysfunction based on the estimated or measured creatinine clearance.

d. Management of fluids, solutes, and nutrition is usually unaffected by nonoliguric ARF.

e. The extent of renal dysfunction is limited and almost always reversible. Use of renal replacement therapy is rarely necessary.

2. Oliguric ARF

a. A postrenal cause should be excluded first (see section IV, B). If a patient has two functioning kidneys, a Foley catheter excludes obstructive uropathy of the bladder outlet. If this does not make the diagnosis, a renal ultrasound should be obtained to rule out upper tract obstruction. Although unilateral upper tract obstruction does not cause ARF, 1% of the population has a solitary kidney and "functionally" solitary kidneys (where one is nonfunctional) are even more common. Removal of the obstruction should return renal function to normal.

b. If a postrenal cause has been excluded, the possibility of a prerenal source should be evaluated (see section IV, B). Treatment of prerenal azotemia consists of administration of a fluid challenge (10% of estimated circulating volume or approximately 500 ml in a 70-kg adult). This will usually result in increased urine output when oliguria is due to hypovolemia. An even larger bolus may be needed in severe hypovolemia. Generally, isotonic solutions such as normal saline or lactated Ringer's solution are the initial volume of choice. From 65% to 75% of the infused fluid will leave the vascular compartment within 30 minutes, so repeat administration may be needed. Patients with evidence of primary myocardial dysfunction should have therapy directed at the underlying cause, for example, ischemia, cardiomyopathy, or valvular disease. In patients with abdominal compartment syndrome, the fascia may need to be opened to reduce intraabdominal pressure.

c. The treatment of intrinsic renal causes of ARF (see section IV, B) is supportive and includes maintaining adequate renal perfusion; avoiding additional renal insults; and management of fluid, electrolyte, and acid-base disorders as they arise.

d. Diuretics, including osmotic agents, have not been shown to decrease mortality from ARF and should generally be avoided because their use will invalidate the use of urine output and electrolyte values as useful tests of renal function for the next 24 hours after administration.

e. Dopamine

(1) Dopamine has diuretic and natriuretic effects, likely mediated via Na/K ATPase inhibition with subsequent impaired sodium reabsorption.

(2) In animal studies, stimulation of DA-1 dopamine receptors appears to decrease renal vascular resistance and increase renal blood flow. However, this has not been shown to translate into increased GFR.

(3) Human studies demonstrating increased renal blood flow either have shown concurrent increases in cardiac output or have not reported cardiac output data.

(4) Studies in surgical patients have shown dopamine to have a diuretic effect. However, any improvements in renal function appear secondary to increased cardiac output.

(5) Dopamine does not appear to prevent the development or limit the progression of ARF in critically ill patients.

(6) Potential adverse effects include increased myocardial oxygen consumption (even with doses $< 5 \mu g/kg/min$) and cardiac arrhythmias.

3. **Electrolyte derangements in ARF** (see Chapter 3)

a. Measure serum electrolytes daily.

b. Hyperkalemia (serum potassium > 6.5 mEq/L) is a medical emergency and a frequent electrolyte disorder with ARF.

(1) Under the conditions of hypercatabolism and tissue necrosis that characterize these patients, large amounts of potassium may be generated and accumulate over a short period of time.

(2) Acute hyperkalemia decreases cardiac excitability, which may ultimately result in asystole. These events are usually preceded by changes in the electrocardiogram that indicate hyperkalemia. These include loss of P waves, widening of the QRS complex, and peaked T waves.

c. Hyponatremia, hyperphosphatemia, hypocalcemia, and metabolic acidosis are also common with ARF and must be monitored closely. Treatment consists of appropriate additions or restrictions to intravenous solutions and effective use of the artificial kidney.

4. **Specific situations**

a. Burns

(1) The burn patient is at risk for developing ARF because of hypovolemia, sepsis, and myoglobinuria.

(2) When a burn injury produces extensive muscle necrosis with myoglobinuria, renal failure is common.

    (3) Hypovolemia and prerenal azotemia should be minimized via aggressive fluid and electrolyte resuscitation.

  b. CPB

    (1) Cardiac surgery requiring CPB places patients at greater risk for ARF than does general surgery. The overall incidence of ARF is approximately 5%, with a 2% incidence of ARF severe enough to require dialysis.

    (2) The incidence of ARF with valve replacement is approximately twice that after CABG.

    (3) ARF after cardiac surgery is due to renal ischemia. Predisposing factors include prolonged CPB, positive-pressure ventilation, increased age, preexisting chronic renal insufficiency, sepsis, and poor postoperative cardiac function.

    (4) Perioperative decreases in cardiac function are the most important cause of ARF.

    (5) There is a linear correlation between the length of CPB and the incidence of ARF. CPB contributes to ARF via a 30% decrease in renal blood flow and GFR by CPB, nonpulsatile flow, and CPB-induced hemolysis with potential pigment nephrotoxicity.

  c. Liver failure

    (1) Patients with jaundice preoperatively have an increased incidence of developing perioperative ARF. The incidence of ARF in patients with jaundice is approximately 8%. The most important predisposing factor is the degree of bilirubin elevation.

    (2) Hepatorenal syndrome: Patients with either acute or chronic liver dysfunction may develop oliguria and rising serum creatinine along with a low urine sodium. This syndrome clinically appears very similar to a prerenal cause of ARF; however, the intravascular volume status is normal, the urine output does not respond to fluid challenge, and the ratio of urine creatinine to plasma creatinine is greater than 30:1 (usually less than 30:1 with prerenal cause). There is no proven treatment for hepatorenal syndrome.

  d. Sepsis

    (1) Sepsis can cause ARF through direct and indirect effects, which cause both renal injury (ATN) and prerenal azotemia.

      (a) Direct effects include endotoxin- and prostaglandin-mediated damage to the renal microvasculature.

      (b) Indirect effects include hypotension, impaired regional Do_2, and metabolic disturbances that may result in ATN.

      (c) In addition, management of septicemia often requires the use of nephrotoxic antibiotics, which may further exacerbate tubular damage.

    (2) Norepinephrine may increase renal blood flow in patients with septic shock via improving MAP.

    (3) Low-dose dopamine, although it has been demonstrated to reverse norepinephrine-induced renal vasoconstriction in normal volunteers,

has not been shown to improve renal function in septic patients treated with vasopressors.

e. Trauma

   (1) Like thermal injury, the development of ARF in the posttraumatic patient is multifactorial, and hypovolemia is a major problem. Rapid fluid resuscitation must be instituted to avoid shock, which may lead to ARF if untreated.

   (2) If after stabilization and restoration of intravascular volume the patient becomes oliguric, the possibility of traumatic injury to the ureter, bladder, or urethra must be ruled out (see section III, D).

   (3) With blunt trauma to large muscle masses, rhabdomyolysis-induced ARF is a significant concern (see section IV, B).

f. Vascular surgery

   (1) The incidence of ARF after aortic surgery is approximately 8%.

   (2) The most common cause of ARF during vascular surgery is ischemic renal injury and ATN. The most significant predictor of perioperative ARF is preexisting renal insufficiency. Other predisposing factors include expanding or ruptured aortic aneurysms, thoracic aneurysms, perioperative hypotension, and suprarenal aortic cross-clamping.

5. Prognosis

a. Mortality in patients with ARF has remained unchanged and currently ranges from 30% to 80%. Mortality (>70%) is highest in patients with ARF as part of the MSOF syndrome. Death is most commonly caused by infection, with pneumonia being the most common fatal infection.

b. Both survival and recovery of renal function are better in patients with nonoliguric versus oliguric ARF.

c. Recovery of renal function depends on patient age, cause of ARF (worst prognosis with prolonged ischemic insults), and urine output during ARF. Younger patients and those with nonoliguric renal failure have a better prognosis. Patients with ARF who survive have a 25% to 30% chance of complete recovery of renal function and a 40% to 50% chance of at least partial recovery.

d. For patients who recover renal function, 80% do so within 30 days.

e. If renal function has not returned after 8 weeks, recovery is unlikely and provisions should be made for long-term renal substitution therapy.

V. RENAL REPLACEMENT THERAPIES

A. GENERAL GUIDELINES

1. **Indications for renal replacement therapy** include fluid overload (e.g., pulmonary edema, CHF), hyperkalemia, other symptomatic electrolyte disorders, metabolic acidosis, uremic encephalopathy, coagulopathy, and acute poisoning. Absolute values of BUN and creatinine are not indicators for dialysis. Initiation of renal replacement early in the course of ARF is associated with improved survival.

2. **Volume** (e.g., IV fluids, TPN) should be given as needed for the patient, independent of method of renal replacement. Priority must be placed on treatment of the underlying disease processes and renal replacement selected and performed to allow usual treatment of the critically ill surgical patient.

3. **Treatment of patients with ARF** requiring renal replacement therapy should still be directed at returning renal function to normal levels or at least those not requiring artificial support. Creatinine clearance should be followed in these patients because improvement in this parameter may signal a return of renal function.

4. **Currently, three modalities of renal replacement therapy are available** for treatment of ARF in the critically ill patient: (1) hemodialysis, (2) peritoneal dialysis, and (3) continuous arteriovenous hemofiltration. The features of these therapies are described and contrasted in Table 8-4.

B. **HEMODIALYSIS**

1. **Description of technique**

   a. The patient's blood is pumped via an extracorporeal circuit through a porous hollow fiber membrane (artificial kidney), which is permeable to solutes less than 2000 daltons. An isotonic solution surrounds the membrane and provides a concentration gradient for the selective removal of solutes, for example, potassium, urea, and creatinine, while maintaining plasma concentrations of sodium, chloride, and bicarbonate.

   b. Vascular access consists of an arteriovenous shunt or a double-lumen venovenous access. Percutaneous venovenous catheters are usually placed at the bedside for initial therapy. The catheter and access site should be changed frequently to prevent sepsis. Placement of permanent access (subcutaneous arteriovenous shunt) is indicated if renal replacement is required for more than 2 weeks with no signs of renal recovery.

   c. Systemic anticoagulation is required for this procedure, although less heparin may be used in patients with baseline coagulopathy.

   d. Hemodialysis is typically performed every other day for a 3- to 4-hour period but will be required more frequently in catabolic patients with a high urea generation rate.

   e. Solute and volume removal is considered very efficient with hemodialysis in comparison with other methods of renal replacement.

2. **Advantages**

   a. Hemodialysis is the method of choice for rapid removal of life-threatening electrolyte imbalances, toxins, and poisons.

   b. Hemodialysis may also be applied to hemodynamically stable surgical patients with isolated ARF where a contraindication to peritoneal dialysis exists (e.g., postoperative laparotomy).

3. **Disadvantages**

   a. In critically ill surgical patients with ARF, hemodialysis can cause hypotension, hypoxemia, and hemolysis and can precipitate cardiac arrhythmias. These events limit the application of hemodialysis in unstable patients.

TABLE 8-4

COMPARISON OF RENAL REPLACEMENT THERAPIES

Description:	Therapy		
	Hemodialysis	Peritoneal dialysis	CAVHD
Assessment:	Rapid-intermittent	Slow-intermittent	Slow-continuous
Vascular access:	Arteriovenous or venovenous	Abdominal catheter	Arteriovenous or venovenous
Anticoagulation:	Usually required	None required	Required
Solute removal:	Excellent	Excellent	Excellent
Fluid removal:	Excellent	Good	Excellent
Hemodynamic instability:	Potentially significant in critically ill patients	None	None
Risks of procedure:	Hypotension, hemorrhage, isoequilibrium syndrome	Infection/peritonitis, intraabdominal adhesions, respiratory distress	Hypovolemia, hemorrhage, electrolyte imbalance
Overall appraisal:	Useful for urgent removal of solutes or proteins; hemodynamic instability limits use in ICU patients	Contraindicated after recent open abdominal operation; useful in burn and cardiac patients and patients with poor vascular access	Broad flexibility with fluid and electrolyte balance; solute removal and fluid management of CAVHD equals hemodialysis

THE RENAL SYSTEM 8

b. Anticoagulation is also required and may be undesirable in the immediate postoperative or posttrauma setting.

c. Acute CNS disturbances ranging from mild stupor to coma can occur with hemodialysis and are described as the "disequilibrium syndrome."

C. PERITONEAL DIALYSIS

1. Description of technique

a. Peritoneal dialysis is performed via infusion of several liters of a sterile electrolyte solution with hypertonic dextrose into the abdominal space. Using the peritoneal membrane as a selective barrier, the dialysate solution creates an osmotic pressure gradient that extracts extracellular fluid and solutes out of the mesenteric circulation and into the peritoneal cavity. This fluid is then drained after an equilibration period of 1 to 2 hours.

b. Fluid removal usually ranges from 0.5 to 2 L/hr, although greater fluid and solute clearance can be accomplished by using larger volumes of dialysate, increasing the frequency of exchange cycles, or using a higher dextrose concentration in the dialysate.

c. Dialysis catheter placement can be performed in the ICU or OR.

2. Advantages

a. Peritoneal dialysis does not require vascular access or systemic anticoagulation, which makes it useful in patients with peripheral vascular disease or risk of hemorrhage. It is the treatment of choice for the post-cardiothoracic surgical patient with ARF.

b. The slow rate of solute and fluid extraction with peritoneal dialysis minimizes the problems of disequilibrium and hemodynamic compromise experienced with conventional hemodialysis.

3. Disadvantages

a. Catheter infection and peritonitis are the most common complications of the technique.

b. Rigid peritoneal catheters inserted percutaneously in the acute setting become colonized within 48 to 72 hours. Subcutaneously tunneled silastic catheters are associated with a lower incidence of peritonitis (1.6 episodes per patient-year) and should be implanted for prolonged use of peritoneal dialysis.

c. Other access-related complications include visceral injury at the time of catheter placement and formation of intraabdominal adhesions.

d. Hyperglycemia can occur as a result of the hypertonic glucose of the dialysate.

e. Respiratory distress may develop from reduced diaphragmatic compliance and increased intraabdominal pressure, as well as the development of hydrothorax via leakage of dialysate into the thoracic cavity.

f. Repeated lavage of the peritoneal cavity causes protein loss of 10 g/day or more and may exacerbate malnutrition in catabolic ARF patients.

D. CONTINUOUS ARTERIOVENOUS HEMODIALYSIS

1. Description of technique

a. CAVHD is specifically intended for the treatment of ARF in the ICU.

b. CAVHD is an extracorporeal ultrafiltration technique that removes extracellular fluid across a synthetic membrane via a hydrostatic pressure gradient created between indwelling arterial and venous catheters.

c. With a systolic BP ≥ 80 mm Hg, blood flows through the porous hollow-fiber capillary membrane at a rate of 50 to 150 ml/min, driving plasma water and solutes of up to 10,000 daltons (ultrafiltrate) out of the hemofilter at 500 to 700 ml/hr.

d. Arteriovenous access is accomplished by percutaneous cannulation of the femoral artery and vein with a low incidence of complications.

e. Heparinization of the extracorporeal circuit is required, usually at a rate of 500 U/hr.

f. CAVHD uses a dialysate solution that circulates in the extracapillary space countercurrent to blood flow. This creates a concentration gradient for selective removal of large amounts of solute. The ultrafiltration rate is regulated to achieve desired net fluid balance and no substitution fluid is necessary (Figure 8-2).

g. CAVHD is run continuously for as many days as renal replacement is required. Hemofilter performance (as monitored by the ultrafiltration rate) decreases over time, requiring replacement with a new hemofilter approximately every 2 days.

2. Advantages of CAVHD

a. Little or no hemodynamic instability is encountered with the treatment of unstable critically ill ARF patients. This is attributable to the slow and continuous fluid and solute removal, in addition to the low blood-activating properties of the hemofilter membrane.

b. CAVHD permits flexibility with volume management and eliminates the need for fluid restriction in oliguric ARF. Fluid balance and serum electrolyte concentrations can be titrated to any value, and optimum amounts of nutrition can be provided.

c. Solute clearance is approximately equal to that achieved with standard hemodialysis.

3. Disadvantages of CAVHD

a. Dehydration and electrolyte imbalance may occur as a result of continuous fluid and electrolyte removal.

b. Hemorrhage may occur as a result of systemic anticoagulation.

4. Management considerations for CAVHD

a. Ultrafiltration rate

(1) The ultrafiltration rate is dependent on the patient's BP, blood flow through the hemofilter, available free water, and the distance between the collection container and the hemofilter.

(2) To prevent excess hemoconcentration of blood at the venous end of the hemofilter (which decreases hemofilter performance and longevity), the maximum ultrafiltration rate (UFR_{max}) should be calculated.

8

THE RENAL SYSTEM

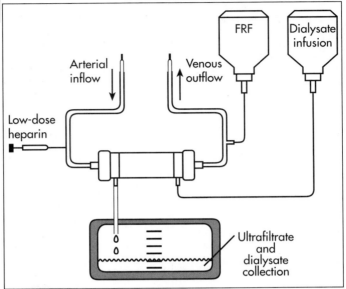

FIGURE 8-2

Continuous arteriovenous hemodialysis. CAVHD combines the advantages of continuous hemofiltration with the selective properties and clearance capabilities of hemodialysis. A sterile dialysate solution is infused countercurrent to hemofilter blood flow and provides a concentration gradient for selective removal of large amounts of uremic solutes. *(From Mault JR et al: Continuous hemofiltration: a reference guide for SCUF, CAVH, and CAVHD, Ann Arbor, Mich, 1990, University of Michigan Printing.)*

First, the hemofilter blood flow rate (BF) is calculated from the circuit time (recorded upon unclamping the hemofilter blood tubing) and the hemofilter circuit volume as follows:

$$\text{BF (ml/min)} = \text{circuit volume (ml)/circuit time (sec)} \times 60 \text{ sec/min}$$

Next, determine the plasma flow (PF) and UFR_{max}:

$$PF \text{ (ml/min)} = BF \times (100\% \ UFR_{max} - \text{hematocrit})/100$$
$$UFR_{max} \text{ (ml/min)} = 0.2^* \times PF$$
$$^*\text{For hematocrit} < 40\%, \text{ use } 0.3.$$

(3) In CAVHD, both the dialysate and ultrafiltrate fluids will drain through the ultrafiltrate line into the collection container. To determine the actual UFR, subtract the dialysate infusion rate (DI) from the total fluid collected (TFC) as follows:

$$UFR_{CAVHD} \text{ (ml/min)} = TFC \text{ (ml/min)} - DI \text{(ml/min)}$$

(4) As described earlier, the clearance capabilities of CAVHD eliminate the need for replacement fluid and limit the use of ultrafiltration to maintenance of a desired fluid balance (DFB). Therefore, by using a Hoffman clamp or volumetric control pump on the ultrafiltrate line, the TFC is limited to the sum of the DI plus total IV fluids (TIV) minus all other fluid output (OFO; i.e., urine output, chest tube, and nasogastric drainage), plus or minus the DFB (for a net negative fluid balance, add DFB; for a net positive fluid balance, subtract DFB) as follows:

TFC (ml/hr) =

$$DI \text{ (ml/hr)} + TIV \text{ (ml/hr)} - OFO \text{ (ml/hr)} + DFB \text{ (ml/hr)}$$

(a) The minimum TFC allowed equals the rate of DI and must not be restricted below that rate.
(b) If the calculated TFC is less than the dialysate infusion rate, then a filter replacement fluid (FRF) should be infused to make up the difference.

(5) Thrombus accumulation in the hemofilter will cause decreased blood flow and a subsequent decrease in UFR. If the systolic blood pressure is greater than or equal to 80 mm Hg and the unrestricted UFR is less than or equal to 100 ml/hr, the hemofilter should be discontinued to prevent thrombosis of the vascular access. Increasing the heparin infusion will not reverse clotting that has occurred in the hemofilter and should not be attempted as a means of "saving the filter."

b. Anticoagulation

(1) The objective of heparinization in CAVHD is to prevent thrombosis of blood in the hemofilter without necessarily producing systemic anticoagulation. This objective may or may not be achieved in an individual patient. In most cases, a continuous infusion of heparin at 7 to 10 U/kg/hr is administered to patients with normal clotting times; hemofilter longevity averages 48 hours. However, a single hemofilter may last several days with little or no heparin in a patient with a coagulopathy.

(2) To monitor anticoagulation status, the ACT (normal range 100 to 120 seconds) should be checked frequently. The ACT is a measure of whole blood clotting and is the preferred method for monitoring heparin therapy (if the ACT is unavailable, TCT or PTT can be effectively substituted).

c. Fluid and electrolyte balance

(1) Strict records of all fluids in and out are essential.

(2) In CAVHD, approximately 8 to 14 L of ultrafiltrate are removed per day according to patient conditions. This ultrafiltrate contains uremic solutes (urea and creatinine) but also essential solutes (e.g., Na^+, Cl^-, HCO_3^-) that must be replaced. The concentrations of these solutes in the ultrafiltrate are identical to those in the plasma. Solute losses can be calculated by multiplying the plasma concentration by the UFR.

d. Drug clearance
   (1) All non—protein-bound drugs will be cleared with the ultrafiltrate. These losses should be compensated by increased dosages to maintain therapeutic levels.
   (2) The drug clearance (DC) can be estimated from the plasma concentration of the drug ($[D]_P$), the percent drug-protein binding (%PB), and the UFR as follows:

$$DC \text{ (amount/min)} = [D]_P \times UFR \times (100\% - \%PB)$$

e. Complications
   (1) For severe hypotension, clamp the ultrafiltrate line but allow blood flow to continue through the hemofilter. The heparin infusion must also be maintained. With CAVHD, the FRF infusion may be continued if required to expand intravascular volume. The dialysate infusion must be discontinued when clamping the ultrafiltrate line.
   (2) If any portion of the extracorporeal circuit becomes disconnected, immediately occlude the arterial and venous cannulae and disconnect the hemofilter circuit.
   (3) Any change in ultrafiltrate color to pink or red indicates rupture of a hemofilter capillary and requires immediate removal and replacement.

f. Discontinuing hemofiltration
   (1) If the maximum unrestricted UFR is at most 100 ml/hr, discontinue hemofiltration.
   (2) If the ultrafiltrate color changes to pink or red, indicating hollow-fiber rupture, discontinue hemofiltration.
   (3) If renal function recovers sufficiently so that all infusions and nutrition can be maintained without fluid restriction, discontinue hemofiltration.
   (4) If renal function is not recovered when all other organ failure(s) have resolved, the patient should be treated with hemodialysis or peritoneal dialysis.

SUGGESTED READINGS

Ahn JH, Morey AF, McAninch JW: Workup and management of traumatic hematuria, *Emerg Med Clin North Am* 16:145-164, 1998.

Badr KF, Ichikawa I: Prerenal failure: a deleterious shift from renal compensation to decompensation, *N Engl J Med* 319:623-629, 1988.

Better OS, Stein JH: Early management of shock and prophylaxis of acute renal failure in traumatic rhabdomyolysis, *N Engl J Med* 322:825-829, 1990.

Kellerman PS: Perioperative care of the renal patient, *Arch Intern Med* 154:1674-1688, 1994.

Muther RS, Barry JM, Bennett WM: *Manual of nephrology,* Philadelphia, 1990, BC Decker.

Perdue PW, Balser JR, Lipsett PA, et al: "Renal dose" dopamine in surgical patients. Dogma or science? *Ann Surg* 227:470-473, 1998.

Rose DB: *Clinical physiology of acid-base and electrolyte disorders,* ed 4, New York, 1994, McGraw-Hill.

Shusterman N: Surgery in the patient with chronic renal failure. In Goldmann DR, Brown FH, Guarnieri DM, editors: *Perioperative medicine,* ed 2, New York, 1994, McGraw-Hill.

Sladen RN, Endo E, Harrison T: Two-hour versus 22-hour creatinine clearance in critically ill patients, *Anesthesiology* 67:1013-1016, 1987.

8

THE RENAL SYSTEM

THE GASTROINTESTINAL SYSTEM

Kirsten Bass Wilkins

I. GASTROINTESTINAL HEMORRHAGE

A. ETIOLOGY

1. Upper GI bleeding

a. Gastric or duodenal peptic ulceration
   (1) Most common cause (40% to 50%) of upper GI bleeding
   (2) Duodenal 4 times more common than gastric
   (3) Association with *Helicobacter pylori* infection

b. Esophageal varices
   (1) Etiology of 10% to 15% of upper GI bleeding
   (2) Most often associated with portal hypertension
   (3) Accounts for 50% to 75% of upper GI bleeding in cirrhotics
   (4) Rupture is related to the size of the varix and to wall tension (Laplace's law)
   (5) High rate of rebleeding (>70% within 6 weeks)

c. Mallory-Weiss tear
   (1) Accounts for 10% to 15% of upper GI bleeding
   (2) Arterial bleeding from a mucosal tear at the GE junction
   (3) Caused by an acute increase in intraabdominal pressure (e.g., vomiting, retching, coughing, seizures)

d. Erosive esophagitis or gastritis
   (1) Esophagitis may be of peptic (gastroesophageal reflux) or infectious etiology.
   (2) Gastritis may be associated with NSAID use, alcohol use, or "stress" (e.g., sepsis, shock, burns, intracranial pathology).

e. Dieulafoy's arteriovenous malformation

f. Esophageal or gastric neoplasms

2. Lower GI bleeding

a. Most lower GI bleeding arises from the colon and rectum, including diverticula, angiodysplastic lesions, neoplasms, inflammatory bowel disease, hemorrhoids, and anal fissures.

b. Small intestinal sources of bleeding are less common but include neoplasms, inflammatory bowel disease, and Meckel's diverticulum.

B. INITIAL MANAGEMENT (Figures 9-1 and 9-2)

Immediate volume resuscitation is the initial priority.

1. Initiate volume replacement

a. Place two large-bore (14- or 16-gauge) peripheral IV catheters.

b. Rapidly infuse 2 L of isotonic crystalloid solution.

c. Blood transfusion if blood loss is greater than 30%.
   (1) PRBC use is based on the amount of initial and ongoing blood loss.
   (2) Use warmed blood to prevent hypothermia and related complications.

9

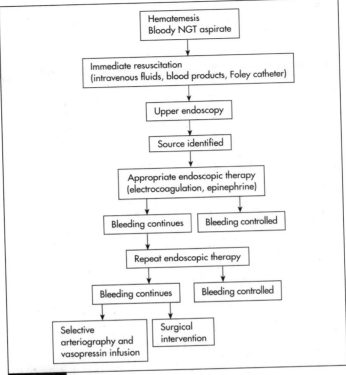

FIGURE 9-1

Management algorithm for upper GI hemorrhage.

    (3) Consider FFP administration after 6 units PRBC and in coagulopathic patients.
    (4) Consider platelet administration after 10 units PRBC and in thrombocytopenic patients.
  d. The initial vital signs and the response to the initial fluid challenge will help estimate initial blood loss:
    (1) From 15% to 30% blood loss: tachycardia, narrow pulse pressure, orthostatic hypotension, and vital signs should return to normal and stabilize with initial fluid challenge.
    (2) Greater than 30% blood loss: hypotension on recumbency, altered mental status, oliguria, and blood pressure will only rise temporarily in response to fluid challenge.

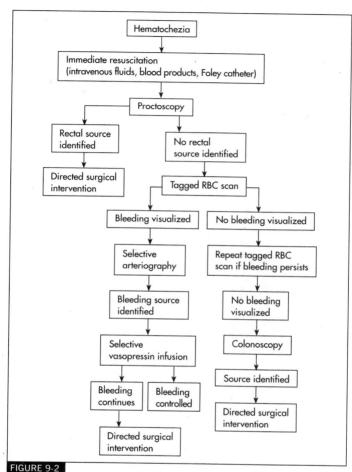

FIGURE 9-2

Management algorithm for lower GI hemorrhage.

2. Laboratory evaluation

a. Send blood specimens for CBC, electrolytes, PT/PTT, type and screen, and crossmatch (have ready 6 units of PRBCs).

b. Serial hematocrits should be performed every 4 hours. Keep in mind that the initial hematocrit may not accurately reflect blood loss because it may take 12 to 24 hours for the hematocrit to equilibrate.

3. Hemodynamic monitoring

a. Placement of a Foley catheter is mandatory and will provide information regarding the adequacy of volume replacement; maintain urine output greater than 30 ml/hr

b. CVP monitoring

c. PA catheter when indicated

C. LOCALIZATION OF BLEEDING

1. History

a. Hematemesis implies bleeding proximal to the ligament of Treitz.

b. Violent emesis before onset of hematemesis suggests a Mallory-Weiss tear.

c. History of alcoholism or cirrhosis implies esophageal varices or alcoholic gastritis.

d. Prior history of GI bleeding (e.g., ulcers, diverticular disease, NSAID use, *H. pylori* infection) may provide clues to etiology.

e. Recent weight loss, anorexia, or adenopathy may suggest a malignant bleeding source.

f. Melena usually reflects an upper GI bleeding source.
 (1) Melena forms because of the effect of gastric acid on hemoglobin.
 (2) Only 50 ml of blood is necessary to produce melena.
 (3) Melena without hematemesis implies a source distal to the pylorus.

g. Hematochezia indicates lower GI bleeding, but massive upper GI bleeding may also cause this.

2. Nasogastric tube placement

a. Lavage and aspiration is mandatory in all cases of GI bleed to evaluate the possibility of an upper GI source.

b. Lavage should be performed with warm saline to prevent hypothermia.

c. Aspirate should be tested for occult blood even if it is not grossly bloody.

3. Rectal examination

a. Mandatory in all patients with GI bleeding.

b. May reveal gross blood or melena.

c. Test all stool for occult blood: a guaiac-positive stool requires only 10 ml/day blood loss.

d. May reveal potential source of bleeding: fissure, hemorrhoid, or neoplasm.

4. Esophagogastroduodenoscopy (EGD) provides an accurate delineation of bleeding site in 90% of ICU patients and allows for therapeutic intervention, as well. If EGD is nondiagnostic, arteriography can be performed and will localize blood loss as low as 0.5 to 2 ml/min.

5. Proctosigmoidoscopy allows evaluation of a rectosigmoid source of bleeding and indicates if blood originates above the level of the rectum.

6. Colonoscopy in the face of massive bleeding is rarely diagnostic. It may be more useful in the hemodynamically stable patient with no evidence of active bleeding.

7. Radionuclide imaging using technetium-labeled autologous RBCs may detect active bleeding at a rate of 0.1 ml/hr.

a. Sensitive for the presence of active bleeding, but is diagnostic of actual site in only 50% of patients because of blood pooling.

b. May be repeated 24 to 36 hours after the initial scan without repeating the labeling process.

c. Is often a precursor to arteriography.

8. Arteriography

a. Diagnostic in 75% to 95% of cases

b. Allows for therapeutic intervention

D. THERAPEUTIC INTERVENTION

1. Upper GI bleeding

a. Duodenal or gastric ulcers

   (1) Histamine receptor antagonists (e.g., cimetidine, ranitidine, famotidine, and nizatidine) and antacids are used as the initial therapy. The proton pump inhibitor, omeprazole, may be used in refractory cases. Appropriate antibiotic treatment of *H. pylori*.

   (2) EGD may reveal bleeding site and allow for intervention.

     (a) Electrocoagulation

     (b) Epinephrine injection

   (3) Operative indications:

     (a) Initial blood loss of 1.5 to 2 L

     (b) Transfusion requirement of 8 to 10 units PRBCs

     (c) Rebleeding requiring more than 1 L blood replacement

   (4) Operative approach to duodenal ulcer:

     (a) Oversew the ulcer

     (b) Perform acid-reducing procedure (vagotomy)

     (c) Perform drainage procedure (pyloroplasty or gastroenterostomy)

   (5) Operative approach to gastric ulcer:

     (a) Excise the ulcer

     (b) Distal gastrectomy if indicated

     (c) Vagotomy and pyloroplasty if duodenal ulcer is also present

b. Esophageal varices

   (1) Pharmacologic intervention

     (a) Correct coagulopathy (FFP, vitamin K, cryoprecipitate)

     (b) Peripheral vasopressin infusion (20 units IV bolus over 20 minutes and continuous infusion of 0.2 to 0.6 units/min; after bleeding stops, decrease by 0.1 unit/min at 6- to 12-hour intervals; do not use vasopressin in patients with ischemic heart disease because of its vasoconstrictive effects)

     (c) Octreotide infusion

   (2) Endoscopic sclerotherapy is the mainstay of treatment and is usually successful in initial control of bleeding

   (3) Tamponade with Sengstaken-Blakemore tube

   (4) Transjugular intrahepatic portosystemic shunt (TIPS)

     (a) Treatment of choice in centers where it is available

     (b) Affords significant splanchnic decompression, similar to side-side shunt

     (c) Preserves portal vein anatomy

9

THE GASTROINTESTINAL SYSTEM

          (5) Operative intervention is needed if the above interventions fail to
              control bleeding
              (a) Direct control of bleeding site via transesophageal ligation and
                  esophageal transection, devascularization procedure (Sugiura), or
                  gastroesophageal resection with interposition graft
              (b) Indirect control of bleeding by reduction of variceal pressures
                  with portocaval shunt
      c. Mallory-Weiss tear
          (1) In the majority of patients, the bleeding will stop spontaneously.
          (2) Use same approach as for nonoperative peptic ulceration.
          (3) Keep NG tube in place to decrease gastric distention and emesis,
              which can aggravate bleeding.
          (4) If operative intervention is necessary, it consists of laparotomy and
              high gastrostomy with oversewing of the linear tear.
      d. Erosive gastritis
          (1) Bleeding usually responds to nonoperative measures discussed above.
          (2) Operative therapy includes oversewing of gastric ulcerations, vagot-
              omy, and pyloroplasty.

2. Lower GI bleeding
      a. Arteriographic intervention
          (1) Selective infusion of vasopressin
          (2) Selective embolization with coils or autologous clot may be used in
              exceptional cases when vasopressin infusion fails to control bleeding
              and the patient is too unstable to be taken to the OR
          (3) Is initially successful in 80% of cases, but rebleeding can occur in as
              many as 50% of patients
      b. Operative intervention is required for persistent hemodynamic instability,
         as well as a transfusion requirement of more than 8 units PRBCs
          (1) Arteriography often allows a "directed" resection, which holds a mor-
              tality rate of 10% to 20% in the emergent situation.
          (2) If a directed approach is not possible, subtotal colectomy is per-
              formed (mortality rate of 30% to 50%).

II. MOUTH

A. PAROTITIS
1. Bacterial infection of the parotid gland is normally prevented by the
   intrinsic bacteriostatic activity of saliva, as well as normal flow of saliva
   through Stensen's duct
2. Risk factors for the development of parotitis include dehydration, poor
   oral hygiene, surgery, malnutrition, presence of nasogastric tube, and
   cholinergic drugs
3. Physical examination reveals the following:
   a. Unilateral pain and swelling over the affected gland
   b. Fever and chills
   c. Pus may be expressed from Stensen's duct, which should be sent for
      Gram's stain and culture

4. Treatment

a. Appropriate antibiotic coverage (because infecting organism is usually *Staphylococcus aureus*, begin treatment with a parenteral penicillinase-resistant penicillin)

b. Follow-up cultures to cover unusual organisms (anaerobes)

c. Adequate hydration

d. Anticholinergic drugs to increase saliva secretion

e. Rarely, surgery may be required for incision and drainage

B. ORAL CANDIDIASIS

1. *Candida* organisms are normal inhabitants of the mucocutaneous body surfaces, but in the proper host, several strains can be quite virulent (e.g., *Candida albicans, C. tropicalis, C. parapsilosis*)

2. Predisposing risk factors for infection

a. Poor oral hygiene

b. Poor nutrition

c. Diabetes mellitus

d. Broad-spectrum antibiotics

e. Immunosuppression (e.g., chronic illness, human immunodeficiency virus [HIV], chemotherapy)

f. Burns

3. Physical examination

a. White, raised, discrete, or confluent patches

b. Reddened tongue that may have deep fissures

c. Patient often complains of burning sensation

4. Diagnosis

a. Lesions are easily scraped off a hyperemic base

b. Budding yeast with pseudohyphae revealed under light microscopy

5. Treatment

a. Nystatin (100,000 units/ml) swish and swallow: 4 to 6 ml q6h

b. Fluconazole (400 mg PO/IV × 1, then 200 mg PO/IV qd) for serious infection, immunocompromised patients, or patients on broad-spectrum antibiotics

III. ESOPHAGUS

A. REFLUX ESOPHAGITIS

1. Predisposing risk factors

a. Prolonged use of NG tube, allowing reflux

b. Lack of appropriate antiulcer prophylaxis and gastric pH monitoring

2. Clinical findings

a. Patient complains of reflux, dysphagia, and back pain

b. Bloody NG aspirate or low NG pH (<5)

3. Endoscopy is used to evaluate reflux esophagitis and grade resulting injury

a. Grade I: hyperemic mucosa without ulceration

b. Grade II: superficial ulceration

c. Grade III: ulceration, transmural fibrosis, dilatable stricture

d. Grade IV: nondilatable stricture

4. **Treatment**
a. Overall goal is to raise gastric pH (>5) using either of the following:
    (1) Antacids (15 to 30 ml PO/via NG q1-2h)
    (2) Histamine receptor blockade (cimetidine 400 mg PO qid or 800 mg PO bid/300 mg IV q6h; ranitidine 150 mg PO bid/50 mg IV q8h; famotidine 20 mg PO bid/20 mg IV q12h)
    (3) Proton pump inhibitor (omeprazole 20 mg PO qd)
    (4) If it is difficult to maintain appropriate gastric pH, continuous infusion of histamine receptor blockers can be used (cimetidine 300 mg IV $\times$ 1, then 37.5 to 100 mg/hr IV infusion; ranitidine 50 mg IV $\times$ 1, then 0.125 mg/kg/hr IV infusion)
b. Second goal is to increase both gastric motility and lower esophageal sphincter tone using the following:
    (1) Metoclopramide 10 mg IV q6h
    (2) Cisapride 10 my PO q6h
    (3) Erythromycin 250 mg IV q6h

B. **INFECTIOUS ESOPHAGITIS**
1. **Candidal esophagitis**
a. Predisposing risk factors
    (1) Immunosuppression
    (2) Broad-spectrum antibiotics
b. Diagnosis is via endoscopic biopsy
c. Treatment
    (1) Nystatin (100,000 units/ml) swish and swallow 4 to 6 ml q6h
    (2) Fluconazole 400 mg PO/qd $\times$ 1, then 200 mg PO/IV qd for 3 weeks
    (3) In refractory cases may use amphotericin B 10 to 20 mg/kg/day
2. **Other infectious causes include cytomegalovirus and herpes**
C. **TRACHEOESOPHAGEAL FISTULA**
1. **Predisposing risk factors**
a. Prolonged ventilatory course
b. High endotracheal or tracheostomy tube cuff pressure predisposing to tracheal erosion
c. Prolonged use of NG tube
2. **Prevention**
a. Use low-pressure cuffs on endotracheal or tracheostomy tubes
b. Early removal of NG tube
c. If early NG tube removal is not possible in a patient requiring prolonged ventilatory support, consider early placement of gastrostomy tube
3. **Treatment**
a. Operative repair or diversion
b. Tracheal stenosis frequently accompanies repair
D. **POSTESOPHAGECTOMY MANAGEMENT**
1. **Secure and keep NG tube in place** until meglumine diatrizoate (Gastrografin) swallow is obtained on postoperative day 5 to 7. Certain surgeons will remove the NG tube before the swallow if the patient is doing well clinically.

2. **Typically, anterior and posterior chest tubes are placed in the OR.** The anterior tube is removed within 24 to 48 hours, but the posterior tube is left in place until the swallow demonstrates no leak.
3. **Routine use of histamine receptor blockers** to decrease the acidity of gastric contents and prevent esophagitis as a consequence of reflux.
4. **Enteral nutrition via jejunostomy feeding tube.**
5. **Chest physiotherapy.**
6. **Anticipate common complications,** including anastomotic leak, reflux esophagitis, aspiration, pneumothorax, chylothorax, and delayed gastric emptying.
   a. Postoperative fever, even within the first 24 hours, may be indicative of an anastomotic leak.
   b. A complete fever workup is necessary even on the first postoperative day.
7. **Management of a documented anastomotic leak:**
   a. Prolonged nutritional support
   b. Posterior chest tube drainage until resolution of leak is documented on repeat swallow study
   c. Operative repair may be required if high-volume leak persists or if the patient becomes septic

E. ESOPHAGEAL PERFORATION

1. **Etiology**
   a. Most cases (45% to 75%) are secondary to iatrogenic disruption (endoscopy and repair of paraesophageal hernia)
   b. Spontaneous perforation (Boerhaave's syndrome) accounts for 15% of perforations
   c. Trauma (20%)
2. **Clinical findings**
   a. Pain
   b. Hematemesis
   c. Dysphagia/odynophagia
   d. Dyspnea and tachycardia
   e. Hypotension and shock
   f. Subcutaneous emphysema with cervical perforation
3. **Treatment**
   a. Immediate intervention includes stopping PO intake, intravenous hydration, broad-spectrum antibiotics, and NG tube decompression of the stomach
   b. Nonoperative management
      (1) Only a few selected patients can be managed in this fashion.
      (2) Perforation must be a walled-off disruption and patient must have only minimal symptoms and no evidence of sepsis.
   c. Operative management
      (1) Necessary for any free perforation
      (2) Basic principles include:
         (a) Debridement
         (b) Closure of the perforation if technically feasible

      (c) Resection of the diseased segment and esophageal exclusion are indicated in certain circumstances

      (d) Drainage of all contaminated areas

IV. STOMACH/DUODENUM

A. STRESS GASTRITIS

1. Description of gastric erosions

a. Almost always multiple, shallow, discrete areas of erythema with areas of focal hemorrhage or clot

b. Usually located in the fundus with sparing of the antrum and duodenum

c. Curling's ulcers: gastric erosions arising in severely burned patients (>35% body surface area)

d. Cushing's ulcers: gastritis encountered in patients with injury to central nervous system

2. Epidemiology

a. Incidence of 60% to 100% in critically ill patients

b. Mortality rate of 50% to 80% when associated with hemorrhage

3. Predisposing risk factors

a. Gastric conditions

    (1) Gastric acid secretion

    (2) Increased gastric mucosal permeability

    (3) Hypoperfusion of gastric mucosa

b. Clinical conditions

    (1) Trauma

    (2) Sepsis

    (3) Thermal burn

    (4) Oliguric renal failure

    (5) Hepatic dysfunction

4. Clinical presentation is typically painless, slow, intermittent bleeding but may progress to rapid hemorrhage

5. Prophylaxis

a. Aggressive treatment of shock regardless of cause.

b. Correct coagulopathy.

c. Reduce gastric luminal acidity with antacids, histamine receptor antagonists, or proton pump inhibitors as described above. Monitor NG tube pH frequently and keep pH greater than 6. Gastric tonometry allows for measurement of intramucosal pH and more accurate assessment of risk of bleeding from stress gastritis.

d. Sucralfate 1 g PO q6h; preferentially binds to denuded epithelium. Requires acidic pH to be effective, so do not administer antisecretory agents simultaneously.

e. Prostaglandins (misoprostol) may be effective in patients who require NSAID use.

f. Regardless of the type of prophylaxis used, the treatment must be initiated early because most bleeding will occur within 48 hours of the initial precipitating event.

6. **Treatment**
a. Gastric lavage and decompression will stop bleeding in 80% of patients.
b. If lavage does not control the bleeding, endoscopy should be performed to identify the bleeding site and attempt control with electrocoagulation, laser, or injection.
c. Angiography with selective embolization may be performed.
d. If all nonsurgical interventions fail, surgical options include oversewing of erosions with vagotomy and pyloroplasty, subtotal gastrectomy, antrectomy and vagotomy, subtotal gastric resection and vagotomy, or gastric devascularization.

B. **DUODENAL STUMP LEAK**

1. **Clinical presentation**
a. Postoperative fever, abdominal pain, and sepsis
b. May rarely present as a controlled fistula without sepsis

2. **Management**
a. In rare circumstances may be managed by percutaneous drainage alone, thereby creating a controlled enterocutaneous fistula.
b. Most patients require operative reexploration and either simple oversewing of the leak or a more extensive intervention, such as bringing up a Roux loop to the leak.
c. Adequate postoperative drainage is essential.

V. HEPATOBILIARY

A. **PORTAL HYPERTENSION**

1. **Etiology**
a. Prehepatic
   (1) Congenital atresia
   (2) Portal, superior mesenteric, or splenic vein thrombosis
b. Hepatic
   (1) Cirrhosis of any cause (alcoholism being the most frequent factor)
   (2) Congenital hepatic fibrosis
   (3) Fulminant hepatic failure
c. Posthepatic
   (1) Budd-Chiari syndrome
   (2) Severe congestive heart failure

2. **Pathophysiology**
a. Increased hydrostatic pressure within the portal vein and its tributaries (normal portal vein pressure is 5 to 10 mm Hg)
b. Development of portosystemic collaterals (gastroesophageal varices, abdominal wall veins via the umbilical vein [caput medusa], hemorrhoidal veins)

3. **Complications**
a. Variceal hemorrhage
b. Ascites

4. **Treatment of complications of portal hypertension**
a. Variceal bleed (management discussed above)

   b. Refractory ascites
     (1) Sodium and water restriction remains the mainstay of treatment
     (2) Diuretics (spironolactone is the first choice because of its potassium-sparing characteristics; thiazide and loop diuretics are the second line used)
     (3) Paracentesis
     (4) Surgery (peritoneovenous shunt)
     (5) TIPS and side-to-side portocaval shunts performed for variceal bleeding are commonly associated with a decrease in ascites

B. HEPATIC FAILURE

1. Etiology

a. Preexisting chronic liver disease with hepatocellular failure
b. Fulminant hepatic failure (defined as the development of acute hepatic encephalopathy within 8 weeks of the onset of hepatocellular disease in a previously healthy person) secondary to:
     (1) Viral hepatitides
     (2) Poisons and drugs (e.g., acetaminophen, halothane, *Amanita* mushroom toxicity)
     (3) Ischemic (e.g., hepatic vascular occlusion, sepsis)
     (4) Miscellaneous (e.g., acute fatty liver of pregnancy, Reye's syndrome)
     (5) Idiopathic

2. Child's classification

a. Class A: bilirubin less than 2, albumin greater than 3.5, no ascites, no encephalopathy, excellent nutrition
b. Class B: bilirubin 2 to 3, albumin 3 to 3.5, easily controlled ascites, mild encephalopathy, good nutrition
c. Class C: bilirubin greater than 3, albumin less than 3, poorly controlled ascites, advanced encephalopathy, poor nutrition

3. Clinical findings

a. Evidence of hepatocellular injury (e.g., elevated transaminases)
b. Hepatic dysfunction (e.g., coagulopathy, hypoglycemia, hyperbilirubinemia, decreased albumin)
c. Encephalopathy
     (1) Altered mental status (Grade I—slightly altered mental status; Grade IV—coma)
     (2) Asterixis
     (3) Elevated blood ammonia levels
     (4) Increased CSF glutamine

4. Treatment

a. Maintain continuous infusion of 10% to 20% glucose and frequent serum glucose monitoring.
b. Correct acid-base and electrolyte abnormalities.
c. Treat hypovolemia with colloid infusion.
d. May need dialysis for renal failure.
e. Provide adequate nutritional support, but control excessive dietary protein.

f. Lactulose and neomycin (to decrease ammonia absorption and production, respectively) should only be used in early stages of encephalopathy.

g. Cerebral edema: Keep head of bed elevated 60 degrees; in late stages, may insert ICP monitor and hyperventilate to $Paco_2$ 25 mm Hg; perform diuresis with mannitol or pentobarbital if previous measures fail to decrease ICP.

h. Correct coagulopathy (FFP, cryoprecipitate, vitamin K).

i. Appropriate antibiotic treatment of infection (prophylactic antibiotic use not a proven benefit).

j. Artificial hepatic support for temporary removal of toxins (exchange blood transfusion, plasmapheresis, hemoperfusion through human cadaveric or animal livers, hemodialysis and ultrafiltration, charcoal hemoperfusion).

k. Orthotopic liver transplantation.

C. JAUNDICE

1. Etiology

a. Unconjugated hyperbilirubinemia
  (1) Hemolysis
  (2) Massive blood transfusions
  (3) Hematoma
  (4) Gilbert syndrome
  (5) Congestive heart failure

b. Conjugated hyperbilirubinemia
  (1) Intrinsic hepatocellular dysfunction
    (a) Hepatitis
    (b) Hepatotoxic drugs
    (c) TPN
    (d) Shock and sepsis
  (2) Biliary obstruction
    (a) Choledocholithiasis
    (b) Biliary stricture
    (c) Pancreatic cancer
    (d) Cholangiocarcinoma

2. Clinical evaluation

a. Obtain history (hemolytic anemia, cholelithiasis, drugs with hepatotoxic potential).

b. Obtain liver function tests, including fractionated bilirubin.

c. Elevated transaminases suggest intrinsic hepatocellular dysfunction.

d. Obtain viral hepatitis panel.

e. Obtain amylase and lipase to rule out pancreatitis.

3. Radiologic evaluation is useful in the workup of conjugated hyperbilirubinemia

a. Abdominal ultrasound is 90% to 95% accurate in distinguishing intrahepatic from extrahepatic causes of jaundice
  (1) Cholelithiasis
  (2) Choledocholithiasis

   (3) Intrahepatic or extrahepatic ductal dilatation
   (4) Pancreatic masses
  b. Abdominal CT scan
   (1) Better method to evaluate the pancreas
   (2) May clarify level of obstruction if not clearly defined on ultrasound
  c. Endoscopic retrograde cholangiopancreatography (ERCP)
   (1) Procedure of choice for further evaluation of obstructive jaundice as
       initially diagnosed clinically or by ultrasound
   (2) Allows for visualization of biliary tree and pancreatic ducts
   (3) Allows for biopsy or brushing of tumors or strictures
   (4) Allows for therapeutic interventions (balloon extraction of stones,
       sphincterotomy, stent placement)
  d. Percutaneous transhepatic cholangiography (PTHC)
   (1) Especially useful in the evaluation of proximal biliary tree lesions
   (2) Greater success rate (>95%) when there is moderate intrahepatic
       ductal dilation
   (3) Allows for therapeutic interventions, including percutaneous biliary
       drain or stent placement

D. POSTHEPATECTOMY MANAGEMENT

1. Liver glycogen stores may be depleted for several weeks after major
   hepatic resection, resulting in hypoglycemia
  a. Monitor blood glucose levels frequently.
  b. Administer 10% dextrose solution for 48 hours or longer if necessary.

2. Liver synthetic function may be reduced for several weeks
  a. Albumin administration 25 to 50 g IV beginning on first postoperative
     day until synthetic function returns
  b. May have coagulopathy secondary to decreased production of factors II,
     VII, IX, and X, as well as proteins C and S (may require correction with
     FFP, cryoprecipitate, vitamin K)

3. Hyperbilirubinemia
  a. Secondary to transient liver dysfunction and blood transfusions
  b. If persists, consider refractory liver failure or possible injury to hepatic duct

4. Hypophosphatemia
  a. Severe problem after major hepatic resection
  b. So common that many surgeons routinely add potassium phosphate
     (15 mmol/L) to maintenance IV fluid

E. POSTOPERATIVE CHOLECYSTITIS

1. Acute calculous cholecystitis
  a. Epidemiology
   (1) Can occur at any age, but highest incidence occurs between fourth
       and eighth decades
   (2) Female-to-male ratio 3:1 up to 50 years of age and 1.5:1 thereafter
   (3) May have history of biliary colic
  b. Pathophysiology
   (1) Gallstones obstruct gallbladder because of impaction in Hartmann's
       pouch or cystic duct

      (2) Results in gallbladder distention, edema, inflammation, venous and lymphatic obstruction, ischemia, ulceration, and necrosis

  c. Clinical findings

      (1) Right upper quadrant or shoulder tenderness

      (2) Murphy's sign

      (3) Fever

      (4) Leukocytosis with left shift

  d. Radiologic evaluation

      (1) Abdominal ultrasound may reveal cholelithiasis, thickened gallbladder wall, or pericholecystic fluid.

      (2) HIDA scan reveals nonfilling of the gallbladder by radiotracer.

  e. Treatment

      (1) IV antibiotics to cover gram-positive and gram-negative aerobes and anaerobes

      (2) Laparoscopic cholecystectomy (may not be appropriate if patient has recently undergone major abdominal procedure with likelihood of multiple adhesions and inflammation)

      (3) Open cholecystectomy

      (4) Tube cholecystostomy in vascular radiology (in a critically ill patient in whom risk of surgery outweighs the benefits) followed by elective cholecystectomy

2. Acute acalculous cholecystitis

  a. Epidemiology

      (1) About 10% of all cases of cholecystitis

      (2) Male-to-female ratio 1.5:1

      (3) Frequently seen in ICU, septic, diabetic, postoperative, and trauma patients

      (4) Predisposing factors: abdominal arterial insufficiency, TPN, cardiac arrest, and congestive heart failure

  b. Pathophysiology

      (1) Gallbladder stasis, exposure of mucosa to stagnant bile, ischemia

      (2) Higher incidence of gangrene and perforation compared with calculous cholecystitis

      (3) High morbidity and mortality rates when it occurs in ICU patient (30% to 50%)

  c. Clinical findings

      (1) Masking of symptoms because associated other serious illnesses often lead to a delay in diagnosis

      (2) Laboratory evaluation may reveal nonspecific results

  d. Radiologic evaluation

      (1) Ultrasound and CT scan are frequently the first radiologic studies obtained. Pericholecystic fluid, adjacent fat stranding, or a sonographic Murphy's sign may be demonstrated.

      (2) Frequently the diagnosis is made by HIDA scan, which reveals cystic duct obstruction (may be nonspecific secondary to hepatic dysfunction, fasting, or TPN).

   e. Treatment
      (1) IV antibiotic
      (2) Emergent cholecystectomy
      (3) If patient's condition precludes surgery, cholecystostomy tube placement followed by elective cholecystectomy

F. CHOLANGITIS

1. Pathophysiology

a. The development of acute cholangitis requires two conditions:
   (1) Bacteria or fungus in the bile (bactibilia)
   (2) An increase in biliary pressure as a result of either partial or complete biliary obstruction
b. Biliary sepsis results from reflux of microorganisms through lymphatics and hepatic veins into the systemic circulation
c. Most common bacteria that are cultured include *Escherichia coli*, *Klebsiella*, and *Enterococcus*

2. Etiology of biliary obstruction

a. Choledocholithiasis
b. Benign or malignant strictures
c. Chronic pancreatitis and pseudocysts
d. Stricture at a biliary anastomosis
e. Obstructed biliary stent or endoprosthesis

3. Clinical findings

a. Charcot's triad: fever, jaundice, right upper quadrant pain (indicative of acute cholangitis, but other diseases can have similar symptoms, including cholecystitis and pancreatitis)
b. Reynold's pentad: fever, jaundice, right upper quadrant pain, altered mental status, shock
c. Leukocytosis with left shift, hyperbilirubinemia, elevated alkaline phosphatase, mild elevations in transaminases
d. Abdominal ultrasound will confirm the presence of a dilated biliary tree and indicate whether obstruction involves the intrahepatic or extrahepatic biliary tree

4. Treatment

a. Aggressive fluid resuscitation
b. Broad-spectrum IV antibiotics
c. Decompression of the biliary tree
   (1) Patients who already have external biliary drains should have drains externalized and then radiologic evaluation of the catheter to confirm patency or to have new drain placed.
   (2) ERCP or PTHC.
   (3) Emergent surgical decompression is reserved for patients in whom ERCP or PTHC are either unsuccessful or unavailable. Surgical decompression in a septic patient carries a mortality rate of 30%.

VI. PANCREAS

A. ACUTE PANCREATITIS

1. Etiology

a. Some 90% of cases are related to alcohol intake or biliary tract disease (gallstone pancreatitis)

b. Hyperlipidemia

c. Hypercalcemia (hyperparathyroidism)

d. Traumatic (blunt, penetrating, or iatrogenic from intraoperative manipulation or ERCP)

e. Ischemia (cardiopulmonary bypass, hypotension)

f. Pancreatic duct obstruction (tumor, pancreas divisum, ampullary stenosis)

g. Infectious (mumps, mycoplasma)

h. Drugs (azathioprine, estrogens, thiazide diuretics)

2. Pathophysiology

a. Release of pancreatic digestive enzymes and subsequent activation of intraparenchymal enzymes, resulting in pancreatic tissue destruction and necrosis

b. Associated with the release of vasoactive amines, resulting in increased capillary permeability and diminished peripheral vascular resistance

3. Clinical findings: Pancreatitis represents a diverse spectrum of illness, ranging from a mild, self-limited disease to a severe disease associated with shock and possible death.

a. Epigastric pain radiating to the back

b. Nausea and vomiting

c. Low-grade fever, tachycardia

d. Abdominal distention

e. Signs suggestive of retroperitoneal hemorrhage

   (1) Turner's sign (bluish discoloration of the left flank)

   (2) Cullen's sign (periumbilical discoloration)

f. Left pleural effusion and possible respiratory failure (tachypnea, dyspnea, hypoxia)

g. Altered mental status

h. Shock (hypotension, hypovolemia, hypoperfusion)

4. Evaluation

a. Laboratory studies: serum amylase

   (1) Hyperamylasemia usually observed within 24 hours of onset of symptoms and returns to normal over the next 7 days

   (2) Elevated in 95% of cases of gallstone pancreatitis

   (3) May be elevated in up to 30% of alcoholics with underlying chronic pancreatitis

   (4) The degree of initial hyperamylasemia is not a reliable predictor of the severity of pancreatitis

   (5) High rate (30%) of false-positive results (hyperamylasemia may be associated with biliary tract disease, intestinal obstruction, mesenteric infarction, perforated peptic ulcer, salivary gland disorders, renal failure, diabetic ketoacidosis, or ovarian disorders)

b. Elevated serum lipase is a more accurate predictor of acute pancreatitis
c. Leukocytosis, hyperglycemia, abnormal liver function tests (indicative of gallstone pancreatitis), hypocalcemia, mild azotemia, and hypoxia
d. Radiologic evaluation
   (1) CXR (left basilar atelectasis, pleural effusion)
   (2) Plain abdominal films ("sentinel loop," nonspecific ileus, obliteration of psoas muscle, gallstones, pancreatic calcifications indicating previous history of pancreatitis)
   (3) Abdominal ultrasound is useful to reveal biliary disease but allows poor visualization of pancreas and retroperitoneum
   (4) CT scan with IV and oral contrast is the most valuable radiologic intervention available (allows accurate diagnosis, as well as follow-up of potential complications, such as abscess, pseudocyst, and phlegmon)

5. **Management**
   a. Medical
      (1) Aggressive intravenous fluid hydration and electrolyte replacement (because of massive fluid sequestration) and Foley catheter insertion (CVP or PA catheter monitoring may be necessary in patients with severe chronic illnesses or signs of shock)
      (2) NPO (NG tube placement is not necessary except in cases of severe nausea and abdominal distention)
      (3) Aggressive respiratory support
         (a) In patients who survive the first 48 hours, 30% to 60% will develop pulmonary complications, ranging from mild hypoxia to ARDS.
         (b) Treat with pulmonary toilet, supplemental oxygen, and possibly intubation.
      (4) Marked hyperglycemia (from endocrine insufficiency) requires careful insulin administration
      (5) Prophylaxis for stress gastritis
      (6) Analgesia (meperidine is used; morphine is associated with sphincter of Oddi spasm)
      (7) Nutritional support
         (a) Patient is allowed gradual resumption of oral intake after abdominal pain has completely resolved and pancreatic enzymes normalize.
         (b) Often the course is prolonged and the patient requires either TPN or enteral support distal to the pancreas.
      (8) Prophylactic antibiotics are not recommended
   b. Surgical indications
      (1) Gallstone pancreatitis: After the acute episode resolves, it is recommended that cholecystectomy be performed during the same admission
         (a) May perform ERCP and sphincterotomy followed by laparoscopic cholecystectomy.

(b) Otherwise, perform cholecystectomy, intraoperative cholangiography, and common duct exploration if indicated.

(2) Treatment of pancreatic sepsis (pancreatic abscess or infectious necrosis) by one of two accepted surgical approaches

(a) Laparotomy with wide debridement and sump drainage

(b) Laparotomy with debridement and open packing

(c) Regardless of which option is chosen, several repeat debridement procedures will be necessary

(3) Progressive clinical deterioration despite optimal supportive care

(4) Uncertainty of the diagnosis

(a) Exploratory laparotomy may be indicated if other conditions that can mimic pancreatitis cannot be excluded.

(b) Such diagnoses include perforated viscus and acute mesenteric ischemia

c. Prognosis: Ranson's criteria aid in the ability to assess the severity of pancreatitis and to predict morbidity and mortality (Box 9-1)

6. Sequelae of pancreatitis

a. Pseudocyst: In patients with pancreatic ductal disruption, extravasated pancreatic juice may be contained as a pseudocyst. Treatment includes:

(1) Surgery 6 to 8 weeks after onset, at which time a mature wall of granulation tissue will be present for anastomosis. Operative management is indicated for pain, inability to eat, infection, and venous hypertension resulting from compression of splenic or portal vein.

BOX 9-1

RANSON'S CRITERIA

ON ADMISSION

Age > 55

WBC > 16,000/mm^3

Serum glucose > 200 mg/dl

SGOT > 250 SF units

LDH > 350 IU/L

DURING INITIAL 48 HOURS

Fall in hematocrit > 10%

Calcium < 8.0 mg/dl

Pao$_2$ < 60 mm Hg

Rise in BUN > 5 mg/dl

Base deficit > 4 mEq/L

Third space fluid loss > 6 L

PROGNOSIS BASED ON NUMBER OF RANSON'S CRITERIA PRESENT:

One to two signs: 1% mortality

Three to four signs: 15% mortality

Five to six signs: 40% mortality

Seven or more signs: 100% mortality

(2) Preferred procedure is internal drainage via cystojejunostomy, cysto-gastrostomy, or cystoduodenostomy.

(3) Ultrasound- or CT-guided percutaneous drainage with an indwelling pigtail catheter may be used for diagnostic purposes and in patients early in the course of disease who require symptomatic relief. As with operative external drainage, this may result in the development of a chronic pancreaticocutaneous fistula if the proximal pancreatic duct is obstructed.

b. Pseudoaneurysm may occur in up to 10% of patients, most commonly involving the splenic or gastroduodenal arteries. An initial attempt at angiographic embolization is the procedure of choice.

c. Exocrine insufficiency.

(1) Symptoms develop when secretion falls to 10% or less.

(2) Affects fat absorption much more than protein or carbohydrate absorption.

(3) Fat malabsorption causes steatorrhea and diarrhea.

(4) Treatment requires pancreatic enzyme supplements to be given with every meal.

B. POSTPANCREATICODUODENECTOMY (WHIPPLE'S PROCEDURE) MANAGEMENT

1. Special considerations

a. Large volume of third space fluid losses are common in the postoperative period because of extensive resection; thus aggressive fluid resuscitation is mandatory.

b. Patients may have trouble with delayed gastric emptying and prolonged ileus, which may be responsive to the routine administration of erythromycin.

2. Complications

a. Bleeding

b. Infection: Pancreatic abscess may develop, which may be diagnosed via CT scan and drained percutaneously or surgically

c. Pancreatic fistula

(1) Diagnosed by excessive drain output that is high in amylase

(2) Routine use of octreotide (100 U SQ q8h) may reduce the incidence of postoperative fistula

(3) Most will close with adequate drainage without need for further operation

VII. SMALL INTESTINE

A. SMALL BOWEL OBSTRUCTION

1. Etiology

a. Adhesions—60%

b. Malignant tumor—20%

c. Hernia—10%

d. Inflammatory bowel disease—5%

e. Volvulus—3%

f. Miscellaneous—2% (gallstone ileus, phytobezoar, pyloric stenosis and intussusception in children)

2. **Pathophysiology**

a. Small bowel distention

b. Distention stimulates physiologic secretion of fluid, electrolytes, and succus entericus into the bowel lumen

c. Further distention results in venous hypertension and ischemia, which may eventually progress to arterial occlusion (associated with extensive third space fluid loss)

d. Bowel necrosis ensues with resultant bacterial translocation and sepsis

3. **Clinical findings**

a. Intermittent colicky pain

b. Nausea and vomiting

c. Abdominal distention

d. Obstipation

e. Hyperactive bowel sounds

f. Must examine the patient thoroughly:

(1) Be sure that hernias are not present.

(2) Perform rectal examination to screen for intraluminal masses, as well as for gross or occult blood.

4. **Laboratory evaluation**

a. CBC with differential

b. Serum chemistry

c. Serum amylase

d. Arterial blood gas (to follow metabolic acidosis)

5. **Radiologic evaluation**

a. Flat and upright plain abdominal films reveal distended (>3 cm) loops of small bowel with air/fluid levels and a paucity of colonic air.

b. A patient with closed loop obstruction may present with a gasless abdomen on plain film (closer evaluation of plain films may reveal "ground glass" haziness in the middle portion of the abdomen or displacement of adjacent bowel).

c. Upper gastrointestinal series with small bowel follow-through may be particularly useful for identifying the presence, location, and degree (partial vs. complete) of obstruction.

d. CT scan can be useful and often reveals the cause of obstruction (particularly extrinsic causes, such as tumor, abscess, hematoma, inflammation). May reveal signs of strangulation (thickened bowel wall, pneumatosis, portal venous gas).

6. **Medical management**

a. All patients with bowel obstruction must receive aggressive fluid resuscitation and correction of electrolyte abnormalities

b. Foley catheter allows close monitoring of urine output

c. CVP or PA catheter monitoring may be necessary in certain patients

d. NPO

e. Bowel decompression with nasogastric tube

f. Serial abdominal examinations (pain medications must not be administered because abdominal pain may be masked)

g. Serial abdominal plain films to follow progress of abdominal distention

7. Surgical intervention

a. The timing of intervention is frequently based on whether the patient has partial or complete obstruction.

b. With both partial and complete obstruction it is paramount to differentiate between simple and strangulating obstruction. Overall, patients with partial obstruction are considered to be at a negligible risk for strangulation. Patients with complete obstruction, however, run a 20% to 40% risk of strangulation. Any sign of strangulation is an indication for emergent surgical intervention.

c. The presence of strangulating obstruction increases the mortality rate from 5% to 20%.

d. Five classic signs of strangulation: continuous pain, fever, tachycardia, peritoneal signs, and leukocytosis.

e. Most patients with partial obstruction benefit from 24 to 72 hours of conservative medical management. With this approach, 60% to 80% of patients will have resolution of the obstruction without the need for surgical intervention.

f. Patients with complete obstruction benefit from an initial 12 to 24 hours of resuscitation and then most will undergo surgical exploration.

B. POSTOPERATIVE ILEUS

1. May persist for 3 to 5 days after surgery

2. Gastrointestinal motility returns as follows:

a. Small bowel (1 to 3 days)

b. Stomach (3 to 5 days)

c. Colon (4 to 7 days)

3. Management

a. NPO until return of bowel function (as evidenced by flatus or bowel movement)

b. IV fluid hydration and electrolyte replacement

c. If prolonged ileus:

(1) Avoid narcotics and calcium channel blockers

(2) Rule out intraabdominal abscess via CT and drain percutaneously as indicated

(3) Encourage patient ambulation

(4) Perform upper GI with small bowel follow-through to rule out possible mechanical obstruction, which may require operative intervention

C. ISCHEMIA

1. Etiology

a. Arterial embolism (25% to 45%)

(1) Most commonly involves superior mesenteric artery or its branches

(2) Predisposing factors include elderly patient with acute MI, atrial fibrillation, mitral stenosis, and ventricular aneurysm

b. Arterial thrombosis (15% to 25%): occurs in patients with chronic occlusive disease of suprarenal aorta or aneurysmal disease of thoracoabdominal aorta

c. Nonocclusive mesenteric ischemia (10% to 30%)
   (1) Prolonged arterial vasospasm
   (2) Vasopressors

d. Venous thrombosis (5% to 15%)
   (1) Trauma
   (2) Mesenteric venous obstruction (portal hypertension, small bowel obstruction)
   (3) Peritoneal inflammation/sepsis
   (4) Hypercoagulable states
       (a) Protein C, protein S, or antithrombin III deficiency
       (b) Oral contraceptives
       (c) Pregnancy
       (d) Malignancy

2. **Clinical findings**
   a. Acute, continuous abdominal pain out of proportion to physical findings
   b. Abdominal distention, tenesmus, bloody diarrhea
   c. History will usually reveal predisposing risk factors

3. **Management**
   a. Diagnosis should be confirmed by angiography.
   b. Angiography allows for therapeutic intervention, as well (urokinase may be selectively injected in cases of thrombolysis or papaverine instilled in cases of vasospasm).
   c. Early vascular surgical consult: abdominal exploration is necessary if abdominal pain worsens despite thrombolytics or patient shows signs of sepsis or possible bowel necrosis.
   d. Intraoperative thrombectomy or embolectomy and possible bowel resection for irreversible ischemic changes.
   e. Aortomesenteric bypass may be required if thrombectomy does not improve arterial inflow.
   f. If venous thrombosis is encountered, patient must be immediately heparinized and then coumadinized for at least 3 to 6 months.

4. **Chronic mesenteric ischemia**
   a. Atherosclerotic occlusive disease of the mesenteric arteries
   b. Symptoms begin when two of the three main mesenteric arteries (celiac, superior mesenteric, inferior mesenteric) are significantly occluded
   c. Symptoms
      (1) Pain after eating (100% of patients)
      (2) Weight loss
      (3) Nausea and vomiting
      (4) Diarrhea or constipation
   d. Angiography confirms diagnosis and allows for balloon angioplasty
   e. Aortomesenteric bypass has excellent results with an 80% to 90% 5-year patency rate

9

THE GASTROINTESTINAL SYSTEM

D. CROHN'S DISEASE

Subtypes:

1. Inflammatory

a. Typically affects long segments of bowel

b. Patients present for surgery because of intractability and the failure of medical management

c. Surgical resection is limited to areas of worst involvement

2. Fibrostenotic

a. Usually occurs years after the initial presentation

b. Muscular hypertrophy and fibrosis lead to a gradual decrease in luminal diameter

c. Eventual partial small bowel obstruction, which will sometimes resolve with conservative management (bowel decompression and steroids) if obstruction is also associated with inflammation

3. Fistulizing

a. Fistulas develop between bowel and skin, other bowel segments, bladder, vagina, and ureter.

b. Patient usually benefits from a period of bowel rest and TPN and then surgical resection.

c. If patient has obvious infection, either percutaneous or surgical drainage is performed to control sepsis.

VIII. COLON

A. LARGE BOWEL OBSTRUCTION

1. Etiology

a. Colorectal cancer (80%)

b. Diverticulitis

c. Ulcerative colitis and Crohn's disease

e. Volvulus

f. Fecal impaction

g. Hernia

2. Clinical findings

a. Nausea and vomiting, abdominal distention and pain, failure to pass flatus and obstipation, feculent breath

b. History is very important and may provide clues to etiology (weight loss, hematochezia, change in bowel habits, prior history of polyps or diverticulosis)

c. Patient may be anemic because of chronic blood loss from carcinoma

3. Radiologic evaluation

a. Plain abdominal film: small and large bowel dilation with variable amounts of distal colonic or rectal air, depending on the location and degree of obstruction

b. Contrast enema will then delineate the level of obstruction, as well as the potential cause (may be valuable to use water-soluble contrast instead of barium because inspissation may occur proximal to the obstruction and barium peritonitis will ensue after perforation)

c. CT scan is helpful in patients with suspected diverticulitis

4. **Management**
a. Colonic obstruction requires emergent surgical intervention
b. Left-sided lesions: if bowel has not been prepped, diverting colostomy with or without resection
c. Right-sided lesion: diverting colostomy or ileostomy either with or without resection (primary reanastomosis may be attempted if minimal soilage and patient stable)

B. **DIVERTICULITIS**
1. **Epidemiology**
a. Diverticula are protrusions of the mucosa and muscularis mucosa through the muscularis propria.
b. Diverticulitis is an inflammatory process involving diverticula.
c. Most common in sigmoid, but may occur anywhere in colon.
d. In patients older than 80, 50% will have diverticula.

2. **Clinical findings**
a. Lower abdominal pain (usually greater on the left side)
b. Fever and chills
c. Leukocytosis
d. Progressive obstipation

3. **Radiologic evaluation:** CT scan may reveal inflammatory mass and possible abscess, which should be drained percutaneously. This is followed by a barium enema to document diverticula or other lesions (carcinoma)

4. **Treatment:** 90% of cases can be managed conservatively
a. Diverticulitis without signs of perforation or obstruction can be managed conservatively: NPO, nasogastric decompression, IV antibiotics, percutaneous drainage of abscess. If successfully treated in this manner, perform elective surgical resection if patient has recurrent symptoms.
b. If perforation, obstruction, sepsis, or bleeding present, perform emergent surgical exploration.
c. In surgery, a one-stage (resection and primary reanastomosis) or two-stage procedure (Hartmann's procedure) may be performed.

C. **OGILVIE'S SYNDROME: NONOBSTRUCTIVE COLONIC DILATION (COLONIC PSEUDOOBSTRUCTION)**
1. **Predisposing risk factors**
a. Elderly patient
b. Electrolyte imbalance
c. Hypothyroidism
d. Diabetes mellitus
e. Neurologic diseases (CVA, paralysis)

2. **Clinical findings**
a. Distended, tympanitic abdomen
b. Peritoneal signs absent (if present, this is surgical emergency)
c. Hypoactive bowel sounds
d. Laboratory findings: electrolyte abnormalities common; normal WBC if no ischemia or perforation

9

THE GASTROINTESTINAL SYSTEM

3. Radiologic evaluation

a. Plain abdominal films: colonic distention. Need to rule out free air and pneumatosis. Serial examinations are necessary to follow changes in bowel diameter. Cecum is at greatest risk of perforation (increased risk as diameter increases beyond 12 cm).

b. Need to be sure that mechanical obstruction is not present. Contrast enema or colonoscopy may be used to document mechanical lesions.

4. Management

a. Fluid resuscitation and correction of electrolyte abnormalities

b. Gastrointestinal decompression (NG tube and rectal tube)

c. Colonoscopic decompression if cecal diameter approaches 12 cm

d. Pharmacologic intervention: intravenous guanethidine (adrenergic-blocking agent) followed by intravenous neostigmine (parasympathomimetic)

e. If cecum cannot be decompressed:
   (1) Percutaneous endoscopic cecostomy
   (2) Surgical intervention
      (a) If perforation, ileocecectomy with end ileostomy and mucous fistula
      (b) If cecum intact, tube cecostomy

D. PERIRECTAL ABSCESS

1. Etiology

a. Cryptoglandular obstruction followed by bacterial overgrowth and suppuration (most common cause)

b. Other causes include carcinoma, trauma, Crohn's disease, radiation, and immunosuppression

2. Clinical findings

a. Dull, aching perianal or deep perineal pain

b. Fever and chills

c. If superficial, may be able to palpate indurated, fluctuant area

3. Management

a. Incision and drainage (I&D; usually best to perform in OR); anal canal should be examined before I&D because an internal opening may be visualized, which will be important in later management of fistula

b. IV antibiotics should not be necessary if abscess has been adequately drained

c. Wound is packed open and dressing changes TID until wound granulates

d. Daily sitz baths

e. Stool softeners

f. Follow-up in clinic in several weeks to evaluate for possible fistulas

E. DIARRHEA

1. Differential diagnosis

a. Osmolar
   (1) Excessive enteral feeding
   (2) Sorbitol and other nonabsorbable medications
   (3) Antacid therapy
   (4) Refeeding after cachexia

b. Anatomic
   (1) Dumping syndrome
   (2) Blind loop syndrome with bacterial overgrowth
   (3) Fistulas (gastrocolic, enteroenteric, enterocolic)
   (4) Partial bowel obstruction
c. Secretory—endocrine
   (1) Hyperthyroidism
   (2) Zollinger-Ellison syndrome
   (3) Watery diarrhea hypophosphatemia acidosis (WDHA) syndrome
d. Secretory—exocrine
   (1) Pancreatic insufficiency
   (2) Impaired bile reabsorption
e. Infection
   (1) *Salmonella* organisms
   (2) *Shigella* organisms
   (3) *Clostridium difficile*

2. Evaluation
a. Rectal examination
b. Stool sample evaluation
   (1) Ova and parasites
   (2) Fat, blood, and mucus
   (3) *C. difficile* toxin
   (4) Reducing substances
c. Review of medication and nutritional therapy
d. Radiologic contrast studies to define GI tract anatomic abnormalities

3. Treatment
a. Therapy is based on diagnosis.
b. Therapy with antidiarrheals is usually contraindicated.

F. COLITIS
1. Pseudomembranous
a. Caused by the endotoxin of *C. difficile*
b. Occurs after systemic therapy with almost all antibiotics
c. Clinical findings
   (1) Acute diarrheal colitis
   (2) Leukocytosis
   (3) May produce septic shock
   (4) May observe pseudomembranes on sigmoidoscopy
   (5) Diagnosis dependent on demonstration of toxin in stool
d. Treatment
   (1) Vancomycin 125 mg PO q6h for 5 to 10 days, or
   (2) Metronidazole 250 mg PO/IV q6h for 5 to 10 days

2. Ischemic
a. Etiology
   (1) Occlusive (embolic, thrombosis, AAA, previous intraabdominal surgery)

(2) Nonocclusive (hypovolemia, hypotension, digitalis toxicity, vasopressin, increased intraluminal pressure)
b. Clinical findings
  (1) Abdominal pain
  (2) Diarrhea
  (3) Hematochezia
  (4) Possibly signs of sepsis
c. Diagnosis
  (1) Clinical suspicion
  (2) Colonoscopy revealing mucosal edema, hemorrhage, ulceration, or patchy necrosis
d. Treatment
  (1) Between 80% and 90% of cases will respond to supportive measures (aggressive fluid resuscitation and bowel rest)
  (2) Serial abdominal examinations, abdominal plain films (pneumatosis, free air), and clinical evaluation to identify those patients who are worsening despite supportive measures; 10% to 20% of patients will require operative intervention

3. Neutropenic
a. Occurs in immunosuppressed patients with neutropenia
b. Presents with abdominal tenderness, diarrhea, and fever
c. Should send stool specimens for fecal leukocytes, culture, ova and parasites, and *C. difficile* toxin
d. Common etiologic agent is *C. difficile,* which should be managed as discussed previously
e. Serial abdominal examinations and plain abdominal films (to rule out free air and detect the presence of intestinal pneumatosis) are indicated
f. Certain manipulations are avoided in neutropenic patients, including placement of nasogastric tubes, rectal tubes, rectal examinations, and contrast enemas (because of risk of inducing bacteremia)
g. Patients are managed conservatively with bowel rest and intravenous fluid hydration and appropriate antibiotics
h. Worsening clinical status or bowel perforation are indications to proceed with surgery

SUGGESTED READINGS

Bass KN, Jones B, Bulkley GB: Current management of small-bowel obstruction. In Cameron JL, Balch CM, Langer B, et al, editors: *Advances in surgery,* vol 31, St Louis, 1998, Mosby.

Giurgiu DIN, Roslyn JJ: Calculous biliary disease. In Greenfield LJ, Mulholland M, Oldham KT, et al, editors: *Surgery: scientific principles and practice,* ed 2, Philadelphia, 1997, Lippincott-Raven.

McIntyre KE: Mesenteric vascular disease of the small bowel. In Cameron JL, editor: *Current surgical therapy,* ed 6, St Louis, 1998, Mosby.

O'Keefe G, Maier RV: Current management of patients with stress gastritis. In Cameron JL, Balch CM, Langer B et al, editors: *Advances in surgery,* vol 30, St Louis, 1997, Mosby.

Vanek V, Al-Salti M: Acute pseudo-obstruction of the colon (Ogilvie's syndrome) An analysis of 400 cases, *Dis Colon Rectum* 29:203-210, 1986.

Yeo CJ, Cameron JL: The pancreas. In Sabiston DC, Lyerly HK, editors: *Textbook of surgery: the biological basis of modern surgical practice,* ed 15, Philadelphia, 1997, WB Saunders.

THE VASCULAR SYSTEM

Paul M. Kirshbom

I. INTRODUCTION

The management of vascular disorders is an important part of the intensive care unit course for patients regardless of their primary diagnosis. The vascular system is an obvious concern in patients admitted to the ICU for primary vascular disease; however, one must remember that many patients who present with nonvascular disease will require subsequent evaluation and treatment of vascular disorders. These patients may have exacerbations of underlying vascular disease, iatrogenic injuries, or complications of their primary disease process. This chapter is designed to provide a framework of information and algorithms for management of these problems.

10

II. GENERAL CARE OF VASCULAR SURGICAL PATIENTS

A. PREOPERATIVE EVALUATION AND PREPARATION

1. **History**
   a. Differentiate symptoms of chronic vs. acute vascular diseases.
   b. Atherosclerotic disease tends to be systemic. Specifically question with regard to history of cardiac, cerebrovascular, and peripheral vascular disease in all patients (e.g., angina, TIA, CVA, claudication).
2. **Physical examination**
   a. Inspection
      (1) Pale or cyanotic extremities with hair loss may indicate poor peripheral perfusion.
      (2) The presence of dark blue or black tissue with or without ulcers is indicative of critical ischemia with irreversible tissue loss.
      (3) Frankly gangrenous extremities typically require amputation.
      (4) Peripheral hyperpigmentation and dependent edema are hallmarks of venous disease.
   b. Palpation
      (1) A complete examination of pulses must be documented to allow for future comparison.
      (2) Capillary refill and temperature can be excellent indicators of peripheral perfusion. Capillary refill greater than 2 seconds or a significant change from prior examinations should be investigated further.
      (3) The abdomen is palpated to detect any pulsatile masses.
   c. Auscultation
      (1) The presence of a bruit over any vascular bed should be documented. It is important to remember that the presence of a bruit indicates vascular turbulence in a nearby vessel, but it may not represent a hemodynamically significant lesion in the vessel of interest.
      (2) If a peripheral pulse is not palpable, the vessel should be evaluated with a Doppler ultrasound device. The ankle-brachial index (ABI)

can be a useful longitudinal measure of the degree of peripheral vascular disease. The ABI is derived by measuring the systolic blood pressure at the ankle and the wrist using a blood pressure cuff and Doppler ultrasound. The pressure at the ankle is divided by the upper extremity pressure. Asymptomatic patients typically have an ABI between 0.6 and 1.1. An ABI below 0.6 typically accompanies claudication, whereas rest pain is common in patients with an ABI below 0.3. The ABI may be inaccurate in patients with calcified vessels that cannot be compressed (common in diabetics).

(3) Noninvasive vascular studies involve Doppler ultrasound examination with pressure and waveform analysis at multiple levels before and after exercise. These studies can be very useful in preoperative evaluation and postoperative follow-up.

3. Laboratory

a. Screening laboratory studies should be performed as for other major surgeries.

b. Particular attention should be paid to rule out hypercoagulable states in patients who have previously thrombosed vascular prostheses or present with deep venous thrombosis.

c. A specimen should be sent to the blood bank for any major vascular procedure. Although there is considerable variability, a reasonable guide is a type and screen for carotid endarterectomy, crossmatch 2 units of blood for infrainguinal surgery, and 4 units for aortic surgery.

4. Radiologic examinations

a. All patients undergoing a major vascular procedure should have a PA and lateral CXR.

b. Arteriography remains the gold standard for the study of vascular anatomy. Other modalities, such as magnetic resonance angiography (MRA) and duplex ultrasound, are useful in specific circumstances (e.g., renal insufficiency, severe contrast allergy) or as screening modalities. These and other studies may play a larger role as the technology involved is refined.

5. Bowel preparation with cathartics or enemas can be helpful for intraabdominal procedures

6. Preoperative antibiotics: although postoperative infections are uncommon after vascular procedures, they can be catastrophic when they occur; therefore administration of a broad-spectrum antibiotic, typically a first-generation cephalosporin, 15 to 30 minutes before skin incision should be part of the routine

7. Assess preoperative risk by organ system

a. It is important to remember that 50% of early postoperative deaths after vascular surgery are due to cardiac disease; thus particular attention must be paid to cardiac evaluation (Figure 10-1).

b. All significant cardiac, pulmonary, renal, infectious, and nutritional issues should be addressed and corrected, if possible, before elective vascular procedures.

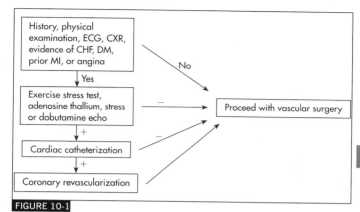

FIGURE 10-1

Evaluation of cardiac risk for elective vascular surgery.

B. POSTOPERATIVE CARE

1. **The patient's history, operative procedure, and intraoperative course** should be reviewed on arrival to the ICU.
2. **A complete physical examination** should be performed and documented with particular attention to peripheral pulses and Doppler signals in vascular grafts.
3. **Routine laboratory evaluation** should be performed, including serum chemistries, CBC, PT, and PTT, as well as an ECG and portable CXR.
4. **Evaluate and follow end-organ perfusion.**
   a. An unstimulated urine output of greater than 0.5 ml/kg/hr generally indicates adequate end-organ perfusion.
   b. Perioperative oliguria is most commonly caused by hypovolemia, and an initial volume challenge will resolve the issue in most cases. If a patient does not respond to an initial volume bolus, invasive monitoring must be considered (see Chapters 1, 2, and 5).
   c. Other indicators of adequate perfusion include heart rate, blood pressure, capillary refill, and mental status if the patient is not sedated.
5. **Hypertension**
   a. Hypertension in the early postoperative period can lead to serious complications, such as graft disruption, myocardial ischemia, and stroke.
   b. Intraarterial line for BP monitoring should be routine for all major vascular procedures.
   c. Systolic BP should be maintained within 10% of preoperative BP for normotensive patients and no higher than 150 mm Hg for baseline hypertensive patients. Another common goal is a mean arterial BP below 75 to 80 mm Hg.

d. The agent most commonly used for BP control during the commonly labile initial postoperative period is a sodium nitroprusside infusion (50 mg in 250 ml D5W) titrated to the desired blood pressure.

e. The preoperative antihypertensive regimen should be restarted as soon as bowel function returns.

6. Myocardial ischemia

a. Patients with known coronary artery disease should be maintained on IV nitroglycerin during the early postoperative period with conversion to topical nitrates on transfer from the ICU.

b. Any acute change in cardiac status should be investigated with a 12-lead ECG, repeat physical and laboratory examination, and serial cardiac isoenzymes.

c. Remember, a common causes of postoperative myocardial ischemia is undiagnosed hemorrhage!

7. Postoperative prophylactic measures

a. Stress ulceration: antacids, histamine antagonists, or sucralfate (Carafate) are all accepted prophylaxis for postoperative stress ulcer

b. Infection
   (1) Perioperative antibiotics should be administered before skin incision with repeated doses to continue for 24 to 48 hours postoperatively.
   (2) Sterile dressings from the operating room should be left in place for 2 to 3 days, provided they remain clean and dry.

c. Deep venous thrombosis
   (1) While in bed, patients should be positioned with their legs above the level of their hearts.
   (2) Patients should be mobilized as soon as possible with progressive ambulation as tolerated.
   (3) Pharmacologic prophylaxis, including subcutaneous low molecular weight heparin or systemic anticoagulation, should be reserved for high-risk patients who have documented DVTs, malignancies, or hypercoagulable states, or who will be immobile for prolonged periods.
   (4) Sequential compression devices are contraindicated in the presence of infrainguinal arterial bypass grafts or with severe peripheral arterial disease.

III. SPECIFIC VASCULAR DISEASES

A. ABDOMINAL AORTIC ANEURYSM

1. Elective repair of AAA

a. Approximately 75% of cases are repaired electively, with an expected mortality of 2%.

b. Elective repair is typically undertaken when AAA is greater than 5 cm or aneurysm is documented to grow more than 1 cm per year.

2. Ruptured AAA

a. Symptoms
   (1) Severe back or abdominal pain
   (2) Tender pulsatile abdominal mass

(3) Hemodynamic instability, which may be sporadic if the rupture is initially contained by the retroperitoneum

b. The majority of patients with a ruptured AAA expire before arrival at a hospital

c. Expected morbidity and mortality are 50%, respectively, for patients who undergo surgery for a ruptured AAA

3. Postoperative issues

a. Initial physical examination with attention to femoral and distal pulses, as well as peripheral perfusion.

b. As discussed, hypertension must be strictly controlled.

c. Considerable intestinal and duodenal manipulation is required for trans-peritoneal AAA repair, so NG decompression is required to prevent emesis and aspiration.

d. Attention must be paid to rewarming the patient and promptly correcting any coagulopathy; reexploration must be considered if there is any evidence of ongoing bleeding in a warm, noncoagulopathic patient.

e. Renal dysfunction.
   (1) Can be expected in 10% and 60% of patients undergoing elective and emergent AAA repair, respectively.
   (2) Adequate volume resuscitation and maintenance of cardiac output are the most effective methods for prevention of renal failure.
   (3) Ureteral injury, although rare, must be considered.

f. Intestinal ischemia.
   (1) Occurs after approximately 5% of AAA repairs.
   (2) Caused by ligation of a patent inferior mesenteric artery, which typically arises from the AAA.
   (3) Symptoms include abdominal pain, diarrhea, and hematochezia with leukocytosis.
   (4) Diagnosis is confirmed by flexible sigmoidoscopy or colonoscopy.
   (5) Most cases are patchy and limited to the mucosa, requiring bowel rest and broad-spectrum IV antibiotics. Transmural ischemia, however, requires exploration and colon resection. If there is uncertainty regarding the degree of ischemia, the abdomen should be re-explored and bowel viability assessed directly.

g. Paraplegia is exceedingly rare after AAA repair (0.1%) but may occur in up to 6% of patients after thoracic aortic aneurysm repair. Documentation of postoperative neurologic examination is essential.

h. Patients can present to the ICU with several late complications of aortic grafting. These include graft infection, which typically requires graft excision and extraanatomic bypass grafting to supply circulation to the lower extremities. One of the most dreaded late complications is the development of an aortoenteric fistula resulting from erosion of the graft into the bowel, most commonly the duodenum. Studies that can aid in the diagnosis include upper GI endoscopy and abdominal CT scanning, which can demonstrate bowel and an inflammatory process directly adjacent to the graft.

10

THE VASCULAR SYSTEM

B. **AORTOILIAC OCCLUSIVE DISEASE**
1. **Symptoms** include fatigue or claudication of the buttocks and thighs, atrophy of leg muscles, and pallor of legs and feet. Men can experience impotence. Less commonly, patients present with atheroembolism of aortoiliac plaque, causing painful, punctate, purple lesions of the toes and feet.
2. **Aortobifemoral bypass grafting** with Dacron or polytetrafluoroethylene (PTFE) grafts has a reported 5-year patency of 90% and a 2% operative mortality. Extraanatomic bypass or iliac angioplasty are also potential treatments.
3. **Very similar to AAA repair with regard to postoperative care.**
C. **INFRAINGUINAL OCCLUSIVE DISEASE**
1. **Patients present with symptoms** ranging from mild claudication to rest pain and finally tissue loss.
2. **The type of surgical revascularization** depends on the anatomy of the lesions and the availability of conduit. Most patients require either femoropopliteal or femorodistal (infrapopliteal) bypass grafting (Figure 10-2). Grafts limited to above the knee can be fashioned from Gore-Tex (PTFE). Saphenous vein grafts, either reversed or in situ, have been shown to have considerably better long-term patency when the graft must extend below the knee.
3. **Five-year graft patency** ranges from 40% to 80% depending on the anatomy and conduit.
4. **Postoperative issues:**
   a. Documentation of the distal pulses and graft flow on a regular basis are mandatory. Many grafts can be salvaged after occlusion if the diagnosis and treatment are prompt. Early graft occlusion should be suspected if the extremity becomes pale and painful with loss of distal pulses.
   b. Patients who experience prolonged limb ischemia either preoperatively or intraoperatively and patients who bleed into the lower extremity are at risk for development of compartment syndrome. A high index of suspicion is critical to the diagnosis of this complication early. A tense calf with loss of distal pulses and increasing pain are suggestive and require investigation, most commonly exploration. Measurement of compartment pressure may be useful. A compartment pressure greater than 30 mm Hg is consistent with an impending compartment syndrome. Treatment is immediate fasciotomy.
   c. Postoperative anticoagulation is used in patients with distal prosthetic grafts, hypercoagulable states, or a history of repeated graft occlusions.
D. **ACUTE ARTERIAL INSUFFICIENCY**
1. **Patients present with one or more of the five Ps:** *p*ain, *p*allor, *p*ulselessness, *p*aresthesia, and *p*aralysis. These patients can often pinpoint the moment when their symptoms began, as opposed to patients with chronic ischemia who experience a gradual progression of symptoms.
2. **Prompt diagnosis and treatment** are required to achieve a successful outcome in patients with acute ischemia. In general, one can expect

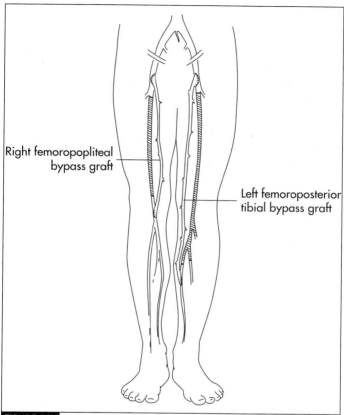

FIGURE 10-2

Patient with right femoropopliteal graft and left femoroposterior tibial graft.

irreversible tissue injury if circulation is not restored within 6 hours. This time limit is somewhat variable, depending on the presence of collateral circulation.

3. **If the diagnosis is clear,** patients should be anticoagulated and taken to the operating room as soon as possible for exploration and thromboembolectomy. If the diagnosis is unclear, arteriography can delineate the anatomy, degree of chronic arterial disease, and the presence or absence of an embolus.

4. **Most patients with embolic disease will require prompt embolectomy.** Thrombolytic therapy may be indicated in certain cases of acute graft

occlusion or distal arterial thrombosis. Most grafts, even if they are reopened with thrombolytics, will require revision to prevent prompt reocclusion.

5. **Postoperative issues:**
a. Reperfusion of an ischemic extremity can result in "wash-out" of ischemic by-products into the systemic circulation. This can lead to lactic acidosis, hyperkalemia, and myoglobinemia.
   (1) Acidosis should be treated with sodium bicarbonate.
   (2) Hyperkalemia should be treated with the usual interventions, including calcium gluconate, insulin and glucose, furosemide and saline, sodium polystyrene sulfonate (Kayexalate; enemas or PO), and hemodialysis, if needed.
   (3) If untreated, myoglobinemia can lead to renal failure. Serial urine specimens should be tested to rule out myoglobinuria. If present, the patient should be treated with aggressive volume resuscitation, osmotic diuresis with mannitol, and urine alkalinization to increase myoglobin solubility. A urine output of greater than 100 ml/hr should be maintained until the myoglobinuria resolves.
b. Reperfusion of an ischemic extremity may result in compartment syndrome as discussed above.

E. **CEREBROVASCULAR DISEASE**
1. **Stroke is the third leading cause of death in the United States,** with an incidence of approximately 160 per 100,000 population per year. Carotid atheroembolism represents the most common cause.
2. **Carotid atheroembolism presents with three syndromes,** differentiated by the duration of symptoms. TIA (less than 24 hours), RIND (1 to 7 days), and stroke (more than 7 days) all may present with hemiparesis, unilateral sensory deficits or paresthesias, unilateral facial droop, aphasia, or monocular visual loss (amaurosis fugax).
3. **Carotid endarterectomy** has been shown to be beneficial in symptomatic patients with ipsilateral internal carotid stenoses greater than 70%. Patients with asymptomatic severe internal carotid stenosis may also benefit from carotid endarterectomy.
4. **Postoperative issues:**
a. The initial evaluation should include a detailed neurologic examination and inspection of the neck. Blood pressure control is critical because hypotension may result in cerebral hypoperfusion and hypertension may cause bleeding.
b. New onset of neurologic symptoms requires radiologic evaluation or re-exploration.
c. Bleeding into the limited compartments of the neck can rapidly lead to airway compression with respiratory compromise. Such a situation requires immediate intubation and cervical exploration. If the airway cannot be secured promptly, the cervical incision should be reopened to release the pressure on the airway and allow intubation.

F. RENOVASCULAR HYPERTENSION

1. **Results from a stenotic lesion in one or both renal arteries, triggering a cascade of hormonal responses.** In brief, decreased perfusion pressure is sensed by the juxtaglomerular complex of the renal cortex, which releases renin. Renin converts angiotensinogen (produced by the liver) to angiotensin I, which is then converted to the vasoactive agent angiotensin II by angiotensin converting enzyme (ACE) in the lung. Angiotensin II triggers several physiologic responses, including increased aldosterone release from the adrenal cortex. The final physiologic effects are sodium and water retention and hypertension.

2. **Renal artery stenosis** should be suspected in young patients with no family history of hypertension who have severe hypertension that is difficult to control.

3. **Diagnostic evaluation** should include both an anatomic study, the gold standard being arteriography, and a functional study to document the physiologic significance of the lesion. The most commonly used functional studies are renal vein renin assays and the enalapril renal perfusion scan.

4. **Results of surgical bypass are excellent** with improvement of hypertension and preservation of renal function in 80% of patients. Angioplasty and stenting are indicated for focal lesions and in patients who represent poor surgical candidates.

5. **Postoperative issues:**

a. Patients tend to be total body fluid overloaded as a result of chronic hyperaldosteronism, so postoperative volume status must be monitored and managed carefully.

b. Antihypertensive medications should not be weaned in the immediate postoperative period because blood pressure control is needed to prevent postoperative bleeding.

c. Sudden return of uncontrollable hypertension or a decrement in renal function may indicate graft failure, which should prompt evaluation with renal scanning or arteriography.

G. DEEP VENOUS THROMBOSIS

1. **DVT occurs in approximately 20% of patients after major abdominal surgery and up to 70% of patients after major lower extremity orthopedic surgery.**

2. **Symptoms are often vague** but classically include unilateral lower extremity edema with a dull ache.

3. **Use of clinical signs and symptoms alone for diagnosis of DVT has been compared with the "tossing of a coin"** with false-positive and false-negative rates of approximately 50%. Classic findings are calf pain on dorsiflexion of the ankle (Homans's sign) with a distinctive "doughy" feel to the muscle.

4. **Duplex ultrasonography and MRI** have become the tests of choice for the diagnosis of DVT. These studies have begun to supplant the prior gold standard, contrast venography, because they are noninvasive and

do not require IV contrast. Ultrasound can be performed quickly, with a portable machine if necessary, is widely available, and is less expensive than MRI. MRI, on the other hand, can better evaluate the deep pelvic veins. The decision of which test to use is typically determined by institutional expertise and individual preferences.

5. **The local effects of the DVT are not the primary concern.** Embolization of venous thrombi to the pulmonary circulation can result in acute respiratory decompensation and even death. Multiple pulmonary emboli, if untreated, can cause progressive pulmonary hypertension.

6. **Patients with documented DVT should be systemically anticoagulated with intravenous heparin.** This therapy does not dissolve the clot, but it does prevent further propagation of thrombus, thus allowing the thrombus to stabilize and undergo fibrinolysis.

a. Patients who suffer pulmonary emboli while fully anticoagulated or who cannot be anticoagulated should be considered for inferior vena cava (IVC) filter placement. IVC filters are percutaneously placed in the infrarenal IVC to trap emboli and hold them in the bloodstream until they lyse. This prevents pulmonary decompensation and chronic pulmonary injury. Risks associated with IVC filters include IVC thrombosis (5%) and migration or misplacement of the filter (4%).

b. When the patient's clinical situation allows, anticoagulation with warfarin (Coumadin) should be initiated for long-term therapy. Most patients with uncomplicated DVT are treated for 3 to 6 months. Recurrent DVT warrants workup for hypercoagulable state and lifetime anticoagulation.

H. VASCULAR TRAUMA

1. **As with all trauma patients, the history and mechanism of injury are important.** Both blunt and penetrating trauma can injure the vascular system. Even patients with palpable pulses distal to an injury can subsequently suffer acute thrombosis resulting from intimal disruption.

2. **Evaluation**

a. Physical examination should document the location of the injury and all entrance/exit wounds. An initial neurologic examination is also critical.

b. Obvious arterial bleeding, expanding or pulsatile hematomas, limb ischemia, or pulse deficits warrant immediate OR for revascularization. Further tests in these patients may result in harmful delays.

c. In patients without obvious indications for OR, pulse examination and peripheral arterial pressures should be documented in all extremities. A pressure difference of greater than 10% between an injured and uninjured extremity suggests a vascular injury, which may require further evaluation with arteriography.

d. Certain orthopedic injuries have a high incidence of associated vascular trauma. These include posterior dislocation of the knee (popliteal artery); supracondylar fracture of the humerus (brachial artery); shoulder dislocation (axillary artery); pelvic fracture (hypogastric vessels); and fractures of the radius, ulna, or tibia, which are associated with delayed compartment syndrome.

e. Remember that 60% of patients with vascular trauma will have associated major injuries. One cannot focus on the vascular injury alone; every patient requires a complete trauma evaluation.

f. Serial examination will often uncover injuries missed during the initial ER evaluation or progression of vascular injuries. Compartment syndrome may develop hours to days after the injury and can rapidly lead to permanent neurologic and muscular damage.

3. Treatment

a. Identification of a significant vascular injury typically requires operative repair or bypass.

b. Intimal injuries resulting from arterial stretching (commonly associated with orthopedic injuries described above) may require bypass to prevent delayed thrombosis and limb ischemia.

c. The diagnosis of compartment syndrome requires prompt fasciotomy to relieve tissue ischemia.

10

THE VASCULAR SYSTEM

SUGGESTED READINGS

Ernst CB, Stanley JC, editors: *Current therapy in vascular surgery,* ed 2, Philadelphia, 1991, BC Decker.

Rutherford, RB, editor: *Vascular surgery*, ed 4, Philadelphia, 1994, WB Saunders.

Sabiston DC Jr, editor: *Textbook of surgery: the biological basis of modern surgical practice*, ed 15, Philadelphia, 1991, WB Saunders.

Schwartz LB: The vascular system. In: D'Amico TA, Pruitt SK, editors: *The handbook of surgical intensive care: practices of the surgical residents at Duke University Medical Center,* ed 4, St Louis, 1995, Mosby.

THE ENDOCRINE SYSTEM

Bryan M. Clary

I. DIABETES MELLITUS

A. COMORBIDITIES

Diabetic patients are at higher risk for coronary artery disease, renal failure, and peripheral vascular disease. They require major surgical procedures more often than nondiabetics and have been shown to have higher morbidity and mortality.

B. GLUCOSE MONITORING

Blood glucose monitoring is an important aspect in the care of most critically ill patients. The stress response may exacerbate underlying glucose intolerance in previously normal patients, as well as in known diabetics.

1. **Blood glucose:** Definitive, but requires time to obtain result. Levels below 175 mg/dl in the stressed patient may be normal. Spuriously high levels may be result when the blood sample is drawn proximal to an IV glucose infusion.
2. **Fingerstick:** Immediate value obtainable. It is recommended that correlation with serum glucose be obtained, which then allows one to follow trends.
3. **Urine sugar and acetone:** Generally not reliable unless correlation with serum glucose is established. May not detect elevated blood glucose in the presence of renal insufficiency.

C. TREATMENT OF HYPERGLYCEMIA

Goal is to prevent dehydration, avoid diabetic ketoacidosis (DKA), and promote the anabolic actions of insulin. Blood sugar levels between 150 and 200 mg/dl are targeted. Care is taken to avoid iatrogenic hypoglycemia, especially in patients who are sedated and unresponsive and thus unable to show signs of hypoglycemia.

1. **Insulin types (human)**
a. Regular: Onset following SQ administration 0.5 to 1 hour, peak effect within 2 to 4 hours, and duration of action of 6 hours.
b. NPH (neutral protamine Hagedorn): Onset following SQ administration 1 to 2 hours, peak effect within 8 to 12 hours, and duration of action 18 to 24 hours.
2. **Insulin delivery**
a. IV bolus: 5 to 10 units of regular insulin is a standard dose providing rapid response. This delivery form will require supplementation or modifications of the basal regimen.
b. IV infusion: Start at 1 to 2 units/hr, titrate according to hourly glucose monitoring.
c. Intramuscular: Intermediate absorption, longer half-life than IV bolus.
d. Subcutaneous: Least reliable in hypoperfused patients. In well perfused is advantageous given the longer half-life.

TABLE 11-1	
INSULIN SLIDING SCALE	
Glucose	Regular Insulin (SQ)
<70	Call HO
71-200	None
201-250	3 U
251-300	6 U
301-350	9 U
351-400	12 U
>400	15 U, call HO

HO, House officer.

This represents a common scale that may need to be modified based on the patient's response to the above parameters.

3. **Sliding scale insulin (SSI)** (Table 11-1): Based on q6h (NPO patients) or qac and qhs (patients tolerating diets) blood glucose levels. Use to estimate the next day's insulin requirements.

D. PERIOPERATIVE MANAGEMENT

1. **Management of non—insulin-dependent diabetes mellitus (non-IDDM) patients undergoing surgical procedures**

a. Preoperative
   (1) Withhold oral hypoglycemic agents beginning the night before. NPO after midnight.
   (2) Check glucose on arrival to preoperative holding.
   (3) Start IV infusion of D5½NS + 20 mEq/L KCl at 75 to 100 ml/hr.
   (4) Administer SSI as necessary.

b. Postoperative
   (1) Maintain blood glucose less than 200 mg/dl.
   (2) Check blood glucose level in recovery room and q6h thereafter.
   (3) Continue D5½NS + 20 mEq/L KCl.
   (4) Administer SSI as necessary.
   (5) As the patient resumes oral feedings, convert to preoperative regimen.

2. **Management of IDDM patients undergoing surgical procedures**

a. Preoperative orders:
   (1) NPO after midnight.
   (2) Decrease the morning dose to one half of the usual morning insulin dose. Patients taking NPH or a combination of NPH and regular should take AM as NPH. In individuals who require large doses of NPH at night, one should consider reducing their nighttime dose by 20% on the night before surgery in addition to decreasing the morning dose.
   (3) Check blood glucose on arrival to preoperative holding.
   (4) Start IV infusion of D5½NS + 20mEq/L KCl at 75 to 100 ml/hr.
   (5) Administer SSI as necessary.

b. Postoperative orders:
  (1) Maintain blood glucose less than 200 mg/dl; avoid ketoacidosis.
  (2) Check blood glucose level in recovery room and q6h thereafter.
  (3) IVF: D5½NS + 20 mEq/L KCl at appropriate rate.
  (4) Basal insulin regimen given SQ q6h. Total daily dose should equal one half the preoperative daily dose and be divided equally q6h. SSI is administered as necessary. The basal regimen should be modified according to the SSI requirements.
  (5) When patient tolerates an oral diet, the preoperative regimen can be resumed (the insulin doses may need to be modified).
  (6) Insulin infusions may be required for difficult to control hyperglycemia. Administer as regular insulin (25 U in 250 ml NS) beginning at an infusion rate of 10 ml/hr (1 U/hr). Titrate as necessary based on hourly blood glucose checks.
  (7) Weaning of insulin infusions:
    (a) NPO: Divide the previous 24 hours' insulin requirements by 4 and administer SQ q6h. After the first SQ dose, wean the infusion to off, checking blood glucose levels every hour.
    (b) PO: In patients able to take oral diets, resume the preoperative regimen, altering the dose as appropriate, taking into account the previous 24 hours' insulin requirement.

E. MANAGEMENT OF DIABETIC KETOACIDOSIS

1. Recognition: hyperglycemia, dehydration, ketosis, anion gap acidosis, altered mental status

2. Precipitating factors: recent reduction of insulin dosing, infection, acute illnesses (e.g., MI, pancreatitis, CVA), medical interventions (e.g., steroids, pentamidine, peritoneal dialysis)

3. Laboratory findings

a. Serum glucose 500 to 800 mg/dl, although milder elevations may occur
b. Metabolic acidosis-elevated lactate, keto acids (10 to 20 mmol/L); acidemia may be attenuated in patients with vomiting, high NG output
c. Electrolytes: mild hyponatremia, total body potassium depleted despite normokalemia seen in most patients

4. Treatment

a. Confirm diagnosis, laboratory evaluation (electrolytes, ABG, phosphorus, magnesium, CBC)
b. Volume/electrolyte replacement
  (1) Anticipate 5- to 10-L volume deficit
  (2) Initiate volume resuscitation with NS + 20 mEq KCl/L, 2 L over 2 hours
  (3) Monitor electrolytes/volume status frequently
  (4) Continue volume resuscitation with NS until serum sodium is greater than 150 mEq/L or volume replete, then switch to ½NS (0.45%)
  (5) Add dextrose (D5) when serum glucose is less than 250 mg/dl
  (6) Supplement potassium further according to the serum level
  (7) Supplement phosphorus (if less than 2 mg/dl) and magnesium (if less than 1.5 mg/dl) as necessary

   c. Insulin
     (1) Initial bolus of 0.1 U/kg
     (2) Begin insulin infusion 0.1 U/kg/hr (50 U/500 ml NS)
     (3) Hourly blood glucose checks
     (4) Double the infusion rate hourly until the blood glucose begins to fall, then titrate according to subsequent levels
     (5) Add dextrose (D5) when serum glucose is less than 250 mg/dl
   d. Bicarbonate: acidosis usually resolves with insulin therapy; bicarbonate should not be routinely administered unless the pH is critically low (less than 7.1), at which point many clinicians will administer 2 ampules of bicarbonate (although this remains controversial)

F. MANAGEMENT OF HYPEROSMOLAR NONKETOTIC DIABETIC COMA (HNDC)

1. Recognition: severe hyperglycemia, dehydration, electrolyte depletion, serum hyperosmolarity, minimal ketosis/acidosis, and altered mental status

2. Neurologic dysfunction: secondary to hyperosmolarity and volume depletion

3. Treatment: same as that for diabetic ketoacidosis (see above); these patients may require more volume than those with ketoacidosis

G. MANAGEMENT OF HYPOGLYCEMIA

1. Etiology

   a. Insulin overdose

   b. Decreased clearance of insulin or oral hypoglycemic agents (liver and kidney dysfunction)

   c. Drug interactions between oral hypoglycemic agents and salicylates, sulfonamides, monoamine oxidase (MAO) inhibitors, insulin, β-blockers, and others

   d. Other: NPO, decrease in TPN/enteral feeds, resolving infection, and emesis

   e. Nondiabetics: alcohol ingestion, liver failure, shock, malignancy, pregnancy, sepsis

2. Recognition: hypoglycemia on routing measurements, mental status changes, sweating, headache, hypothermia, and tachycardia

3. Treatment

   a. Severe (symptomatic, less than 50 mg/dl): Administer IV one ampule of D50, address etiology, decrease insulin dose. PO intake of juice if tolerating diet. Continue to recheck levels until normalized.

   b. Mild (asymptomatic, greater than 50 mg/dl): Decrease insulin/oral hypoglycemic dose, PO intake of juice if tolerating diet. If NPO, then begin/increase dextrose-containing IV fluids. Continue to recheck levels until normalized. Address etiology.

II. ADRENAL DISORDERS IN THE CRITICALLY ILL

A. TESTS OF ADRENAL FUNCTION

1. Serum cortisol: AM normal 8 to 25 μg/dl, PM normal 5 to 15 μg/dl.

2. ACTH stimulation: Measure the plasma cortisol concentration before and 30 to 60 minutes after a parenteral dose of 250 μg of synthetic

ACTH (cosyntropin). A rise above 20 μg/dl or an absolute increase of more than 7 μg/dl is normal.

B. CHRONIC ADRENAL INSUFFICIENCY (ADRENAL AXIS SUPPRESSION)

1. **Suspect in any patient who has taken supraphysiologic doses** (more than 7.5 mg prednisone) for more than a week in the year preceding surgery.
2. **ACTH stimulation test to detect suppressive state.**
3. **In patients with abnormal ACTH stimulation tests** or those who have not been tested and require major surgery, steroid coverage is commonly provided (controversial) and tapered as follows:

a. Preoperative (midnight before if in-house) 100 mg hydrocortisone IV.
b. Postoperative day (POD) 0: hydrocortisone 100 mg IV q8h.
c. POD 1: hydrocortisone 50 mg IV q8h.
d. POD 2: hydrocortisone 25 mg IV q8h.
e. POD 3: hydrocortisone 25 mg IV q12h.
f. POD 4: hydrocortisone 25 mg IV q24h.
g. POD 5: Discontinue if patient not taking immediately preoperatively. Patients who were taking steroids preoperatively are placed back on their preoperative regimen (or IV equivalent if NPO). Switch to oral prednisone at equivalent dose may be made at any time in patients able to tolerate oral feeds.
h. The above regimen is a common regimen, although others exist and are likely just as effective. Table 11-2 details the equivalent potencies between the different steroid preparations.
i. H_2 blockers are routinely administered for GI prophylaxis during high-dose steroid replacement.

C. ACUTE ADRENAL INSUFFICIENCY

1. **Signs and symptoms:** weakness, apathy, anorexia, nausea, vomiting, abdominal pain, diarrhea, fever, and hypotension
2. **Laboratory findings:** hyponatremia, hyperkalemia, acidosis, hypoglycemia, eosinophilia, lymphocytosis, low cortisol, hypercalcemia, and subnormal ACTH response

TABLE 11-2

RELATIVE STEROID POTENCY

Steroid	Relative Glucocorticoid Potency*	Relative Mineralocorticoid Activity*	Equivalent Dose (mg)
Cortisol	1	1	20
Cortisone	0.8	0.8	25
Prednisone	4	0.8	5
Prednisolone	4	0.8	5
6α-methylprednisolone	5	0.5	4
Betamethasone	10	0	2
Dexamethasone	25	0	0.6

*Relative to cortisol (given reference value of 1).

3. Treatment
a. Aggressive fluid and electrolyte repletion.
b. Empiric therapy before definitive diagnosis in critical clinical situations. Dexamethasone does not cross-react with the serum cortisol assay and thus can be the initial glucocorticoid replacement given while performing the ACTH stimulation test.
c. Glucocorticoid and mineralocorticoid replacement: Should match the expected 300 to 400 mg/day of cortisol that is secreted by the normal adrenal gland during stress. The replacement regimen should possess mineralocorticoid activity, that is, hydrocortisone alone (most commonly given) or dexamethasone plus fludrocortisone are acceptable alternatives. An acceptable regimen is as follows:
   (1) Hydrocortisone 200 mg IV stat
   (2) Hydrocortisone 100 mg IV q6h thereafter
d. Monitor blood glucose and electrolytes frequently, and supplement as needed.
e. Identify and treat the precipitating illness/cause.
f. Maintenance therapy: After stability is achieved, longer-acting preparations are then instituted (prednisone 7.5 to 10 mg per day + fludrocortisone acetate 0.1 to 0.2 mg PO qAM).

D. PHEOCHROMOCYTOMA
1. Signs and symptoms: hypertension (sustained or paroxysmal), sweating, cutaneous flushing, fever, weight loss, glucose intolerance, headache, tachycardia, palpitations, panic attacks, and anxiety
2. Diagnosis
a. 24-hour urine showing elevated
   (1) Vanillylmandelic acid (VMA)
   (2) Metanephrine/normetanephrine
   (3) Free catecholamines
b. Elevated plasma catecholamine levels (<1400 ng/L in patients with hypertension)
c. Clonidine suppression (administer 0.3 mg PO)
   (1) Serum catecholamine levels measured at baseline and 3 hours after clonidine. Normal response is a decrease in the catecholamine levels.
   (2) Urine: 10-hour collection with normal epinephrine and norepinephrine productions of less than 20 and 60 nMol/mol creatinine, respectively.
3. Treatment
a. Acute hypertensive crisis: nitroprusside drip (1 mg/250 ml D5W) titrated to effect; phentolamine (5 mg/500 ml D5W) as an infusion can be used, as well
b. Perioperative management
   (1) Minimize preoperative invasive studies
   (2) Preoperative fluid repletion
   (3) Preoperative pharmacologic blockade
      (a) Prevents immediate complications
      (b) α-Adrenergic blockade: Phenoxybenzamine 10 mg PO tid initiated more than 7 days preoperatively. Increase the dose until hyper-

tension is controlled and the patient experiences mild orthostatic hypotension. Prazosin beginning at 2 mg PO bid is an alternative.
(c) β-Adrenergic blockade: Propanolol initiated at 10 mg PO q8h. Thought to provide control of intraoperative arrhythmias (β-blockade is controversial and not critical in most instances).

III. THYROID DISORDERS IN THE CRITICALLY ILL

A. GENERAL CONSIDERATIONS

1. Tests of thyroid function

a. Thyroid-stimulating hormone (TSH): Release of TSH indirectly controlled by thyroid hormone levels via thyrotropin-releasing hormone (TRH). TSH is the major regulator of thyroid hormone production. Most effective measure of thyroid activity. A normal TSH excludes hypothyroidism and hyperthyroidism.

b. Free T_3 and T_4 (FT_3, FT_4): T_3 is the active form and is derived from peripheral conversion of T_4 secreted by the thyroid gland. In the presence of a low TSH, high or normal levels of FT_3 and FT_4 indicate overt and subclinical hyperthyroidism, respectively. In the presence of a high TSH, low or normal levels of FT_4 indicate overt and subclinical hypothyroidism, respectively. FT_3 conversion from FT_4 can be impaired during illness (euthyroid sick syndrome). These individuals are euthyroid.

c. Resin T_3 uptake (RT_3U): Measures unoccupied thyroid hormone binding sites on thyronine-binding globulins (TBGs). It is directly proportional to the fraction of free T_4 in the serum. RT_3U is high in thyrotoxicosis and low in hypothyroidism. This test is cheaper and easier to perform than direct T_4 measurements.

d. Serum thyroglobulin: Elevated in goiter, hyperthyroidism, thyroiditis, and thyroid tumors. It is suppressed in factitious thyrotoxicosis.

2. Effect of illness on thyroid hormone metabolism

a. Many drugs used in the ICU patient affect thyroid hormone metabolism, including steroids, cimetidine, metoclopramide, opiates, salicylates, diazepam, propranolol, phenobarbital, heparin, and nitroprusside.

b. Starvation: Decrease in total and FT_3 levels.

c. Postoperatively: Transient (1 week) decrease in T_3. Brief fall in TSH.

d. Chronic illness: Decreased conversion of T_4 to T_3 (euthyroid sick syndrome).

e. Nonthyroidal diseases: Including hepatic dysfunction can reduce the level of TBG and consequently total T_4 levels. FT_4 usually remains normal.

f. Acute illness: Often have decreased T_3. T_4 levels are more useful in this population of patients. Hypothyroidism can be excluded in these patients by TSH measurements (low levels).

B. HYPOTHYROIDISM

1. Contributing factors

a. Previous radioactive iodine treatment

b. Prior neck surgery

c. Prior exogenous thyroxine therapy

2. **Signs and symptoms**
a. Cold intolerance
b. Constipation
c. Dry, scaly skin
d. Lethargy, weakness
e. Bradycardia
f. Delayed deep tendon reflexes
g. Peripheral and periorbital edema
h. Decreased hypoxic and hypercapnic ventilatory drives

3. **Laboratory abnormalities**
a. Elevated TSH
b. Low free thyroxine index

4. **Treatment:** thyroxine 100 to 200 mg PO qd

5. **Myxedema coma**
a. Caused by a severe deficit in circulating thyroid hormones
b. Usually seen in individuals with a long history of hypothyroidism
c. As many as 50% of the cases have occurred after hospitalization
d. Common precipitating factors
   (1) Pulmonary infection (most common) or other infection
   (2) Surgery or trauma
   (3) Hypoglycemia and hypovolemia
   (4) CVA
   (5) CHF
e. Diagnosis is made on the clinical grounds of a precipitating event followed by:
   (1) Altered mental status
   (2) Profound hypothermia
f. Treatment
   (1) Treat the precipitating cause.
   (2) Passively warm the patient.
   (3) Administer crystalloid fluid if the patient is hypovolemic.
   (4) Administer hydrocortisone 100 mg IV q6h.
   (5) Administer T_4 300 to 500 mg IV loading dose then 100 mg IV qid.
   (6) Supportive treatment: Hyponatremia may require hypertonic solutions. Ileus, urinary retention, and hypoglycemia should be treated appropriately. Pericardial and pleural effusions usually resolve spontaneously.

6. **Euthyroid sick syndrome**
a. Most common thyroid abnormality seen in critically ill patients
b. Thought to be due to a deficiency in the enzyme that converts T_4 to T_3
   (1) T_4 is preferentially degraded into reverse T_3 (rT_3), which is physiologically inactive.
   (2) Diminished active T_3 production limits the utilization of protein and oxygen.
c. Signs and symptoms consistent with hypothyroidism

d. Laboratory abnormalities
   (1) TSH is normal.
   (2) Free thyroxine index is low.
   (3) Serum T_4 and T_3 are low.
   (4) rT_3 is elevated.
e. Treatment: not indicated and may be deleterious

C. MANAGEMENT OF THYROTOXIC CRISIS

1. An acute exacerbation of an underlying hyperthyroid condition

2. Etiology

a. Graves' disease is the most common etiologic factor.
b. Other thyroid diseases may also precipitate a thyroid crisis.

3. Precipitating factors

a. Surgery
b. Radioactive iodine treatment
c. Parturition
d. Stressful illness or infection

4. Signs and symptoms

a. Heat intolerance, hyperthermia, sweating, and cutaneous flushing
b. Diarrhea, nausea, and vomiting
c. Weakness and weight loss
d. Dyspnea
e. Nervousness, agitation, restlessness, and delirium
f. Hyperkinesis and hyperreflexia
g. Tachycardia and atrial fibrillation

5. Laboratory abnormalities

a. TSH usually undetectable in serum
b. Increased serum T_4 and T_3

6. Treatment

a. Inhibition of hormone synthesis: propylthiouracil 800 to 1200 mg PO loading dose, then 200 to 300 mg PO q6h; or methimazole 25 mg PO q6h
b. Inhibition of thyroid hormone release using one of the following:
   (1) Sodium iodide 0.5 g IV q12h
   (2) Saturated solution of potassium iodide (SSKI) 1 to 10 drops PO tid
c. Block conversion of T_4 to T_3: dexamethasone 2 mg PO/IV q6h; or hydrocortisone 50 to 100 mg IV q8h
d. Symptomatic treatment of excess T_4
   (1) Propranolol 40 to 60 mg PO or 1 to 2 mg IV q6h
   (2) Reserpine 1 mg PO/IM/IV q6-12h in patients with heart failure or asthma that cannot tolerate β-blockade

IV. PARATHYROID DISORDERS IN THE CRITICALLY ILL

A. MANAGEMENT OF HYPERCALCEMIC CRISIS

1. Etiology

a. Primary hyperparathyroidism
b. Malignancy: PTH-related protein, direct osteolytic disease, and hematologic malignancies

c. Others: granulomatous diseases, factitious, Paget's disease, thyrotoxicosis, acromegaly, and hypoadrenalism

2. **Signs and symptoms**
a. Symptoms almost always present when serum calcium is greater than 14.5 mg/dl
b. Malaise and lethargy
c. Anorexia
d. Polyuria
e. Dehydration
f. Nausea and vomiting
g. Mental status changes
h. Cardiac arrhythmias (shortened QT, bundle branch block, bradycardia, heart block)

3. **Laboratory evaluation**
a. Serum calcium: ionized is most accurate (45% of serum calcium); elevated
b. Hypercalciuria (urine calcium greater than 280 mg/24 hours in men, 200 mg/24 hours in women)
c. Alkaline phosphatase: elevated in 75% of patients with crisis
d. Parathyroid hormone level (intact): elevated in the presence of hypercalcemia is diagnostic of hyperparathyroidism

4. **Treatment**
a. Aggressive volume resuscitation with normal saline
b. Loop diuretic (e.g., furosemide 40 to 80 mg IV) once normovolemic
c. Frequent calcium and other electrolyte measurements
d. Parathyroidectomy in primary hyperparathyroidism once stabilized
e. Refractory hypercalcemia may require osteoclast inhibitors
   (1) Mithramycin: 25 μg/dl IV qd for 3 to 4 days, repeat weekly as necessary
   (2) Corticosteroids: hydrocortisone 250 to 500 mg IV q8h (takes several days to see effects)
   (3) Calcitonin: 4 IU/kg and increase to 8 IU/kg q6h
   (4) Phosphate: final option; Neutra-Phos 250 mg tid to qid or as a 100-ml Fleet retention enema

B. **MANAGEMENT OF HYPOPARATHYROIDISM**

1. **Etiology**
a. Iatrogenic after head and neck surgery
b. Hypomagnesemia
c. Genetic defects in PTH synthesis
d. Autoimmune destruction of PTH glands

2. **Signs and symptoms**
a. Chvostek's sign: contraction of facial musculature in response to tapping the facial nerve
b. Trousseau's sign: carpopedal spasm after blood pressure cuff inflation above systolic blood pressure for more than 3 minutes
c. Tetany

d. Laryngeal stridor
e. Seizures
f. Circumoral tingling/numbness
g. Muscle cramps and numbness of the extremities
h. ECG abnormalities: QT prolongation, T-wave peaking/inversion

3. Laboratory evaluation
a. Hypocalcemia
b. Check electrolytes
c. Low PTH levels

4. Treatment
a. Asymptomatic: manage expectantly
b. Symptomatic
   (1) Calcium supplementation: Initial 1 ampule of calcium gluconate (90 mg) administered over 15 minutes. Follow with constant infusion of calcium (10 ampules of 10% calcium gluconate in 1000 ml of normal saline) at 20 to 100 ml/hr. Oral calcium instituted once the serum calcium level has stabilized.
   (2) Calcitrol: 0.5 to 2 μg/day in divided doses (oral or IV)

V. DIABETES INSIPIDUS

A. GENERAL CONSIDERATIONS
Diabetes insipidus (DI) is the failure of water homeostasis. Pituitary DI is due to ADH deficiency in response to increased serum osmolality. Some 70% of patients with DI have an intracranial neoplasm or head trauma.

B. SYMPTOMS
polyuria, polydipsia, thirst

C. LABORATORY
1. Hypernatremia
2. Urine specific gravity less than 1.005
3. Urine osmolality less than 200 mOsm/L
4. Serum osmolality greater than 290 mOsm/L
5. Normal GFR
6. Increase in urine osmolality of greater than 10% with vasopressin (5 U SQ) after overnight fluid deprivation

D. TREATMENT
1. Initial therapy: vasopressin 5 U SQ q4h
2. Access to water
3. Desmopressin for long-term management: 2 to 4 μg intranasally bid, titrated to prevent nocturia

SUGGESTED READINGS

Clark OH, Duh Q, editors: *Textbook of endocrine surgery,* Philadelphia, 1997, WB Saunders.

Goldmann DR, Brown FH, Guarnieri DM, editors: *Perioperative medicine,* Philadelphia, 1994, McGraw-Hill.

Moylan JA, editor: *Surgical critical care,* St Louis, 1994, Mosby.

11

THE ENDOCRINE SYSTEM

THE HEMATOLOGIC SYSTEM

Jeffrey H. Lawson

I. PATIENT EVALUATION

A. ROUTINE PREOPERATIVE EVALUATION

1. History

a. Unusual bleeding with prior trauma or surgery, including dental procedures

b. History of epistaxis, easy bruising, DVT/PE, unusual menstrual bleeding, liver disease, malignancy, or renal disease

c. Family history of bleeding

d. Medications (e.g., warfarin, aspirin, NSAIDs)

2. Physical examination: Contusion, telangiectasia, jaundice, hepatomegaly, splenomegaly, and hemarthrosis

3. Laboratory data: Decision to obtain additional laboratory tests depends on the history, physical examination, and nature of the planned procedure; patients grouped into the following three categories:

a. Category I: negative history and physical examination, minor procedure—no additional laboratory tests

b. Category II: negative history and physical examination, major procedure—CBC to evaluate hematocrit and platelet count; may obtain additional tests, such as PT and APTT, although in the setting of an unremarkable history and physical examination, the benefit of these tests is unproved, and they are probably not cost effective

c. Category III: positive history, physical examination, procedures that cause alteration of coagulation (CPB or liver resection), or procedures in which the consequences of unexpected bleeding may be catastrophic (neurosurgical or ophthalmologic procedures)—additional tests warranted, including platelet count, PT, APTT, and bleeding time

4. Considerations for patients on chronic warfarin anticoagulation who present for elective surgery

a. Some minor procedures can be performed without significant risk, even with the PT prolonged to 1.3 to 1.5 times the control.

b. Warfarin treatment for DVT can be substituted with pneumatic compression devices, subcutaneous heparin, or placement of a vena caval filter.

c. Bioprosthetic valves are less prone to thrombosis than mechanical valves; valves in the aortic position are less prone than those in the mitral position.

d. Treatment

    (1) Hold warfarin (do not reverse with vitamin K).

    (2) When PT is less than 1.2 to 1.5 times the control, start heparin infusion.

    (3) Hold heparin 4 to 6 hours before surgery.

    (4) Resume heparin infusion immediately after procedure (do not bolus).

    (5) Resume warfarin several days postoperatively.

12

B. LABORATORY TESTS

1. Prothrombin time

a. Tissue thromboplastin (tissue factor) and calcium are added to plasma and the clotting time is determined. The PT evaluates the extrinsic co-agulant pathway and is sensitive to deficiencies in factor VII, and factor X may be prolonged with deficiencies in factor V, prothrombin, and fibrinogen.

b. Prolongation is seen with liver insufficiency, vitamin K deficiency, and warfarin ingestion.

2. Activated partial thromboplastin time

a. Plasma is incubated with a platelet membrane substitute (phospholipid), a factor XII activator, and then recalcified. The APTT evaluates the intrin-sic coagulation pathways and is sensitive to deficiency in all factors except VII and XIII.

b. APTT is prolonged with congenital factor VIII or IX deficiency or heparin therapy.

3. Thrombin clotting time

a. A standard concentration of thrombin is added to plasma and the clot-ting time is measured, assessing the functional rate of fibrinogen conver-sion to fibrin.

b. TCT is prolonged by hypofibrinogenemia, dysfibrinogenemia, and heparin.

4. Fibrinogen assay

a. Fibrinogen is measured using a modified TCT (normal 160 to 360 mg/dl).

b. Fibrinogen decreases with DIC, fibrinolysis, liver insufficiency, and mas-sive transfusion.

5. D-dimers (fibrin fragments): D-dimers are specific fibrin fragments that are detected by immunoassays. These fragments are only released dur-ing states of fibrinolysis. Elevated D-dimers are seen in DIC, thromboem-bolism, and liver disease.

6. Specific factor assay

a. Specific factor–deficient plasma is incubated with the patient's plasma.

b. Failure of clotting time to correct indicates a specific factor deficiency (available for factors II, V, VII, VIII, IX, X, XI, and XII).

7. von Willebrand factor: ristocetin cofactor assay

a. Platelets are mixed with ristocetin (normally triggers vWF-induced plate-let activation) and plasma is added. Platelet agglutination is monitored by measuring changes in light transmission. The time required for agglu-tination is prolonged in patients with vWF deficiency.

b. This test is a sensitive and specific test for von Willebrand's disease (vWD).

8. Bleeding time

a. A blood pressure cuff is placed on the arm and inflated to 40 mm Hg. A commercial instrument is then used to perform a small skin incision on the anterior surface of the forearm. The incision is dabbed with filter paper every 30 seconds, and the bleeding time is determined as the time required for bleeding to stop. The normal range is 3 to 10 minutes, but considerable variability exists.

b. Prolonged bleeding time occurs with abnormal platelet function. Platelet counts greater than 50,000 may induce prolonged bleeding time; therefore the test is most useful in assessing platelet function in patients with normal platelet counts.

9. **Lupus anticoagulant panel**

a. Initial studies include PT, APTT, incubated mix test, and TCT. With the incubated mix test, the test plasma is incubated with normal plasma containing appropriate coagulation factors; correction of clotting times indicates specific factor deficiencies, and failure of clotting times to correct suggests the presence of inhibitors. TCT is performed to exclude heparin therapy as the possible inhibitor. In patients whose clotting times fail to correct with mix and who have a normal TCT, more sensitive assays (such as the Russell viper venom time) are performed to confirm the presence of inhibitors. Although some inhibitors impede normal coagulation and predispose to bleeding, the lupuslike anticoagulant has been associated with increased risk of thrombosis.

b. Lupus anticoagulant panel is often obtained to help explain an abnormally elevated PT or APTT. It should also be obtained on patients suspected of having a hypercoagulable state.

10. **Activated whole blood clotting time**

a. ACT is used to monitor heparin anticoagulation during cardiac surgery.

b. The ACT correlates with heparin dose in a linear manner.

11. **Indirect and direct antiglobulin (Coombs') tests**

a. Detect the presence of RBC antibodies in the patient's serum (indirect Coombs') or on the patient's RBCs (direct Coombs').

b. Useful in evaluating delayed transfusion reactions, autoimmune hemolytic anemia, and hemolytic disease of the newborn.

C. EVALUATION OF BLEEDING IN THE POSTOPERATIVE PATIENT

The first and most important question is whether or not a mechanical source of bleeding is present that could be corrected surgically. Bleeding from a single region of an incision implies a mechanical source. Alternatively, multiple bleeding sites, such as needle punctures, IV sites, the endotracheal tube, or hematuria, imply a nonmechanical systemic disorder of coagulation.

1. **History**

a. Consider any preoperative or intraoperative use of anticoagulants.

b. A preoperative history of liver or renal disease may also be significant.

c. Certain procedures, such as liver resection or those involving CPB, also result in distinct coagulation deficits.

2. **Physical examination**

a. Evaluation of all potential sites of bleeding: all wounds, mucosal surfaces, and intravascular catheters

b. Body temperature: normal coagulation impeded by hypothermia (particularly common in trauma or CPB patients)

c. Elevated BP: may contribute to bleeding in patients after vascular surgery

3. **Laboratory data**
a. Hematocrit: losses replaced with PRBCs and isotonic saline
b. Platelet count
    (1) If the platelet count is less than 50,000/mm^3, platelet transfusion in an actively bleeding patient is warranted.
    (2) Abnormal platelet function can be assessed with bleeding time; patients actively bleeding with a prolonged bleeding time may require platelet transfusion even if the platelet count is greater than 50,000/mm^3. Patients with renal failure, vWD, and aspirin usage may have normal platelet counts but impaired platelet function.
c. Coagulation system
    (1) Obtain PT, APTT, fibrinogen level, and D-dimer assay.
    (2) If the PT is prolonged and the APTT normal, consider hepatic insufficiency, vitamin K deficiency, and malnutrition as possible causes. Treat with FFP, 2 U initially, and vitamin K 10 to 15 mg IM/IV q12h. Follow serial PT to monitor correction.
    (3) If the APTT is prolonged and the PT normal, consider heparin administration or congenital factor VIII or IX deficiency as possible causes. Heparin effect may be reversed with protamine sulfate 25 to 50 mg IV over 10 minutes (doses greater than 50 mg are seldom required); repeat the APTT or ACT to assess complete reversal. A specific factor deficiency is treated with either cryoprecipitate or factor concentrate.
    (4) If both the PT and APTT are prolonged, obtain fibrinogen level and D-dimer assay.
        (a) If there is a low fibrinogen level (<100 mg/dl), consider DIC, primary fibrinolysis, massive transfusion, recent fibrinolytic therapy, or severe liver disease as possible causes.
        (b) A positive assay for D-dimers signifies increased fibrin degradation, as seen in DIC and primary fibrinolysis. Treatment for both DIC and primary fibrinolysis involves addressing the primary cause of these conditions. Administration of FFP or cryoprecipitate replaces fibrinogen and other factor losses. ε-Aminocaproic acid (5 g IV load, 1 g/hr IV maintenance) may also play a role in the treatment of primary fibrinolysis. However, definitive treatment for DIC requires identification and removal of source of procoagulant activity (i.e., sepsis).

II. SPECIFIC HEMATOLOGIC CONDITIONS
A. **SICKLE CELL DISEASE AND SICKLE CELL TRAIT**
1. **Sickle cell trait affects approximately 8% of African-Americans, and 0.15% suffer from sickle cell disease.**
2. **A diagnosis can be made** by demonstrating sickling of patient's RBCs under conditions of reduced oxygen tension. If this screening test is positive, hemoglobin electrophoresis can be conducted, which definitively distinguishes sickle cell trait from sickle cell disease.

3. **Patients with sickle cell trait are generally asymptomatic** and their overall life expectancy and frequency of hospitalization are unchanged. Patients with sickle cell disease have impaired development, a severe hemolytic anemia, and a variety of serious clinical problems that begin as early as 6 months of age.

a. Acute infections: There is an increased risk for overwhelming infection by encapsulated organisms, such as *Streptococcus pneumoniae* and *Haemophilus influenzae*. Sickle cell patients should receive the pneumococcal and influenza vaccines.

b. Aplastic crisis: This occurs when decreased RBC production, usually following a viral or bacterial infection, is superimposed on the preexisting shortened RBC survival. Treatment is supportive and includes PRBC transfusions as needed. It is important to exclude a concomitant folate deficiency, which may develop in these patients.

c. Sequestration: Large volumes of blood rapidly accumulate in the sinusoids of the spleen, which produces hypovolemia, shock, and, if not reversed, death.
   (1) Sequestration usually occurs in patients under the age of 5 years; older patients develop autoinfarction and are functionally asplenic.
   (2) Symptoms include pallor, listlessness, abdominal fullness, and abdominal pain.
   (3) Physical examination reveals a large, tender spleen.
   (4) Treatment is hemodynamic support with IV fluids and PRBC transfusions. Because recurrence is common, splenectomy is recommended after a second episode.

d. Painful crisis: Microvascular occlusion secondary to RBC sludging causes painful crisis.
   (1) Painful crisis usually involves the extremities, but abdominal pain and abdominal distention are common and often difficult to distinguish from an acute abdomen.
   (2) Treatment includes IV hydration, supplemental O_2 therapy, analgesics, and correction of any acid-base disorder.

4. **Preoperative care for sickle cell disease patients**

a. For major surgery, preoperative transfusion to hematocrit 30% to 35% is indicated; many sickle cell disease patients may have developed alloantibodies to RBCs, making it difficult to obtain compatible blood.

b. Hydrate liberally with 1.5× maintenance throughout the perioperative period because dehydration is a major predisposing factor for RBC sickling and sludging.

c. Avoid hypoxia; supplemental O_2 may be helpful.

B. **HEMOLYSIS**

1. **Hemolysis may occur in severe burn patients, with electrical injuries, or with sepsis and DIC.**

2. **Any intravascular prosthesis or device in contact with blood may induce hemolysis** (e.g., cardiac valve prostheses, ventricular assist devices, IABP, or ECMO circuits).

12

THE HEMATOLOGIC SYSTEM

3. **Diagnostic signs of hemolysis include the following:**
   a. Falling hematocrit
   b. Low serum haptoglobin
   c. Elevated serum and urine-free hemoglobin
   d. Elevated LDH
4. **Treatment** involves addressing the underlying cause and avoiding hemoglobin-induced renal failure.
   a. Urine output should be maintained at a level greater than 1 ml/kg/hr with saline infusion.
   b. Diuretics may be used as needed.
   c. Sodium bicarbonate may be added to the IV fluids to maintain the urinary pH at a level greater than 6 and that facilitates excretion of the hemoglobin.

C. **CONGENITAL DISORDERS OF COAGULATION**

1. **Hemophilia A**
   a. Hemophilia A is a deficiency of normal factor VIII activity secondary to a molecular defect in the coagulant portion of factor VIII.
   b. Symptoms depend on the level of functional factor VIII present.
      (1) Patients with levels greater than 25% have normal hemostasis.
      (2) Patients with levels between 5% to 25% of normal do not suffer spontaneous bleeding but develop serious problems after surgery or trauma.
      (3) The majority of patients have levels less than 5% and suffer recurrent spontaneous bleeding, which includes intracranial, intraarticular, and urinary tract hemorrhage.
   c. Diagnosis often can be made based on personal or family history. Elevated PTT occurs with factor VIII levels less than 30%. Definitive diagnosis requires measurement of factor VIII levels.
   d. Treatment:
      (1) Spontaneous hemarthrosis or retroperitoneal bleeding requires transfusion several times per day or continuous transfusion of factor VIII to maintain levels of 25% to 50% for at least 72 hours.
      (2) Patients undergoing elective surgical procedures should be screened for circulating inhibitors (present in approximately 6% of severe hemophiliacs), which prevent the correction of factor VIII levels necessary for surgery. In the absence of inhibitors, factor VIII levels are corrected with recombinant factor VIII. Before surgery, levels are corrected to 100% and maintained postoperatively above 40%.
      (3) The following formula estimates the number of units required to raise levels:

$$\text{Dose (U)} = (\text{desired \% activity} - \text{initial \% activity}) \times \text{weight (kg)}/2$$

      (4) Because the half-life of factor VIII is 8 to 12 hours, two thirds of the initial replacement dose should be repeated every 12 hours to maintain the desired level.

2. Hemophilia B

a. Hemophilia B results from the deficiency or absence of factor IX activity.

b. Symptoms are similar but less severe than hemophilia A. Prolongation of APTT is an initial finding, and the diagnosis is confirmed with measurement of factor IX levels.

c. Replacement therapy is required for factor IX–deficient patients undergoing surgery. Either FFP or recombinant factor IX may be used. Preoperative replacement to 60% and postoperative maintenance of greater than 20% to 30% of normal for 10 to 14 days are adequate. The half-life and dosing interval of factor IX is 16 to 24 hours.

D. ACQUIRED DISORDERS OF COAGULATION

1. Vitamin K deficiency

a. Vitamin K serves as a cofactor in the hepatic synthesis of factors II, VII, IX, and X, as well as protein C and protein S. Most of the vitamin K that is used by the body is produced by the microbial flora of the gut and is absorbed as fat in the ileum. Vitamin K deficiency is suggested by the clinical history and a prolonged PT. Deficiency of vitamin K can result from obstructive jaundice, hepatic insufficiency, use of antibiotics that suppress gut flora, prolonged inanition, short-gut syndrome, and any other causes of fat malabsorption.

b. Treatment for vitamin K deficiency includes the following:

(1) Correct underlying disorder whenever possible.

(2) Administer vitamin K 10 mg IM/IV daily × 3 days; failure of the PT to correct suggests causes other than vitamin K deficiency.

(3) For emergent surgery, begin factor replacement with FFP, monitor correction of PT, and continue infusion as needed to maintain complete correction.

2. Liver disease

a. The liver plays a complex role in the maintenance of normal hemostasis. With hepatic insufficiency, there is a decrease in the synthesis of prothrombin, fibrinogen, and other coagulation factors. Liver disease may cause reduced vitamin K absorption, which further complicates the problem of decreased synthesis. The liver is also a major site of clearance of activated clotting factors, and the reduced clearance that results with liver failure may trigger uncontrolled fibrinolysis and DIC. Platelet number may also be reduced in cirrhotics with portal hypertension and splenomegaly, whereas platelet function is impaired by liver failure and alcohol. Finally, the liver is also the site of production for endogenous anticoagulants—plasminogen, antithrombin III, and protein C—therefore liver insufficiency may result in both hemostatic and hypercoagulable disorders.

b. Management of the bleeding patient with liver disease includes the following:

(1) Directed, specific treatment is indicated if an isolated bleeding point can be identified.

(2) Obtain PT, PTT, fibrinogen level, bleeding time, and platelet count; obtaining factor VIII level may be helpful diagnostically to distinguish

DIC from a primary problem with hepatic synthesis. (Because factor VIII is not synthesized in the liver, its level would be normal for hepatic synthesis defect but decreased for DIC.)

(3) Administer vitamin K 10 mg IM/IV daily × 3 days; a response to vitamin K should be evident within 1 to 2 days. Failure of PT to correct after vitamin K suggests severe hepatic synthetic impairment.

(4) Transfuse platelets for counts less than 50,000 to 75,000/mm^3. If bleeding time is prolonged, a platelet transfusion may be indicated, even with normal counts.

(5) FFP is the best factor replacement; care should be taken to avoid volume overload.

(6) Severely depressed fibrinogen levels with marked elevation of the FDPs implies DIC or primary fibrinolysis. Sources of sepsis should be evaluated. Fibrinogen should be replaced with cryoprecipitate, and ε-aminocaproic acid may help inhibit ongoing fibrinolysis.

3. Hemostatic disorder of uremia
a. Patients usually have normal factor levels and normal platelet counts. The defect lies in platelet adhesion and aggregation; transfused platelets rapidly become dysfunctional. It is also important to consider the possibility of residual heparin from dialysis.

b. Management includes the following:

(1) Preoperatively, obtain PT, APTT, bleeding time, and platelet count.

(2) Perform dialysis immediately preoperatively because dialysis has a beneficial effect on platelet dysfunction. If the bleeding time is prolonged, infuse 0.3 to 0.4 μg/kg desmopressin (DDAVP) 1 hour before surgery. If unexpected bleeding develops intraoperatively or postoperatively, repeat DDAVP infusion and start infusion of cryoprecipitate.

4. Massive transfusion
a. Definition: Replacement of greater than one blood volume (5000 ml for a 70-kg patient) in a 24-hour period. The majority of these patients will demonstrate laboratory evidence of coagulopathy, and at least half demonstrate clinical evidence of a hemostatic defect.

b. Platelet loss: This is perhaps the most significant consideration. PRBCs fail to replace the loss of platelets that occur with bleeding; furthermore, there may be loss of platelet hemostatic function resulting from acidosis, hypothermia, or drug infusions. Generally, transfuse 2 U of platelets for every 10 to 12 U of PRBCs.

c. Factor deficiencies: Factor levels are much less labile during massive transfusion because of endogenous stores. Nevertheless, serial PT/APTT should be obtained during massive transfusions. Generally, 2 U FFP should be administered for every 10 U PRBCs transfused.

d. Hypothermia: Patient exposure, hypoperfusion, and the administration of unwarmed intravenous fluids all contribute to the development of hypothermia, which may itself inhibit normal hemostasis. All fluids and blood products must be warmed before infusion, and in addition, overhead lamps and warming blankets should be used.

e. Citrate toxicity: PRBCs contain citrate, which is added as an anticoagulant. Rapid infusion of PRBCs (several units over less than 1 hour) may result in reduced ionized calcium secondary to calcium complexing with citrate. Therefore calcium gluconate (10%) 10 ml IV may be administered during massive transfusion and ionized calcium levels monitored.

f. Acidosis may occur initially during massive transfusion secondary to citrate but rarely requires treatment. The citric acid is rapidly converted to pyruvate and bicarbonate, which may produce metabolic alkalosis. Acidosis in this patient group is more likely secondary to hypoperfusion.

g. Transfused RBCs have depleted amounts of 2,3-diphosphoglycerate, which normally enhances release of oxygen at the tissues. Therefore, during massive transfusion, oxygen delivery may be reduced and a higher hematocrit may be required to provide adequate tissue oxygenation.

5. Disseminated intravascular coagulation

a. Definition: DIC is unregulated activation of the coagulation cascade by tissue thromboplastin or other agents with subsequent consumption of both platelets and coagulation factors. Clinical manifestations may be either bleeding or thrombosis.

b. Common causes include sepsis, massive trauma, pancreatitis, liver disease, peritoneovenous shunts, disseminated malignancy, and obstetric catastrophes.

c. Diagnosis: Laboratory manifestations include thrombocytopenia, presence of schistocytes on peripheral smear, prolongation of both the PT and APTT, diminished fibrinogen levels, and increased D-dimers. The amount of fibrinogen decrease may be the best gauge of the clinical severity.

d. Treatment:

    (1) Correct underlying cause (sepsis, shock, trauma, retained fetal products).

    (2) In bleeding patient, administer FFP (2 U initially) for general factor replacement, and follow PT/APTT.

    (3) Severe depletion of fibrinogen less than 100 mg/dl in actively bleeding patient warrants replacement with cryoprecipitate.

    (4) Platelet transfusion for bleeding if count is less than 50,000/mm^3.

    (5) ϵ-Aminocaproic acid is only indicated for life-threatening hemorrhage with evidence of marked fibrinolysis (elevated D-dimers).

6. Primary fibrinolysis

a. Clinical manifestations and laboratory data are very similar to DIC. There may be a relatively greater decrease in fibrinogen and increase in FDPs, with more normal PT/APTT and platelet counts.

b. Causes include liver disease, inherited disorders (e.g., α_2-antiplasmin inhibitor deficiency), and metastatic prostate cancer.

c. Fibrinogen replacement with cryoprecipitate and administration of ϵ-aminocaproic acid should be considered as part of the treatment when bleeding develops.

7. **Coagulopathy after CPB**
   a. Coagulation defects that may arise during CPB are diverse and include DIC and primary fibrinolysis.
   b. The most important question to ask is still whether there is a surgical site that could account for the bleeding and if reoperation is necessary.
   c. Determine whether heparin administered before CPB has been fully reversed.
   d. Most patients have mild hypothermia after CPB, which contributes to coagulation defects; body temperature can be normalized with heating lamps, heating blankets, and infusion of warmed IV fluids.
   e. Systemic hypertension can aggravate mediastinal bleeding and should be addressed with afterload-reducing agents.
   f. Platelet destruction and impairment are more common after CPB than defects in coagulation factors. The platelet count does not reflect platelet function, and platelet transfusion may be appropriate even when counts are greater than 50,000/mm^3.

E. **PLATELET DISORDERS**
Normal platelet counts range from 150,000 to 450,000/mm^3, and normal surgical hemostasis requires between 60,000/mm^3 and 100,000/mm^3. Thrombocytopenia results from decreased production (marrow failure), sequestration (hypersplenism), or increased destruction (autoantibody, prosthetic valves, DIC). Rapid decreases in platelet count (>25% in 24 hours) suggests destruction rather than decreased production. Decreased platelet production is confirmed by bone marrow aspiration demonstrating decreased megakaryocytes.

1. **Immune thrombocytopenia purpura**
   a. ITP is a result of platelet destruction caused by autoantibodies. The disease is self-limiting in children, with near total recovery seen within 6 months. Adults suffer a more chronic form.
   b. The medical treatment is prednisone 1 to 3 mg/kg/day. Intravenous immunoglobulin (IVIG) may also help maintain platelet counts. The majority of patients, however, will relapse on medical treatment and will require splenectomy.
   c. Preoperative preparation for splenectomy in ITP includes the following:
      (1) Administer pneumococcal and *Haemophilus influenzae* vaccine preoperatively.
      (2) Transfuse platelets intraoperatively to obtain a platelet count greater than 50,000/mm^3.
      (3) Continue steroids postoperatively until platelet counts return to normal, then taper gradually.
   d. Accessory spleens are a cause of recurrence after splenectomy.

2. **Thrombocytic thrombocytopenia purpura**
   a. TTP is a rare syndrome caused by inappropriate, unregulated aggregation of platelets.
   b. Characteristic findings include microvascular deposition of hyaline thrombi, microangiopathic hemolytic anemia, thrombocytopenia, fever,

renal failure, fluctuating levels of consciousness, and focal neurologic deficits.

c. Treatment involves the use of exchange transfusion and intensive plasmapheresis; only half of the patients recover.

3. Drug-induced thrombocytopenia

a. Any patient with unexplained thrombocytopenia should have all medications carefully reviewed.

b. Certain medications inhibit platelet production, whereas others trigger an immune response in which the platelets are innocent bystanders.

c. Common agents that cause thrombocytopenia include most chemotherapeutic agents, alcohol, thiazide diuretics, diphenylhydantoin, numerous antibiotics, cimetidine, ranitidine, quinidine, and estrogens.

4. Splenic sequestration

a. Splenic enlargement from any cause results in a greater fraction of total platelets residing in the spleen.

b. Therefore the absolute number of circulating platelets declines.

5. Heparin-induced thrombocytopenia

a. Heparin-induced thrombocytopenia is thought to be caused by an immunoglobulin G (IgG)-heparin immune complex, which causes platelet activation and aggregation.

b. Although most cases have occurred with patients receiving large doses of heparin, small doses (such as line flushes) may induce thrombocytopenia.

c. Thrombocytopenia usually begins between 3 and 15 days after heparin therapy and is more common with heparin derived from bovine lung than from porcine gut.

d. Although patients remain asymptomatic in most cases, the syndrome of HATT may develop, which is characterized by diffuse arterial thrombosis (0.4% in patients receiving therapeutic doses of porcine heparin).

e. Management of HATT includes the following: Daily platelet counts should be performed on patients receiving heparin. If the platelet count falls below $100,000/mm^3$ or has an abrupt decline, heparin should be discontinued and warfarin therapy begun. If warfarin therapy cannot be initiated, the use of low molecular weight heparin should be considered.

6. Decreased platelet function

a. Aspirin and NSAIDs inhibit the platelet enzyme cyclooxygenase and reduce the production of thromboxane A_2, which mediates platelet secretion and aggregation.

b. Aspirin irreversibly acetylates cyclooxygenase; a single dose impairs hemostasis for 5 to 7 days.

c. NSAIDs inhibit in a competitive, reversible fashion and the effect is more transient.

7. von Willebrand's disease

a. vWD is the most common inherited bleeding disorder. It is an autosomal dominant disorder in which there is a deficiency of vWF, which normally facilitates platelet adhesion and acts as a carrier for coagulant factor VIII.

12

THE HEMATOLOGIC SYSTEM

b. Classifications include types I, IIa, IIb, and III. Types I, IIa, and III represent progressively more severe deficiencies of vWF function. Type IIb represents a form in which there is an excess of abnormal vWF, which results in increased platelet aggregation and may result in thrombocytopenia.

c. Clinical manifestations are heterogeneous, ranging from abnormal bleeding only after surgery or trauma to spontaneous bleeding.

d. Laboratory diagnosis includes prolonged bleeding time, reduced vWF, reduction in ristocetin cofactor activity, and reduced factor VIII activity.

e. Before surgery or after major trauma, patients should be treated with cryoprecipitate. After minor trauma or in patients with mild vWD, DDAVP 0.3 μg/kg IV may be sufficient. DDAVP is contraindicated in patients with type IIb vWF.

8. Thrombocytosis

a. Thrombocytosis is classified as primary (myeloproliferative disorders) or secondary (in response to inflammation, acute bleeding, iron deficiency, splenectomy, or neoplasm).

b. In primary thrombocytosis, platelet function is invariably impaired and patients may develop bleeding or thrombotic complications. Hydroxyurea or alkylating agents can be used to reduce platelet counts in symptomatic patients with primary thrombocytosis.

F. HYPERCOAGULABLE STATES

Hypercoagulable states are a result of congenital or acquired defects in the biochemical mechanisms that normally inhibit thrombus formation. As many as 10% to 20% of patients with recurrent thromboembolism, DVT, or PE have a hypercoagulable state. Any patient with recurrent arterial or venous thrombosis or any thromboembolism in the first or second decade of life should be evaluated for the presence of a hypercoagulable state.

1. Antithrombin III deficiency

a. Inherited or acquired deficiency of antithrombin III, which functions as the major inhibitor to activated serine protease coagulation factors.

b. Antithrombin III activity is augmented 1000-fold by heparin.

c. Patients with mildly decreased antithrombin III levels can be anticoagulated with heparin. Patients with a severe deficiency cannot be anticoagulated with heparin unless antithrombin III is first administered. These patients should be maintained chronically on warfarin.

2. Protein C deficiency

a. Protein C is a vitamin K–dependent factor synthesized in the liver, which is normally activated by thrombin and inactivates factors Va and VIIIa.

b. Patients may be heterozygous or homozygous for the defect, with the latter representing a much less common, more severe form of the disease. Patients who are heterozygous may be anticoagulated with heparin or warfarin; those who have experienced recurrent thrombotic episodes should remain on warfarin for life.

c. Warfarin therapy, however, may further decrease protein C levels and must be approached with caution; some of these patients may be resistant to warfarin anticoagulation and may develop warfarin-induced skin necrosis.

3. Protein S deficiency

a. Protein S, like protein C, inhibits thrombosis by participating in the inactivation of activated factors Va and VIIIa.

b. Patients with protein S deficiency may be homozygous or heterozygous for the defect. Although protein S deficiency is less common than protein C deficiency, the symptoms, diagnosis, and treatment are similar.

4. Lupuslike anticoagulants

a. This disorder is a result of heterogenous antiphospholipid antibodies that prolong phospholipid-dependent coagulation assays and can be detected in various pathologic conditions other than SLE.

b. Despite the term *anticoagulant* and the characteristic prolongation of the APTT with this disorder, clinically, these patients experience increased episodes of thrombosis.

c. Any patient with recurrent thrombosis should be evaluated for lupuslike anticoagulants; patients with lupuslike anticoagulants and venous thrombosis should be maintained on warfarin.

5. Factor V Leiden

a. A molecular defect in factor Va that renders the activated cofactor (Va) resistant to inactivation by activated protein C; thus the active form of the cofactor persists, resulting in a hypercoagulable state

b. The most common genetic hypercoagulable state

c. Long-term treatment with warfarin

III. BLOOD COMPONENT THERAPY

A. WHOLE BLOOD

1. Whole blood contains RBCs and plasma components; anticoagulated with any one of several solutions, including citrate phosphate dextrose.

2. Whole blood is indicated in patients with impaired oxygen-carrying capacity and hypovolemia, such as trauma patients with massive blood loss.

3. If ABO group and Rh type are not known, transfuse O-negative blood.

4. If ABO group and Rh type are known, transfuse type-specific blood.

B. PACKED RED BLOOD CELLS

1. PRBCs are prepared by removing supernatant plasma from whole blood. The hematocrit is 65% to 70%, and the volume is about 300 ml/U.

2. PRBCs are the product of choice for improving oxygen-carrying capacity without extensive blood volume expansion.

3. The indications for transfusion are not absolute and depend on individual patients; an asymptomatic young patient recovering from uncomplicated surgery may tolerate a hematocrit less than 20% without the need for transfusion. Conversely, an elderly patient with cardiopulmonary insufficiency and a complicated postoperative course may show improved Vo_2 and Do_2 after transfusion, even if the hematocrit is as high as 35% to 40%.

4. **In an adult, 1 U PRBCs should raise the hemoglobin 1 g/dl or the hematocrit by 3%.**

C. **FRESH FROZEN PLASMA**

1. **FFP is separated from whole blood by centrifugation;** it is frozen within 8 hours and stored frozen until used. The activity of labile factors (V and VIII) rapidly declines after thawing; therefore it should be used as soon as possible.

2. **FFP contains factors II, VII, IX, X, XI, and XII** in concentrations similar to those in normal plasma. Although FFP provides a broad spectrum of coagulation components, rather large volumes are required to raise levels appreciably in recipients.

3. **FFP is indicated** in the management of patients with multiple coagulation defects, such as hepatic insufficiency, coagulopathy associated with massive transfusion, or DIC.

4. **FFP contains anti-A, anti-B and anti-Rh antibodies;** type- and Rh-specific plasma should be used.

5. **Because FFP is a single-donor product,** 1 U carries the same risk of virally transmitted disease as 1 U of whole blood.

D. **CRYOPRECIPITATE**

1. **Cryoprecipitate is prepared** by thawing FFP to 1° to 6° C and recovering the precipitate, which is then refrozen and stored. Cryoprecipitate from several different donors may be pooled before refreezing.

2. **After thawing,** it should remain at room temperature and never be refrozen.

3. **Contains 150 mg fibrinogen per bag,** 80 U coagulant factor VIII per bag, large amounts of vWF, and moderate amounts of factor V.

4. **Indications** include hemophilia A, vWD, primary fibrinolysis, or DIC when fibrinogen levels are markedly depressed (<100 mg/dl).

E. **RECOMBINANT FACTOR VIII**

1. **Very high concentration of factor VIII derived from genetically engineered cells,** which has eliminated the risk of viral transmission.

2. **Indicated primarily for hemophilia A.**

F. **RECOMBINANT FACTOR IX**

1. **Contains factor IX derived from genetically engineered cells,** which express high levels of human factor IX.

2. **Indicated in hemophilia B.**

G. **PLATELETS**

1. **A concentrate of platelets is separated from a single unit of whole blood** and suspended in a small amount of the original plasma; units are generally pooled before transfusion.

2. **Because some donor plasma is present, the platelets must be ABO compatible.**

3. **Each unit of platelets can be expected to raise the platelet count** of the normal 70-kg adult 5000 to 10,000/mm^3 and that of an 18-kg child by 20,000/mm^3.

4. **Active bleeding in a patient with a platelet count less than 50,000/mm^3 is the primary indication for transfusion.** Platelet transfusion may be indi-

cated for patients with higher counts who are bleeding if they have abnormal platelet function.

H. AUTOTRANSFUSION

1. **Autologous blood may be donated 1 month before elective surgery,** which allows the patient time to regenerate red cells. This blood is processed and stored similarly to standard blood products.

2. **Intraoperative collection of shed blood with immediate reinfusion** is commonly used with cardiac surgery. With noncardiac surgery, shed blood usually is treated with citrate or heparin before reinfusion. Such recovery systems may result in activation of the clotting system with subsequent reinfusion of fibrin fragments, which may actually have a negative effect on normal coagulation.

I. COMPLICATIONS OF TRANSFUSIONS

1. **Acute hemolytic transfusion reaction**

a. Occurs when donor's RBCs and recipient's plasma are incompatible. Undetected serologic incompatibilities can cause these reactions; however, most are due to ABO mismatches secondary to clerical error.

b. Manifestations include shock, chills, fever, dyspnea, chest pain, back pain, headache, or abnormal bleeding. In an anesthetized patient, fever, tachycardia, or hypotension may be signs of transfusion reactions. DIC and renal failure may ensue.

c. Treatment:

   (1) Stop the transfusion.

   (2) Send both patient blood and donor blood for typing.

   (3) Support the circulation; pressors may be initially required, but crystalloid or colloid infusion should be the primary treatment.

   (4) Maintain a high urine output with saline infusions or diuretics. Saline may be supplemented with sodium bicarbonate to maintain urine at a pH greater than 6 and facilitate excretion of hemoglobin.

   (5) Treat DIC and bleeding with factor or platelet replacement.

2. **Delayed hemolytic reaction**

a. A delayed hemolytic reactions rarely occurs and is usually a result of recipient antibodies undetected at the time of transfusion.

b. Signs may occur 4 to 14 days after the transfusion and include a progressive fall in the hematocrit, fever, hemoglobinuria, hyperbilirubinemia, and renal failure.

c. Treatment is similar to treatment for an acute hemolytic reaction.

3. **Transmission of viral disease**

a. Viral hepatitis

   (1) Viral hepatitis is the most important infectious complication of blood product transfusions.

   (2) Serologic tests to screen donors are now available for both hepatitis B and hepatitis C; however, donors may have very low but infective levels of these viruses that are not detected.

   (3) The incidence of contamination is estimated to be less than 1 in 103,000 U for hepatitis B and less than 1 in 63,000 U for hepatitis

    C. The incidence of posttransfusion hepatitis (all types) in patients who have received multiple transfusions is now well below 1%.

    (4) A small fraction of patients who become infected with either hepatitis B or C will develop chronic hepatitis, cirrhosis, and liver failure.

    (5) The development of recombinant clotting factors has greatly reduced the risk of viral transmission once associated with factor replacement therapy.

  b. HIV-1 and HIV-2

    (1) An antibody test is currently used to help screen out infected donors; however, donors may be infectious for a period of time before seroconversion.

    (2) The incidence of contaminated units is approximately 1 in 676,000 U, and not all patients who receive contaminated units will become infected.

  c. CMV

    (1) Transmission of this pathogen is significant only in CMV-negative, immunosuppressed patients (e.g., transplant recipients).

    (2) Because CMV is predominantly intracellular, transmission with non-cellular products is not a concern. Furthermore, leukofiltration of PRBCs and platelet products markedly reduces transmission and should be used in seronegative immunosuppressed patients.

4. Bacterial contamination of blood products

a. Contamination is rare and usually occurs with older, stored products.

b. Organisms are often gram-negative bacilli, and recipients may develop severe endotoxin reactions. Manifestations include a sudden, high fever; chills; and hypotension.

c. If contamination is suspected, discontinue transfusion, culture the product being transfused, and start broad-spectrum antibiotics.

5. Febrile reactions

a. Febrile reactions occur in about 1% of transfusions and are a result of antibodies that agglutinate leukocytes.

b. Patients with these reactions should be examined to rule out a more serious complication, but in most instances the fever may be treated symptomatically (acetaminophen [Tylenol]) and the transfusion completed.

c. Patients with recurrent febrile reactions will benefit from leukocyte-reduced products.

6. Allergic reactions

a. Allergic reactions are manifested as hives or pruritus and occur with 1% of transfusions.

b. These reactions are triggered by plasma proteins in the transfusion.

c. Antihistamines (diphenhydramine [Benadryl] 25 to 50 mg PO/IM) may ameliorate symptoms, and usually the transfusion may be completed.

7. Citrate toxicity

a. Immediately after the transfusion, citrate anticoagulants may result in a small acidosis, but the ultimate effect is a metabolic alkalosis as citrate is metabolized.

b. In addition, citrate binds serum calcium and may result in a transient hypocalcemia. Although not a concern with small transfusions, the development of sudden tetany, hypotension, and decreased cardiac output in a patient receiving a massive transfusion may signal hypocalcemia. Calcium gluconate (10%) 10 ml IV should be administered to massively transfused patients to avoid hypocalcemia; if transfusion continues, periodic measurement of ionized calcium is recommended.

8. Pulmonary edema

a. The majority of infused blood products remain intravascular and therefore may rapidly expand intravascular volume.

b. Elderly patients with impaired cardiac function are at risk of developing cardiopulmonary edema; in these patients, slower infusion is indicated when possible, and concomitant administration of a diuretic may be indicated.

c. Noncardiogenic pulmonary edema may also occur with a massive transfusion.

IV. PHARMACOLOGIC THERAPY

A. HEPARIN

1. Heparin is a glycosaminoglycan that complexes with antithrombin (AT III), accelerating the inhibition of thrombin, factor Xa, and factor IXa. By this mechanism, heparin inhibits thrombus formation and permits the endogenous fibrinolytic system to take effect.

2. Indications include PE, DVT, peripheral arterial thrombus or embolus, and acute coronary thrombosis.

3. Intravenous heparin considerations include the following:

a. The onset of action is virtually immediate. The biologic half-life varies between 30 and 90 minutes.

b. The average 70-kg patient should be loaded with 5000 to 10,000 U IV bolus and continued on an infusion of 1000 U/hr. A convenient preparation consists of 25,000 U in 250 ml of either D5W or normal saline (10 U/ml).

c. The APTT should be obtained in 6 hours; a value of 1.5 to 2.5 times control has been shown to inhibit thrombus formation in DVT models. If the APTT is higher than desired, decrease the infusion to approximately 800 U/hr; if it is less than desired, increase to approximately 1200 U/hr. An APTT should be repeated every 6 hours until stable and then daily.

d. Heparin 5000 U SQ q8h is effective DVT prophylaxis.

4. In general, all patients should be adequately anticoagulated with heparin before beginning warfarin. Warfarin therapy may result in an initial hypercoagulable state secondary to inhibition of protein C and S synthesis.

5. Side effects of heparin:

a. Bleeding: Minor bleeding may be managed by temporarily holding the infusion or reducing the dose. Major bleeding requires that the heparin be stopped. In addition, protamine sulfate 25 to 50 mg IV may be used

12

THE HEMATOLOGIC SYSTEM

to reverse heparin. The protamine dose should be given slowly over at least 5 to 10 minutes.

b. Heparin-induced thrombocytopenia: Daily platelet counts should be obtained on all patients receiving heparin; an absolute platelet count less than 100,000/mm^3 or a rapid decline in platelet count warrants discontinuation of heparin.

c. Osteoporosis can develop in patients receiving moderate doses of heparin for several months.

B. LOW MOLECULAR WEIGHT HEPARINS

1. **Low molecular weight heparins (LMWHs) are fractionated heparins** that have been selected for a low molecular weight subfraction. This low molecular weight fraction of heparin has preferential anti–factor Xa activity, thus decreasing the bleeding potential associated with standard heparin therapy.

2. **Low incidence of heparin-associated thrombocytopenia (HAT).**

3. **Therapy monitored with chromogenic factor Xa assays.**

4. **Dose ranges between 30 to 60 mg IV/SQ, q12h to q24h.**

C. WARFARIN

1. **Warfarin inhibits hepatic conversion of vitamin K to an active form** and therefore prevents its function as a cofactor for the modification of protein C; protein S; and factors II, VII, IX, and X. Without this modification, these factors are inactive and the net result is an inhibition of thrombus formation. Like heparin, warfarin does not dissolve clots that have already formed.

2. **Warfarin produces an anticoagulant effect in 24 to 48 hours,** resulting from a reduction of factor VII (half-life 6 hours). Several more days of therapy may be required for full anticoagulation. Depletion of proteins C and S occur even before factor VII; therefore a brief hypercoagulable state may precede warfarin-induced anticoagulation. The initial warfarin dose is 5 to 10 mg PO daily × 2 days; subsequent daily doses should be approximately half the initial dose and as indicated by the PT.

3. **Methods for monitoring warfarin therapy include the following:**

a. Warfarin anticoagulation is monitored with the PT. Because institutions use different thromboplastin reagents, the same PT value at different institutions may represent different degrees of anticoagulation.

b. An international normalized ratio (INR) has been developed to standardize measurements:

$$INR = (patient's\ PT/control\ PT) \times C$$

where the value C is unique for each institution's thromboplastin reagent, and reflects the international sensitivity index (ISI). The ISI is a measure of the responsiveness of a given thromboplastin to reduction of vitamin K–dependent factors relative to an international standardized thromboplastin. In North America, the ISI ranges from 1.8 to 2.8.

c. The recommended INR for prophylaxis of DVT or treatment of DVT/PE or chronic atrial fibrillation is 2 to 3; this corresponds to a PT ratio of 1.4 to 1.6.

d. In patients with a mechanical heart valve, an INR of 2.5 to 3.5 is recommended (PT ratio of approximately 1.5 to 1.7).

4. Reversal considerations:

a. After stopping warfarin, a change in the PT ratio does not occur for at least 2 days, and normalization requires approximately 1 week.

b. High-dose vitamin K (10 to 15 mg IV q12h) will result in a reversal of the PT ratio in as rapidly as 6 hours; however, patients who have received such doses become refractory to warfarin anticoagulation for at least 1 week.

c. Low-dose vitamin K (0.5 to 1 mg IV daily) will result in a slower reversal of warfarin anticoagulation (over 24 hours) but without subsequent warfarin resistance.

d. FFP rapidly reverses warfarin anticoagulation.

5. Side effects of warfarin include the following:

a. Bleeding
   (1) Bleeding is affected by the intensity of anticoagulation (much higher risk of bleeding with an INR of 3 to 4 compared with an INR of 2 to 3).
   (2) Patients who have a high risk for bleeding while receiving warfarin therapy include those with renal insufficiency, atrial fibrillation, previous stroke, previous GI bleed, and advanced age.
   (3) Concomitant use of antiplatelet agents (particularly aspirin) increases the risk of bleeding.
   (4) For minor bleeding, temporarily withholding or reducing the warfarin dose may be acceptable. For major bleeds, reversal of warfarin is indicated.

b. Skin necrosis
   (1) Rare complication that develops during the first week of therapy, as a result of thrombosis of the microvasculature within the subcutaneous fat.
   (2) Treatment involves discontinuing warfarin and heparinizing the patient.

c. Pregnancy
   (1) Warfarin crosses the placenta, is teratogenic, and may produce fetal death.
   (2) Heparin is an acceptable anticoagulant during pregnancy.

D. ASPIRIN

1. Aspirin irreversibly inhibits the enzyme cyclooxygenase, blocking platelet generation of thromboxane A_2, which normally induces platelet aggregation and vasoconstriction. Patients treated with aspirin have dysfunctional platelets and increased bleeding times.

2. The dosage is 160 to 325 mg PO daily. The effect of a single dose is for the life span of the platelets (7 to 10 days), with platelet replacement occurring at 10% per day.

3. Indications include coronary artery disease, s/p CABG, TIA, thrombotic stroke, peripheral arterial disease, pregnancy-induced hypertension, and placental insufficiency.

12

THE HEMATOLOGIC SYSTEM

4. **Side effects of aspirin include the following:**
   a. Allergic reactions occasionally necessitate the discontinuation of aspirin.
   b. GI complications result from the ability of aspirin to inhibit prostaglandin synthesis by the gastric mucosa, with a subsequent increase in acid-induced mucosal injury, erosion, and potential bleeding. This complication is dose dependent and is significantly reduced when the dose is lowered to 160 mg/day.

5. **Ticlopidine:** Widely used as a platelet antagonist following intravascular stenting. Dose: 250 mg PO bid.

E. **FIBRINOLYTIC AGENTS**

1. **Activate plasminogen to plasmin, which dissolves fibrin;** unlike heparin and warfarin, fibrinolytic agents are able to dissolve clot that has already formed.
   a. rt-PA activates plasminogen associated with thrombus and causes fibrin degradation.
   b. Urokinase and streptokinase are not fibrin-specific. They affect the degradation of fibrinogen and several other plasma proteins in addition to fibrin, with subsequent large rises in D-dimer levels.

2. **Indications for fibrinolytic agents include the following:**
   a. Acute MI (resulted in a reduction of the in-hospital and 1-year mortality rates)
   b. Life-threatening DVT/PE
   c. Acute peripheral arterial occlusion

3. **Absolute contraindications** include the presence of aortic dissection, acute pericarditis, and active bleeding; any hemostatic wound (surgical incision, IV, arterial line site, trauma, or organ biopsy site) may potentially rehemorrhage with fibrinolytic therapy.

4. **Complications of fibrinolytic agents include the following:**
   a. Bleeding
      (1) The most devastating complication is intracranial hemorrhage; in patients with MI treated with fibrinolytics the incidence is approximately 0.5%.
      (2) Management for severe bleeds includes discontinuing infusion and fibrinogen replacement with cryoprecipitate and ϵ-aminocaproic acid.
   b. Allergic reactions
      (1) Most patients have antibodies to streptokinase, which occurs naturally as a foreign protein produced by type B streptococci; following treatment with streptokinase, titers rise significantly and may neutralize repeat treatments.
      (2) Allergic manifestations (e.g., fever, rash, rigor, or bronchospasm) occur in approximately 5% of patients being treated with streptokinase. Anaphylactic shock occurs in less than 0.5%.
      (3) No serious allergic reactions occur with urokinase or rt-PA.

5. **Methods for monitoring fibrinolytic therapy include the following:**
   a. The systemic fibrinolytic state induced by urokinase or streptokinase is manifested by prolongation of the APTT and TCT, marked rises in D-dimers, and a decrease in the fibrinogen level.

b. These measures indicate induction of fibrinolytic activity with streptokinase or urokinase; rt-PA induces much more modest alterations. However, the risk of bleeding in individual patients does not clearly relate to any of these parameters, and the dose is not titrated according to these values. Concomitant heparin therapy is monitored with the APTT.

F. ε-AMINOCAPROIC ACID

1. **ε-Aminocaproic acid inhibits fibrinolysis by blocking t-PA binding to fibrin.**

2. **Dose 5 g IV load (given over 30 minutes), then 1 g/hr IV;** may also be given orally.

3. **Indications are unclear** and limited by the incidence of complicating thrombotic events; may be administered in severe DIC, post-CPB coagulopathy, or with bleeding complicating fibrinolytic therapy. In these situations, uncontrolled fibrinolysis is suggested by increased FDPs.

G. APROTININ

1. **Nonspecific inhibitor of fibrinolysis isolated from bovine lung.**

2. **Widely used in redo cardiac surgery requiring bypass.**

3. **Standard dose for cardiopulmonary bypass:** 2×10^6 U loading dose, 2×10^6 U pump prime dose, 500,000 U/hr $\times$ 4 hours.

H. DDAVP (1-DESAMINO-8-D-ARGININE VASOPRESSIN)

1. **DDAVP is a synthetic analog of ADH** that stimulates the release of endogenous vWF from endothelial stores.

2. **The dose is 0.3 μg/kg IV;** this may be repeated at 12- to 24-hour intervals, but tachyphylaxis may occur.

3. **Indications** include minor hemophilia A, vWD, and minor bleeding in patients with uremia.

I. ANCROD

1. **Ancrod is used for systemic anticoagulation of patients with heparin-induced thrombocytopenia.**

2. **It is a thrombinlike enzyme that depletes the α-fibrinopeptides from fibrinogen,** rendering subsequent fibrin polymers more susceptible to degradation.

3. **The initial dose is 2 U/kg IV over 6 hours,** with subsequent dosing based on the fibrinogen level.

J. DEXTRAN

1. **A high molecular weight polysaccharide that functions as a volume expander** and thereby decreases blood viscosity; may also reduce platelet adhesiveness and reduce factor VIII activity.

2. **May improve early patency rates in some types of lower extremity arterial bypass procedures.**

3. **The dosage** is two 500-ml bottles on the day of surgery and then one bottle on each of the succeeding 3 postoperative days at 75 ml/hr.

K. GP IIB/IIIA ANTAGONISTS

1. **Antibodies or peptides that bind to and block the platelet fibrogen receptor (GP IIb/IIIa).**

THE HEMATOLOGIC SYSTEM

12

2. **Widely used in acute coronary syndromes and interventional cardiac stenting procedures.**
3. **Dose varies depending on the specific peptide or antibody used.**

SUGGESTED READINGS

American Red Cross 1751, *Circular of information,* Arlington, Va, August 1, 1992.

Bick RL: Disseminated intravascular coagulation: objective criteria for diagnosis and management, *Med Clin North Am* 78:511, 1994.

Dyke C, Sobel M: The management of coagulation problems in the surgical patient, *Adv Surg* 24:229, 1991.

Fakhry SM, Sheldon GF: Blood transfusions and disorders of surgical bleeding. In Sabiston DC Jr, editor: *Textbook of surgery,* ed 15, Philadelphia, 1997, WB Saunders.

Greenfield LJ: Lupus-like anticoagulant and thrombosis, *J Vasc Surg* 7:818, 1988.

THE CENTRAL NERVOUS SYSTEM

John C. Wellons III

I. NEUROLOGIC EVALUATION

A. HISTORY

1. **Aim:** To define global and focal deficits with particular attention to causes of impairment treatable by medical or surgical means.

2. **Of note, specific situations require focused neurologic history taking.** For example, primary neurologic admissions (closed head injury, subarachnoid hemorrhage) mandate questioning salient to the admission reason (trauma, headache), whereas the onset of secondary neurologic symptoms in the critical care patient necessitates a different line of questioning. In the former situation, family members may assist with the history and specifics of the presenting illness because often the patient may be unable to communicate an adequate history, whereas in the latter, the nursing staff may be best suited to identify and communicate a significant neurologic change.

3. **History taking.**

a. Characterize the reason for ICU admission or new neurologic finding: chief complaint, onset, length, neurologic modalities involved, intensity, what makes the symptoms better, what makes the symptoms worse, constant or variable findings, and whether the neurologic disturbance is the primary or secondary reason for ICU admission

b. Has the patient, family member, or nursing staff noticed other neurologic disturbances?

(1) Mental status (disturbed level of consciousness [LOC], disorientation, aphasia)

(2) Cranial nerves (abnormal smell, sight, double vision, facial sensation and symmetry, hearing, balance, swallowing, talking, shoulder shrug, tongue movement)

(3) Motor (weakness, increased tone)

(4) Sensation (pain, light touch, position sense)

(5) Cerebellar (coordination, tremor)

(6) Gait (instability, abnormal base)

c. Associated current medical findings

d. Past medical history

(1) Systemic illness

(2) Prior trauma

(3) Prior CNS events

e. Past surgical and anesthetic history with special attention on those identified as neurologic (craniotomy, laminectomy) or those more likely to have neurologic sequelae (cardiopulmonary bypass, carotid endarterectomy)

    f. Recent drugs/medications
- (1) Psychoactive: benzodiazepines, antiepileptics, antipsychotics, antihistamines
- (2) Coagulopathic: warfarin, aspirin, heparin, ticlopidine
- (3) Abuse: alcohol, tobacco, cocaine, PCP, LSD, heroin, marijuana
- (4) Anesthetic: barbiturate, propofol, inhalational agents
- (5) Paralytic: succinylcholine, pancuronium, vecuronium, atracurium
- (6) Analgesic: opioid- and non−opioid-based pain relievers
- (7) Other: steroids, atropine, naloxone, flumazenil, digoxin, theophylline, thyroid replacement, antihypertensives, nitroglycerine

    g. Family history

B. PHYSICAL EXAMINATION

1. Airway, Breathing, Circulation

2. General physical examination

3. Neurologic examination of the conscious patient

    a. Level of consciousness: alertness (unarousable, sleepy, confused, awake), orientation (person, place, time, and situation)

    b. Mental status
- (1) Language: naming (pen, flashlight, thumb), repetition ("no ifs ands or buts about it"), fluency, comprehension (can patient follow simple and complex tasks?)
- (2) Memory: short-term (name three objects immediately and after 5 minutes)
- (3) Cognition: concrete (grass is always greener on the other side is interpreted literally . . .) or abstract (. . . as to mean that things always seem better elsewhere)
- (4) Attention ("world" forwards and backwards, serial 7's)
- (5) Calculation (simple addition)

    c. Cranial nerves
- (1) Optic nerve (II): visual acuity (Snellen's chart), visual fields (count fingers in four quadrants of each visual field), pupillary light reaction (shine a light in both eyes and observe for primary and consensual response), funduscopic examination (observe for papilledema)
- (2) Oculomotor, trochlear, and abducens nerves (III, IV, VI): extraocular muscle integrity (following object in all cardinal directions and observing for conjugate movement)
- (3) Trigeminal nerve (V): facial sensation (pain and light touch using pin and cotton wisp) and jaw clasp symmetry
- (4) Facial nerve (VII): upper and lower facial symmetry at rest and with movement (raise eyebrows, smile, show teeth)
- (5) Vestibulocochlear nerve (VIII): Weber's (tuning fork to midline forehead, sound should stay in midline) and Rinne tests (tuning fork touched to mastoid process followed by placing it next to ear, sound should be louder next to ear)
- (6) Glossopharyngeal and vagus nerves (IX, X): gag (cotton swab lightly touched to back of throat) and midline palate elevation

(7) Spinal accessory nerve (XI): trapezius (shoulder shrug) and sterno-cleidomastoid (head turn to opposite side)

(8) Hypoglossal nerve (XII): intrinsic tongue musculature (protrude tongue)

d. Motor

  (1) Bulk (hypotrophic, normal, hypertrophic)

  (2) Tone (hypotonic, normal, rigid, spastic), including anal sphincter tone

  (3) Power

   (a) Muscle grading: 5—against full resistance, 4—against partial resistance, 3—against gravity, 2—perpendicular to gravity, 1—flicker, 0—no movement

   (b) Upper extremity (main root contribution): Deltoid (C5), biceps (C5, C6), triceps (C7), wrist extensors (C6), finger extensors (C7, C8), wrist flexors (C6, C7), distal finger flexors (C8), thenar muscle group (C7, C8, T1), hypothenar muscle group (C8, T1), first and second interossei (T1)

   (c) Lower extremity (main root contribution): iliopsoas (L1, L2), adductors (L2, L3), quadriceps femoris (L3, L4), dorsiflexors (L4), toe extensors (L5), toe flexors (S1), plantar flexors (S1, S2), hamstrings (S1)

e. Sensation (Figure 13-1)

  (1) Pain (tested with the broken end of a cotton swab)

  (2) Temperature (tested with warm and cold objects)

  (3) Proprioception (position of index fingers or second toes in space and Romberg test)

  (4) Vibrioception (tested using tuning fork placed on bony prominences)

f. Coordination

  (1) Extremity coordination (heel to shin and finger to nose testing)

  (2) Axial coordination (observe for postural instability)

g. Gait

h. Reflexes

  (1) Standard: biceps (C5), brachioradialis (C6), triceps (C7), patellar (L4), ankle (S1), and bulbocavernosus (S2, S3, S4)

  (2) Pathologic: Babinski (toes up indicative of upper motor neuron lesion)

4. Neurologic examination of the comatose patient

a. The level of consciousness is quickly determined by the Glasgow Coma Scale (GCS) (Box 13-1)

b. Brain stem examination

  (1) The pupillary light reflex reveals the integrity of the midbrain.

   (a) Afferent limb: II

   (b) Efferent limb: III

  (2) The corneal reflex reveals the integrity of the pons.

   (a) Afferent limb: V

   (b) Efferent limb: VII

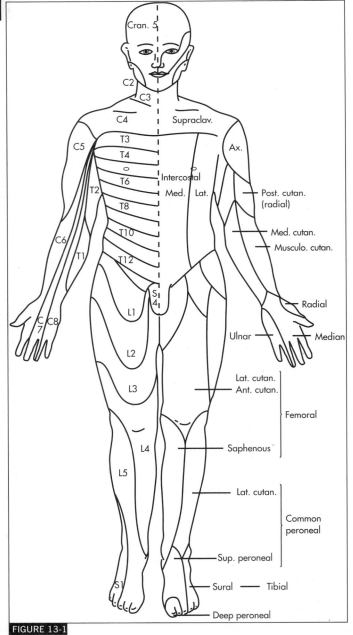

FIGURE 13-1

Anterior and posterior sensory chart.

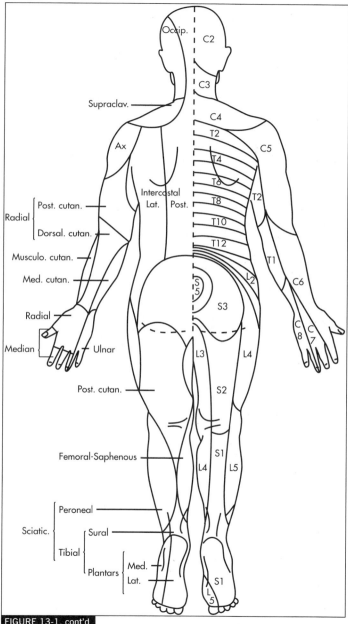

FIGURE 13-1, cont'd

Anterior and posterior sensory chart.

BOX 13-1

THE GLASGOW COMA SCALE

EYE OPENING

E4: Spontaneous

E3: To voice

E2: To pain

E1: No eye opening

VERBAL RESPONSE

V5: Oriented

V4: Confused

V3: Inappropriate words

V2: Incomprehensible sounds

V1: Nothing

MOTOR RESPONSE

M6: Follows commands

M5: Localizes pain

M4: Withdraws from pain

M3: Decorticate (arm flexion and leg extension)

M2: Decerebrate (arm and leg extension)

M1: No response

(3) The gag reflex reveals the integrity of the medulla.
  (a) Afferent limb: IX
  (b) Efferent limb: X
(4) The oculocephalic reflex (doll's eyes) demonstrates the integrity of II, III, VI, the vestibular system, the pons, and neck proprioception.
  (a) This is performed by rapidly turning the head and observing eye movements.
  (b) The eyes should stay midline with the initial turn, followed by a slow drift away from the direction of the head turn.
  (c) Never perform doll's eyes on a patient with an unstable or un-cleared cervical spine.
(5) The oculovestibular reflex (cold calorics) demonstrates the integrity of the same structures as the oculocephalic reflex except neck proprioception.
  (a) This is performed by infusing cold water into the external canal. In the conscious individual, the normal response is slow deviation towards the stimulation, followed by nystagmus with the rapid component away from the lesion; in the comatose individual, there should be slow tonic deviation toward the stimulation.
  (b) Always check the integrity of the canal first.
c. Motor
  (1) Extremity and facial movement to painful central (sternal rub) and peripheral (nail bed pressure) stimulation is examined.
  (2) Apply the GCS motor score (see Box 13-1) to each limb.

d. Sensation
  (1) Wincing of the face to orbital rim pressure indicates functioning facial pain sensation.
  (2) The limb response to central and peripheral stimulation indicates the integrity of the body's pain-conducting system.
e. Reflexes (see section I, B, 3, h)
f. Respiratory patterns
  (1) Cheyne-Stokes respirations are waxing and waning and usually indicative of bilateral hemispheric dysfunction.
  (2) Central neurogenic hyperventilation is sustained, rapid, deep, and usually indicative of lower midbrain injury.
  (3) Apneusis has a prolonged inspiratory pause and is indicative of pontine dysfunction.
  (4) Ataxic breathing has a completely irregular pattern and is indicative of medullary dysfunction.

C. CNS IMAGING AND DIAGNOSTIC MODALITIES
1. Computed tomography
a. General
  (1) Bone is white (hyperdense), brain and soft tissue are various shades of gray (isodense), and CSF is black (hypodense).
  (2) New blood (1 to 3 days) is hyperdense, subacute blood (4 days to 3 weeks) is isodense, and old blood (>3 weeks) is hypodense.
  (3) Bone is better defined on CT than MRI.
b. Head CT
  (1) A head CT is much quicker and more useful in an acute setting (trauma or rapid neurologic change).
  (2) Contrast enhances areas of blood-brain barrier breakdown (traumatic contusion, infection, and various tumors), as well as cerebral blood vessels.
c. Spine CT
  (1) This is necessary for evaluation of vertebral damage in patients with suspected spinal cord injury.
  (2) Intrathecal contrast (CT myelogram) enables examination of intrathecal contents (shift or enlargement of spinal cord, hematoma formation, disk herniation) but does not delineate spinal cord anatomy itself.
  (3) It is impossible to clear a cervical spine from a spine CT because each image is independently placed in the center of the screen by the technologist.

2. Magnetic resonance imaging
a. General
  (1) T1-weighted means that CSF is dark (hypointense) and white matter is white (hyperintense). This is better for delineating anatomic lesions.
  (2) T2-weighted means that CSF is white (hyperintense) and white matter is dark (hypointense). This is better for evaluating early ischemia or edema.

13

THE CENTRAL NERVOUS SYSTEM

(3) Some patients are ineligible because of pacemakers, recently implanted orthopedic devices, or some surgical clips.

b. Brain MRI

(1) Mainly used when evaluating patients for stroke or tumor involvement, and it is especially useful for suspected posterior fossa lesions.

(2) Gadolinium is given to enhance areas of blood-brain barrier breakdown.

(3) No true indication in acute trauma.

c. Spine MRI

(1) Necessary for evaluation of patients with suspected spinal cord injury.

(2) Also used in patients with an acute presentation of radiculopathy (herniated disk), paraplegia (spinal metastases, infection), or other presentations of myelopathy.

3. Cerebral arteriogram

a. This is the gold standard for imaging of cerebral aneurysms and arteriovascular malformations (AVMs). Therefore this is the logical next step in the evaluation of nontraumatic subarachnoid hemorrhage (SAH).

b. In the trauma setting, the arteriogram is extremely useful in evaluating patients for carotid dissection.

4. Lumbar puncture

a. A CT scan of the brain to rule out a posterior fossa lesion or impending herniation is mandatory before lumbar puncture (LP) when focal signs or papilledema are present. The absence of either lowers the risk of iatrogenic tonsillar herniation, but not entirely.

b. One of the most common indications for LP is to rule out meningitis when a patient presents with acute neurologic changes and a fever. The LP is also used when suspicion of SAH is high despite the absence of evidence on CT or in routine evaluation for undiagnosed neurologic disease.

c. Values: See Table 13-1.

5. Electroencephalogram

a. Performed acutely to rule out seizures, especially status epilepticus, in an unresponsive patient. Other indications include seizure characterization.

TABLE 13-1

PERTINENT CSF VALUES

	Protein	Glucose	Cell Count	Appearance
Normal	<45	2/3 serum	0-5	Clear
Viral meningitis	Normal to increased	Normal	20-800	Normal
Bacterial meningitis	Markedly increased	Decreased	>1000	Cloudy
TB, fungal meningitis	Markedly increased	Decreased	200-800	Opalescent
SAH	Increased	Variable	High RBCs	Xanthochromic

b. An EEG is also used to monitor for burst suppression during barbiturate or propofol-induced therapeutic coma.

II. NEUROPHYSIOLOGY
A. CEREBRAL HEMODYNAMICS
1. Cerebral blood flow (CBF)
a. 15% of cardiac output goes to the brain
b. CBF values
   (1) The average adult CBF is approximately 50 ml/100 g brain/min.
   (2) EEG changes are seen as CBF is reduced to 12 to 15 ml/100 g/min.
   (3) Further reduction disrupts cellular ionic pumps and membrane structure, leading to cell death.
c. Regulation of CBF
   (1) Autoregulation causes CBF to be constant when mean arterial pressure (MAP) remains between 60 and 160. Chronically hypertensive adults elevate the upper and lower limits of the MAP within which CBF is maintained (Figure 13-2).
   (2) The H+ ion concentration increases as lactate and pyruvate build up from increased metabolism, elevation of $Paco_2$ (>40 mm Hg), and decreased Pao_2 (<50 mm Hg). This causes cerebral vessels to vasodilate, in turn increasing CBF.
   (3) Causes of loss of autoregulation include hypoxia, hypercapnia, ischemia, trauma, tumors, and CNS infection.

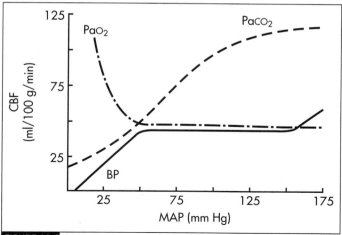

FIGURE 13-2
CBF changes resulting from alterations in Pao_2, $Paco_2$, and blood pressure. *(Modified from Shapiro HM:* Anesthesiology *43:447, 1975.)*

13

THE CENTRAL NERVOUS SYSTEM

(4) When outside of MAP parameters (60-160) or in areas of autoregulatory absence, CBF becomes a passive function of cerebral perfusion pressure (CPP).

2. Cerebral perfusion pressure

a. CPP = MAP − ICP
b. CPP values
   (1) Normal value: 70 to 100 mm Hg
   (2) Goal in refractory raised ICP: 50 to 70 mm Hg
c. This value, easily determined at the bedside, serves as a guide for therapeutic intervention (reduction of ICP or elevation of MAP) in the event of brain injury

3. Cerebral metabolism

a. Best reflected in the cerebral metabolic rate of oxygen consumption ($CMRO_2$)
   (1) Normal value is 3.5 ml/100 g/min
   (2) $CMRO_2$ = CBF × (Ca_{O_2} − Cv_{O_2}); or CBF × AVD_{O_2}; Ca_{O_2} is arterial oxygen content, Cv_{O_2} is mixed venous oxygen content, and AVD_{O_2} is arteriovenous oxygen content difference.
b. Reducing brain metabolism reduces CBF requirement and therefore becomes neuroprotectant.
c. $CMRO_2$ is reduced with inhalational anesthetics, barbiturates, propofol, and hypothermia. The latter three may have preventative or therapeutic implication in brain injury.
d. The jugular bulb catheter
   (1) The jugular venous oxygen saturation (Sjv_{O_2}) and serum lactate levels may be followed by the utilization of the jugular bulb catheter.
   (2) The catheter is placed via a retrograde internal jugular approach until it rests in the jugular bulb and is verified by skull x-rays.
   (3) Sjv_{O_2} replaces Cv_{O_2} in the above equation so that:

   $$CMRO_2 = CBF \times (Ca_{O_2} - Sjv_{O_2})$$

   (4) $CMRO_2$ is indirectly revealed by the AVD_{O_2} or Ca_{O_2} − Sjv_{O_2}. More simply, with a relatively constant CBF and Ca_{O_2}, $CMRO_2$ may be extrapolated by monitoring the Sjv_{O_2}.
   (5) Normal values for the Sjv_{O_2} are 60% to 70%. Lower values indicate increased O_2 extraction and may be indicative of cerebral ischemia.
   (6) Drawbacks include placement proximal to the jugular bulb, which contaminates the Sjv_{O_2} with facial vein drainage. This would elevate the final value and misrepresent the true value of the Sjv_{O_2}. Also, the placement of the catheter into one jugular bulb may only be reflective of that hemisphere's physiology. The risks of thrombosis and infection exist, as well. The efficacy of the jugular bulb catheter is still under review.

B. INTRACRANIAL PRESSURE

1. Cerebrospinal fluid

a. General

    (1) 150 ml in circulation

    (2) 350 to 500 ml produced in one day

b. Production

    (1) 0.3 ml/kg/hr

    (2) CSF is mainly produced in the choroid plexus via active transport of Na and is affected very little by alterations in ICP.

c. Absorption

    (1) Absorption occurs mainly in the arachnoid granulations, which protrude into the superior sagittal sinus from the subarachnoid space.

    (2) This is a function of a passive pressure-based gradient.

2. ICP physiology

a. General

    (1) Monro-Kellie doctrine: The three main components of the intracranial space are brain (1400 ml), CSF (100 ml), and blood (75 ml). A change in the volume of one of the components causes a change in the other two.

    (2) In the event of an intracranial mass lesion, the brain provides an unknown amount of compensation. Intravascular volume can be manipulated to some extent through hyperventilation, and CSF volume (the main physiologic buffer) can be reduced.

b. ICP values

    (1) Normal is relative but usually thought to be 5 to 20 in the adult.

    (2) ICP is equal throughout the neuraxis in the horizontal position, but in the vertical position, the ICP is higher in the lumbar cistern than in the ventricular system. (Therefore opening pressure during a lumbar puncture should always be measured in the horizontal position.)

c. Intracranial dynamics

    (1) Compliance

        (a) This term refers to the ratio of the change in intracranial volume to the resulting change in intracranial pressure (Figure13-3)

        (b) At normal volumes, ICP remains within normal limits and compliance is high. As the volume increases, the ICP changes slowly until compensatory mechanisms are surpassed. At this point the ICP increases rapidly for little changes in volume and compliance is low.

    (2) Elastance

        (a) Elastance is the reciprocal of compliance. It is the slope of the curve of Figure 13-3.

        (b) As the pressure increases, the ability of a system to accept more volume decreases and the elastance is high.

    (3) Example

        (a) If a rubber band is held loosely, it has a great deal of compliance, but it is not very elastic.

13

THE CENTRAL NERVOUS SYSTEM

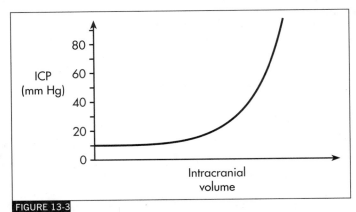

FIGURE 13-3
Relationship of intracranial volume and pressure. *(Modified from Shapiro HM:* Anesthesiology *43:447, 1975.)*

        (b) If that same rubber band is held taut, it is less compliant to change, but it is now very elastic.

3. ICP management

a. Indications

   (1) ICP management is initiated when clinical suspicion of raised intracranial pressure exists, such as in traumatic brain injury, SAH, severe ischemic or hemorrhagic stroke, or radiographic evidence of raised ICP.

   (2) In general, ICP monitoring is instituted when the GCS is less than or equal to 8. This, however, is not always the case and clinical judgment continues to play a crucial role.

b. Methods

   (1) General

      (a) 30-degree head elevation

      (b) Neck in midline position

   (2) Hyperventilation

      (a) Pco_2 initially between 27 and 35

      (b) After the first 24 hours, hyperventilation is no longer of benefit. The jugular bulb monitor may extend this period but is controversial.

   (3) Diuretics

      (a) Mannitol: 25 to 50 g IV q3h, hold if serum osmolarity is greater than 315

      (b) Furosemide (Lasix): 20 to 40 mg IV q6h used in concert with mannitol

(4) ICP monitoring and CSF drainage
  (a) Ventriculostomy
    (i) This is placed into the lateral ventricle ideally at the foramen of Monro.
    (ii) The ventriculostomy is the preferred monitor because the value is directly calculated from a fluid column and the catheter may be used to drain CSF.
    (iii) Strict sterile techniques must be adhered to during placement, as well as daily maintenance.
  (b) Intraparenchymal monitor or subarachnoid bolt
    (i) These monitors are placed approximately 1 cm into the brain parenchyma and into subarachnoid space, respectively.
    (ii) The ICP value is determined from fiberoptics and not direct transduction.
    (iii) Drainage to reduce ICP is impossible, but these catheters are easier to insert especially if significant midline shift or slit ventricles are present.
(5) Sedation: Propofol (best for frequent neurologic examinations) or midazolam infusions help lower ICP
(6) Hypothermia
  (a) This is reserved for refractory cases of raised ICP.
  (b) A cooling blanket is used to lower the core temperature in an effort to decrease the $CMRO_2$.
  (c) Paralytics are used to eliminate shivering associated with induced hypothermia.
(7) Steroids
  (a) Steroids are detrimental in head trauma and intracranial hemorrhage.
  (b) They are, however, efficacious in reducing brain edema associated with brain tumors.
(8) CPP
  (a) It is uncommon for a neurologic process to lower the blood pressure; therefore when the CPP drops, it is usually the function of an increasing ICP.
  (b) Conventional wisdom dictates preserving CBF in the damaged brain. It has been stated above that in areas that have lost autoregulation, the CBF is proportional to the CPP. Therefore, if the CPP falls and the ICP is unable to be lowered by conventional means, a pressor (phenylephrine or dopamine) may be instituted in an effort to preserve CBF.
  (c) The target CPP is 50 to 70.
  (d) Never acutely lower MAP in the setting of acute ischemic stroke unless: (1) the systolic blood pressure (SBP) is greater than 220 or diastolic blood pressure (DBP) is greater than 120, at which point the blood-brain barrier may be compromised and the patient is at risk for hypertensive enceph-

13

THE CENTRAL NERVOUS SYSTEM

alopathy; or (2) the patient is determined to be a candidate for thrombolytic administration.

    (9) Induced coma (EEG burst suppression)

        (a) Propofol or barbiturate infusions may be used to induce burst suppression on continuous EEG monitoring.

        (b) The end point should be guided by the ICP.

4. Herniation syndromes

    (1) Transtentorial herniation—associated with third nerve palsy and hemiparesis.

    (2) Central herniation—associated with Cushing's triad (hypertension, bradycardia, and an abnormal respiratory pattern).

    (3) Subfalcine herniation—radiographic entity in which the medial surface of a cerebral hemisphere herniates underneath the falx cerebri.

III. COMA

A. ETIOLOGY

(AUTHOR'S NOTE: Clearly, this section does not presume to list every possible cause of coma. This will touch on the main causes only. Please consult appropriate sources, such as Plum and Posner's *The Diagnosis of Stupor and Coma* [1982] for a more detailed catalog.)

1. Structural (either from the lesion itself or the ensuing edema and/or herniation; in general, coma-inducing structural lesions must either affect both hemispheres or the brain stem)

a. Vascular—stroke (bilateral hemispheric, thalamic), SAH, or intracranial hemorrhage (ICH)

b. Trauma—subdural hematoma (SDH), epidural hematoma (EDH), contusion, or diffuse axonal injury

c. Posterior fossa lesions—brain stem infarct or cerebellar mass lesion (infarct, tumor, hemorrhage, or abscess)

d. Supratentorial tumor or abscess

e. Hydrocephalus—communicating or noncommunicating

2. Metabolic, multifocal, and diffuse brain diseases (of note, a metabolic process may be associated with focal neurologic findings)

a. Epileptic—status epilepticus or a postictal state

b. Electrolyte disturbances—hypernatremia, hyponatremia, or hypercalcemia

c. Endocrine abnormalities—DKA, nonketotic hyperosmolar state, hypoglycemia, addisonian crisis, or myxedema

d. Toxic—pharmacologic (illicit and iatrogenic), alcohol, poison, or carbon monoxide

e. Infectious—meningitis or encephalitis

f. Nutritional

g. Inherited metabolic diseases

h. Nonneurologic organ failure—renal failure, hypoxia, or hepatic dysfunction

3. **Psychogenic**
B. EVALUATION
See section I, B, 4.
C. TREATMENT
1. **ABCs**
2. **Laboratory evaluation:** CBC with differential, Chem 7, ABG, toxicology screen, anticonvulsant level, calcium, magnesium, phosphorus, ammonia, lactate, PT, PTT, CPK, MB fraction
3. **Initial drugs to administer before continuing workup**
a. Thiamine—100 mg IV
b. D50—1 ampule IV
c. Naloxone—1 ampule IV
d. Flumazenil (if benzodiazepine overdose suspected)—0.2 mg IV over 30 seconds and then 0.3 mg over 30 seconds every 30 seconds until total of 3 mg reached
4. **If patient shows sign of increased ICP** (fixed pupil[s], hemiparesis, rapid decrease in LOC, or posturing) or posterior fossa lesion (vomiting, ophthalmoplegia, multiple cranial nerve abnormalities, or abnormal respiratory pattern), institution of means of ICP control (hyperventilation, head elevation, and mannitol) may be necessary before CT scan
5. **CT brain imaging**
6. **If meningitis suspected,** LP may be performed in CT-proven absence of intracranial mass lesion or herniation
7. **If status epilepticus suspected,** obtain EEG and follow guidelines in section V, D, 1
8. **Continue with specific treatments** as history, physical examination, neurologic examination, laboratory test results, and CT imaging dictate
D. BRAIN DEATH CRITERIA
1. **Neurologic examination**
a. Absent brain stem function
    (1) Absent pupillary, corneal, and gag reflexes
    (2) Absent oculocephalic and oculovestibular reflexes
    (3) Failed apnea test (no spontaneous respirations despite hypercapnia)
b. No motor response to deep central pain
2. **No complicating factors**
a. Core temperature greater than 32.2° C
b. No evidence of any residual drugs affecting neurologic examination (benzodiazepine or phenobarbital)
c. Shock or anoxia not present
d. Patient is not in an immediate postresuscitation state

IV. DELIRIUM AND ICU PSYCHOSIS
A. GENERAL
1. **Diagnosis of exclusion:** Must differentiate from seizures, psychotic disorders, effects of systemic disease, and anatomic CNS pathology

13

THE CENTRAL NERVOUS SYSTEM

2. **Delirium:** Defined as a global, transient impairment of cognition; a common disorder occurring in 10% to 15% of all surgical patients

B. CLINICAL FEATURES

Include confusion, disorientation, agitation, anxiety, combativeness, hallucinations, delusions, paranoia, irritability, hyperexcitability, altered motor behavior, incoherent speech, insomnia, a decreased LOC, inappropriate behavior, disinhibition, and varying symptoms from one time to another; often worse at night.

C. PREDISPOSING FACTORS

1. **Over 50 years of age**
2. **Baseline impairment:** CVA, dementia, blindness, deafness, malnutrition, or underlying psychotic or depressive disorder
3. **Renal or liver disease resulting in metabolic derangement**
4. **Recent episodes of hypoperfusion or hypoxemia**

D. ETIOLOGY

1. **Drugs and drug interactions that affect metabolism of CNS active agents:** Common agents include lidocaine, digoxin, aminophylline, and H_2 blockers
2. **Period for ethanol or benzodiazepine withdrawal:** 24 to 72 hours; often corresponds to the acute postoperative period
3. **Hyperthyroid or hypothyroid states**
4. **Corticosteroid insufficiency or excess**
5. **Abnormalities in glucose metabolism**
6. **Respiratory disturbances,** including hypoxemia, poor oxygen-carrying capacity, and hypercapnia
7. **Toxins related to acute renal or hepatic failure**
8. **Sepsis, with or without fever**
9. **Nutritional/cofactor deficiencies** (thiamine, vitamin B_{12}, nicotinic acid)
10. **Environmental displacement, noise, or sleep deprivation** (or sleep pattern disruption)

E. MANAGEMENT

1. **General**
   a. Withdrawal of nonessential medications and simplification of regimen
   b. Correction of all abnormal metabolic and endocrine findings
   c. Empiric: folate 1 mg and thiamine 100 mg qd for 3 days
   d. Treatment of hypoxemia, acid-base disorders, anemia, and shock
   e. Treatment of sepsis with appropriate definitive therapy directed at primary source of infection in addition to systemic antibiotics
   f. Environmental changes
      (1) Provide outdoor sources of light (patient's bed placed near or facing a window).
      (2) Obtain familiar personal objects for the patient's room.
      (3) Keep a calendar and clock in the patient's range of view.
      (4) Minimize invasive lines and procedures.

2. **Pharmacotherapy**
a. Administer diphenhydramine 50 mg PO or 25 to 50 mg IV to help normalize sleep-wake cycles.
b. Haloperidol is the agent of choice for refractory delirium. If extrapyramidal side effects develop, use diphenhydramine. Administer 2 to 5 mg IV or IM; this dose may be repeated in 10 minutes. Double the dose and administer q20min until therapeutic effect obtained. Use on a scheduled (not PRN) basis to prevent therapeutic escape.

F. **ETHANOL WITHDRAWAL THERAPY**
1. **Multivitamins, thiamine 100 mg, and folate 1 mg qd for 3 days**
2. **Magnesium and potassium supplementation**
3. **Benzodiazepines titrated to obtain adequate sedation using short-acting agents** (midazolam or lorazepam); tapered over 4 to 5 days
4. **May use clonidine to control tachycardia and hypertension;** clonidine 0.2 mg PO initially followed by placement of transdermal patches (patches removed on third and fourth days to obtain taper effect)

V. SEIZURE

A. **ETIOLOGY**
1. **Infants:** perinatal injury, congenital (metabolic and anatomic) defects, or infection
2. **Children:** infection, inherited diseases, or trauma
3. **Adults:** tumor, traumatic mass lesions, infarcts, drug withdrawal, hyponatremia, or vascular lesions

B. **CLASSIFICATION**
1. **Focal seizures are caused by a focal cortical lesion,** with the anatomic site of the lesion usually determining the initial presentation. The description may be modified as focal complex if there is altered consciousness or secondarily generalized if there is progression to a generalized seizure after an initial focal phase.
2. **Complex partial seizures often begin with focal temporal lobe symptoms** and then progress with déjà vu, automatism, hallucinations, or mood changes. Awareness may be present during these episodes, but by definition complex seizures have an alteration in LOC.
3. **During generalized seizures,** the patient is unconscious and unresponsive to stimuli from the environment, and after the event (postictal) is confused, drowsy, and disoriented.
a. Generalized tonic-clonic seizures: Patient exhibits synchronous tonic-clonic motor activity of all muscle groups.
b. Absence seizures: Patient has a brief loss of consciousness, appears to stare aimlessly into space, and is unresponsive. This usually affects children.

C. **EVALUATION**
1. **Exclusion of metabolic derangement;** evaluation of serum electrolytes, glucose, divalent ions, and ABG

2. **Review of medications, recent withdrawal of drugs, and history of drug abuse**
3. **Brain CT scan** to rule out mass lesion in trauma and postoperative patients
4. **CSF sampling** to rule out infection (lumbar puncture performed after CT)
5. **EEG** for localization of a focus

D. **TREATMENT**

1. **Initial protocol for managing status epilepticus**
   a. Airway secured by endotracheal intubation
   b. IV access and blood samples
   c. Lorazepam 2 to 4 mg IV × 1
   d. Fosphenytoin or phenytoin 15 to 20 mg/kg IV × 1 (no faster than 50 mg/min; fosphenytoin may be bolused)
   e. If seizures persist, repeat lorazepam up to a total of 0.1 to 0.15 mg/kg
   f. If seizures persist, phenobarbital up to 20 mg/kg IV at less than 100 mg/min until cessation of seizure or maximum dose; hypotension is a significant side effect, and pressors should be available
   g. If seizures persist, consider pentobarbital or versed drip, titrated to seizure control or burst suppression
   h. If seizures persist, consider general inhalational anesthesia

2. **Individual antiepileptics**
   a. Phenytoin
      (1) Loading dose is 15 to 20 mg/kg at a rate not to exceed 50 mg/min (bolus). ECG monitoring is used to observe for prolongation of PR interval.
      (2) Maintenance dosing 3 to 5 mg/kg/day divided tid and titrated for a serum level 10 to 20 mg/ml.
      (3) Sample dosing for 70-kg man is 1 g IV followed by 100 mg IV q8h.
   b. Phenobarbital
      (1) Loading dose is 20 mg/kg slow IV (<100 mg/min) followed by 30 to 250 mg/d maintenance (divided bid or tid), aiming for serum levels of 15 to 30 μg/ml.
      (2) Be aware that the diagnosis of brain death must be postponed until phenobarbital is metabolized.
   c. Carbamazepine
      (1) Maintenance dosing is 600 to 1200 mg/day PO, dosed tid to qid. The goal serum level is 4 to 8 mg/ml.
      (2) After initiation of carbamazepine, induction of liver enzymes occurs and levels drop over the initial week.
      (3) No role in acute therapy of status epilepticus.
   d. Lorazepam
      (1) Used in short-term control of status epilepticus: 2 to 4 mg IV bolus over 2 minutes
      (2) May repeat every 5 minutes if seizures persist, to maximum of 9 mg

VI. GENERAL NEUROSURGICAL POSTOPERATIVE CARE

A. **GENERAL CONSIDERATIONS**

1. **Routine postoperative care** in neurosurgical patients undergoing craniotomy generally requires overnight stay in a more intensely moni-

tored bed, such as in a step-down unit (for the less complex patients), a postanesthetic unit, a general surgical ICU, or a specialized neurologic ICU. The vast majority of stable patients will spend 24 hours in this setting before being transferred to the floor. Those patients who remain ventilated or with special situations (see section VII) mandate longer stays.

2. **The main purpose** is close observation for worsening of examination in an environment in which rapid identification and intervention exists.

3. **Anesthetic recovery**

a. Identifying patients who have an ongoing pathologic neurologic process from those whose are slow to recover from anesthesia remains a difficult task.

b. Symptoms that point more towards a pathologic process include increasing severe headache, increasing drowsiness, vomiting, or focal findings (e.g., hemiparesis, paresthesia, pupillary changes, or ophthalmoplegia). Any patient with these findings or other reasons of concern deserves rapid CT scanning to either allay fears or confirm pathologic processes.

B. SPECIFIC CONSIDERATIONS

1. **Blood pressure control**

a. Hypertension (SBP > 160 or MAP > 110) is to be avoided in routine postcraniotomy patients unless the patient is extremely hypertensive preoperatively.

b. Failure to adequately control postoperative blood pressure may cause hematoma formation either in the surgical resection bed (in the case of a tumor resection), SDH formation, or EDH formation.

c. Antihypertensives include those listed in Table 13-2.

2. **DVT/PE prophylaxis:** DVT with resultant pulmonary emboli are common problems in the postoperative and traumatic brain-injured patient. Lower extremity compression devices are commonly used for prophylaxis.

3. **Peptic ulcer/GI bleeding prophylaxis:** H_2 blocker (ranitidine) or sucralfate may be used.

TABLE 13-2

COMMON ANTIHYPERTENSIVES AND THEIR EFFECT ON ICP

Drug	Mechanism	Effect on ICP
Nitroprusside	Direct vasodilation	Mild increase
NTG	Direct vasodilation	Increase
Hydralazine	Direct vasodilation	Increase
Propanolol, esmolol, metoprolol	Cardiac selective β-blockade	No effect
Labetalol	α_1- and β-blockade	No effect
Nifedipine, nicardipine	Calcium channel blockade	No effect
Clonidine	Central acting sympatholytic	No effect
Enalaprilat	ACE inhibitor	No effect

NTG, Nitroglycerin.

4. **DIC:** This bleeding disorder is relatively common in association with brain injury. Treatment consists of correction of the underlying deficit using FFP and cryoprecipitate.

5. **Pulmonary care:** Frequent pulmonary toilet must be performed to avoid pneumonia or atelectasis. To avoid raising ICP with ET suctioning, sedation may be used near the time of suctioning.

6. **Sodium management**
   a. Hyponatremia—SIADH and cerebral salt wasting are both best managed by close monitoring of fluid status, including judicial use of hypertonic IVF. SIADH is associated with euvolemia or a volume-overloaded state, whereas cerebral salt wasting is associated with intravascular depletion. Fluid restriction, although beneficial in SIADH, worsens the hypovolemia associated with cerebral salt wasting.
   b. Hypernatremia—Diabetes insipidus is diagnosed by the inability to adequately concentrate the urine in the face of a high serum osmolarity. Treatment consists of high-volume fluid replacement along with the use of DDAVP.

7. **Infarction**
   a. General—Postoperative brain infarction may be associated with a multitude of reasons, including retractor placement, intraoperative fluid management, presenting clinical picture, distal vascular supply of cerebrovascular disorder (diseased carotid, aneurysm, AVM), or overaggressive tumor resection. Hemorrhagic stroke (intracranial hemorrhage) is usually associated with uncontrolled hypertension or inadequate hemostasis.
   b. Specific territorial symptoms associated with ischemic infarction (Table 13-3).

8. **Intracranial hypertension**
   a. General—Raised ICP in a routine postoperative patient is rare. In certain cases, including trauma, aneurysms associated with a large SAH, and posterior fossa tumor resection (the latter usually adequately managed by ventricular drainage), increased ICP may be an issue.
   b. Management: See section II, B, 3.

9. **Infection**
   a. Wound infection—This is uncommon in the immediate postoperative period. Wound infection manifests mainly by fever and erythema near the incision site, is caused usually by intraoperative contamination, and is treated by using the appropriate antibiotics. Untreated or undertreated infections run the risk of seeding the bone flap, which necessitates removal.
   b. Meningitis—The persistence of an unexplained fever with a temperature higher than 38.5°C in the postoperative period suggests the presence of bacterial meningitis and necessitates a lumbar puncture, especially in the face of a CSF leak. This is clearly clinically driven. Broad-spectrum antibiotic coverage may be narrowed after the identification of the offending organism.

TABLE 13-3

SPECIFIC CEREBROVASCULAR TERRITORIAL SYMPTOMS

Artery	Symptoms/Syndromes
Anterior cerebral artery	Contralateral leg weakness, clumsiness, hemisensory loss, and urinary incontinence
	Proximal ACA: contralateral face and arm weakness also
	Bilateral: abulia, akinetic mutism, and rigidity
Middle cerebral artery (dominant)	Contralateral hemiplegia of lower face, trunk, and upper and lower extremities
	Contralateral hemisensory loss
	Homonomous hemianopsia
	Global, Broca's, or Wernicke's aphasias
Middle cerebral artery (nondominant)	Contralateral hemiplegia of lower face, trunk, and upper and lower extremities
	Contralateral hemisensory loss
	Homonomous hemianopsia
	Contralateral neglect
	Asomatognosia (failure to recognize patient's own arm)
	Prosopagnosia (difficulty with face recognition)
	Constructional apraxia
Posterior cerebral artery	Contralateral homonomous hemianopsia
	Memory loss (controversial)
	Proximal PCA: contralateral hemisensory loss progressing to hemihypalgesia (thalamic syndrome)
	Bilateral PCA: cortical blindness
Rostral basilar artery	Contralateral hemiparesis and ipsilateral third nerve palsy (Weber's syndrome, superior alternating hemiplegia)
	Intranuclear ophthalmoplegia
	Severe: coma, pinpoint pupils, locked-in syndrome
Midbasilar artery	Contralateral hemiparesis and ipsilateral sixth nerve palsy (middle alternating hemiplegia)
	Severe: coma, pinpoint pupils
Posterior inferior cerebellar artery	Contralateral body hemisensory loss, ipsilateral facial hemisensory loss, dysarthria, ipsilateral hearing loss, nystagmus, ipsilateral Horner's syndrome and ataxia (lateral medullary syndrome, Wallenberg's syndrome)
Anterior spinal artery	Contralateral hemiplegia, contralateral loss of proprioception and vibrioception, and ipsilateral tongue paresis (inferior alternating hemiplegia)

Data from Haines DE: *Correlative neuroanatomy, the anatomic basis of some common neurologic deficits*, Baltimore, 1985, Urban & Schwarzenberg; and Rowland LP, editor: *Merritt's textbook of neurology*, ed 8, Philadelphia, 1989, Lea & Febiger.

13

THE CENTRAL NERVOUS SYSTEM

VII. ANEURYSMAL SAH

A. GENERAL

1. **Aneurysmal subarachnoid hemorrhage occurs secondary to aneurysmal rupture,** which, because of the subarachnoid location of the circle of Willis and other cerebral vessels, dissects directly into the subarachnoid space.

2. **More than 15 per 100,000 suffer from aneurysmal SAH per year.** Approximately one third will be functional survivors.

3. **Diagnosis** is based on symptoms of headache and acute onset of neurologic symptoms. A major life-threatening hemorrhage is often preceded by a "sentinel bleed," which the patient describes as a severe, unremitting headache and as the "worst in their life."

B. ETIOLOGY OF ANEURYSMAL SAH

1. **Anterior circulation** (85% of total aneurysms)
a. Anterior communicating artery 30%
b. Posterior communicating artery 25%
c. Middle cerebral artery 20%

2. **Posterior circulation** (15% of total aneurysms)
a. Basilar artery 10%—most commonly a basilar tip aneurysm
b. Vertebral artery 5%

C. SYMPTOMS

The symptoms include severe and sudden headache, photophobia, meningeal signs (stiff neck, Kernig's and Brudzinski's signs), vomiting, syncope, coma, and focal weakness or cranial nerve palsy (third nerve palsy).

D. TREATMENT

1. **Medical**
a. Preoperative admission orders to the ICU should include the following:
    (1) General
        (a) Vital signs and neurologic checks q1h
        (b) SAH precautions (quiet environment with restricted visitation)
        (c) Head of bed elevated 30 degrees with bed rest
        (d) NPO if immediately preoperative, NG tube if lethargic (placed under sedation to reduce risk of re-rupture), clear liquids if neither
        (e) IVF: NS + 20 mEq KCl at 100 ml/hr
    (2) Laboratory tests
        (a) Preoperative laboratory tests (CBC, Chem 7, PT, PTT, type and cross 4 units, urinalysis [U/A])
        (b) Initial ABG, CXR, and ECG
        (c) ABG, CBC, Chem 7 at least qd, ABG q6h if unstable, Chem 7 q8h if Na balance abnormal
    (3) Monitors
        (a) Arterial line insertion (with local anesthesia) to monitor BP if unstable (SBP should rise no further than 120 to 150 systolic before surgical clipping).
        (b) Intubation if patient unable to adequately oxygenate, ventilate, or protect airway.

(c) Cardiac monitor is essential because SAH is associated with sub-endocardial ischemia and frequent ECG changes.

(d) PA catheter is usually reserved for postoperative fluid management.

(e) Ventriculostomy may be needed for patients who develop symptomatic hydrocephalus. Excessive loss of CSF during placement or from overdrainage is associated with rehemorrhage.

(f) Pulse oximetry.

(4) Medications

(a) Nimodipine 60 mg PO/NG q4h (reduces morbidity from vasospasm)

(b) Ondansetron 4 mg IV q4-6h PRN

(c) Docusate 100 mg PO/NG bid to prevent constipation and straining

(d) Ranitidine 150 mg PO/NG bid

(e) Codeine 30 to 60 mg PO/NG q4h PRN

(f) Phenytoin (see section V, D, 2 for dosing)

(g) Antihypertensives (see Table 13-2)

(h) Acetaminophen

b. Postoperative issues specific to aneurysmal SAH

(1) General

(a) Postoperative ICU care is maintained for 2 weeks to avoid the complications of cerebral vasospasm. Exceptions to this include patients who presented with only mild headache or nuchal rigidity and a minimal amount of SAH by CT scan. These patients have a much less significant chance of experiencing cerebral vasospasm and may be transferred to the floor before the end of the 2-week period.

(b) These patients remain management challenges because the clip ligation of the offending aneurysm signals only the beginning of a 2- to 3-week period during which the patient may suffer cerebral vasospasm, hydrocephalus, hyponatremia, and seizures, as well as routine postoperative complications (e.g., pneumonia, DVT).

(2) Vasospasm

(a) General

(i) A clinical and radiologic entity during which the blood vessels of the brain constrict, partially occluding the vessel diameter. This usually occurs between post-SAH days 3 and 12. Curiously, one may exist without the other (i.e., the patient may have vasospasm by angiogram and not clinically).

(ii) Approximately 25% of patients with SAH will suffer from vasospasm, and in 7% of patients with SAH it will be fatal.

(iii) Despite much effort to specifically ascertain the etiology, the overall pathophysiology is unknown. It is thought that the inflammatory response plays a role in vasospasm, as well as blood products released into the subarachnoid space. The larger the amount of clot burden, the higher likelihood of occurrence.

13

THE CENTRAL NERVOUS SYSTEM

(b) Symptoms include drowsiness, loss of levels of orientation, and focal neurologic signs consistent with the vessel (or vessels) affected (see Table 13-3). The endpoint of severe vasospasm is stroke or death.

(c) Symptomatic cerebral vasospasm is a clinical diagnosis. However, the presence of vasospasm on cerebral arteriogram (the gold standard) or transcranial Doppler contributes to or confirms the diagnosis.

(d) Current treatment methods concentrate on prevention. This includes the use of "triple-H" therapy (hypertensive, hypervolemic, and hemodilutional), which is guided by the use of the PA catheter. Of note, hypertensive therapy has become controversial and is often left out of the treatment protocols. If instituted, the MAP is increased using pressors if necessary (the goal SBP is controversial but in general has been 160 to 200 mm Hg). Volume expanders, including vasopressin (Pitressin), isotonic and hypertonic saline, colloids, and whole blood, are used to increase cardiac output, and the hematocrit is maintained at approximately 33 to decrease viscosity. The calcium channel blocker nimodipine has been shown to improve outcome in this patient population.

(e) Occasionally, patients become symptomatic despite the above measures and balloon angioplasty must be performed after diagnostic angiography. Papaverine has been used in the past but seems to have only temporary dilatory effects. Balloon angioplasty is not without risk. The complications include vessel rupture, hemorrhage, and infarction.

(3) Hydrocephalus

    (a) Communicating hydrocephalus occurs from occlusion of the arachnoid granulations.

    (b) This is rectified by serial lumbar punctures, continuous lumbar drainage, or ventricular drainage. Some of these patients will ultimately need CSF shunting.

(4) Seizure

    (a) Seizures occur in approximately 13% of patients after SAH.

    (b) Prophylaxis on admission is recommended. Treatment during acute seizure follows the outlines put forth in section V, D, 1.

(5) Hyponatremia

    (a) Cerebral salt wasting occurs (thought to be secondary to atrial natriuretic factor release) in which body salt and volume is depleted, thereby causing dehydration, hypovolemia, and worsening of ischemia if present. Severe hyponatremia and overrapid correction are concerning for seizure induction, as well.

    (b) Management includes administration of fludrocortisone 0.1 mg IV q12h and hypertonic IVF.

2. **Surgical and/or endovascular intervention:** The isolation of a cerebral aneurysm from the circulation may be done via craniotomy in the OR or endovascularly in the interventional suite.

VIII. NEUROTRAUMA
A. HEAD
1. General

a. Approximately 150,000 people in the United States die of trauma-related injury each year. Nearly half are secondary to head injury.

b. Approximately one fourth of all severe head injuries are operative.

c. Severe head injury has been defined as a GCS less than or equal to 8 according to the Guidelines for the Management of Severe Head Injury put forth by The Brain Trauma Foundation, The AANS, and The Joint Section on Neurotrauma and Critical Care in 1995.

d. It is crucial to note that cerebral contusions or diffuse axonal injury (DAI), by themselves subcategories of closed head injury (CHI), may occur concomitantly with a traumatic intracranial mass lesion. After surgery for the traumatic intracranial mass lesion, the management is then dictated by the patient's neurologic examination and ICP.

e. Severe head injury has a 5% association with cervical spine injury specifically, as well as multisystem trauma in general.

2. Diagnosis

a. Commonly, there is an immediate loss of or change in consciousness at the scene of the accident in patients with DAI, a progressively worsening of neurologic examination in patients with severe contusion or SDH, and a "lucid interval" in patients with an EDH. These are far from strict rules, however.

b. Upon arrival to the ER, focal neurologic signs (hemiparesis or a "blown" pupil), as well as altered LOC, including coma, may be found.

c. The patient undergoes a full multisystem trauma evaluation in the ER. Neurosurgery becomes involved early in the management of suspected head injury. The ICU is not the place for initial neurologic evaluation. See section I, B, 4 for the method of evaluating a patient with an altered LOC.

d. Included in the neurologic examination is a head and neck examination for signs of skull fracture (linear, depressed, basilar, temporal bone), midface instability, gunshot wound (GSW) entrance or exit, spinal instability, or other facial and/or head injury.

e. After stabilization and neurologic evaluation, the patient must be rapidly taken for CT scanning of the head followed by other appropriate neurologic (see section I, C) and nonneurologic imaging.

3. Types

a. Closed head injury: This term refers to a broad spectrum of clinical entities, ranging from the mild concussion to severe bitemporal contusions. Concussions (brief losses of consciousness associated with anterograde and retrograde memory loss, headaches, and drowsiness) are not dis-

13

THE CENTRAL NERVOUS SYSTEM

cussed in depth here because these patients are not routinely admitted to the ICU.

(1) Cerebral contusion: Contusions ("hemorrhagic contusions") are radiographic entities defined as areas near the cortex where the brain is "bruised." They commonly occur near bony ridges (frontal lobe contusions occur from impaction on the orbital roofs and temporal lobe contusions occur from impaction on the petrous ridges). It also represents an area of axonal disruption, as well as breakdown of the blood-brain barrier. These in and among themselves may not be the cause of an altered neuroexamination. It is the size and location of the contusion, as well as the simultaneous occurrence of DAI, that may be the true culprit.

(2) Diffuse axonal injury: DAI occurs as a result of rotational forces that shear axons away from their cell body. Often this is diagnosed by the presence of a poor neurologic examination despite relatively little evidence of traumatic brain injury on CT. Radiographic evidence does include the presence of "salt and pepper" hemorrhages on CT scanning.

b. Intracranial mass lesion

(1) Epidural hematoma (EDH): This is a collection of blood located between the dura and skull that usually arises after a fracture of the squamous part of the temporal bone and resultant rupture of the middle meningeal artery. CT imaging reveals the classic lenticular pattern. Common wisdom teaches the concept of the "lucid interval"; however, this is *not* always the case. Treatment consists of surgical evacuation.

(2) Subdural hematoma (SDH): This is a collection of blood between the dura and arachnoid membrane that results from tearing of the bridging veins; it may be acute, subacute, or chronic. Acute subdurals are associated with a worse outcome than EDH and form a crescent-shaped collection on CT imaging. Treatment consists of surgical evacuation.

(3) Gunshot wounds (GSW): Over 90% of these patients die at the scene. Worse outcome is associated with a bihemispheric or intraventricular bullet path.

4. General principles of management

a. Surgical: Epidural or subdural hematomas must be rapidly evacuated. Patients suffering GSWs to the head may undergo a craniotomy to debride nonviable tissue, remove accessible bullet and bone fragments, or prevent CSF leakage. Depressed skull fractures more than the width of the skull need operative correction to reduce the possibility of infection, CSF leak, and seizure focus formation.

b. ICU care

(1) Admission

(a) General

(i) Vital signs and neurologic checks q1h

(ii) Head of bed elevated 30 degrees and neck midline

   (iii) NPO until abdomen is cleared for tube feeding
   (iv) IVF: NS with 20 mEq KCl at 100 ml/hr
   (v) Maintain normal glucose and electrolytes
  (b) Laboratory tests
   (i) CBC, Chem 7, PT, PTT, Ca, Mg, PO_4, anticonvulsant level daily
   (ii) Serum osmolarity q3h if mannitol therapy instituted
   (iii) ABG q6h if unstable or managing raised ICP within the initial 24 hours
  (c) Monitors
   (i) Cardiac monitor
   (ii) Arterial line
   (iii) Foley catheter
   (iv) Intubation and ventilation if patient unable to adequately ventilate, oxygenate, or protect airway, also for initial management of raised ICP
   (v) ICP monitor (see section II, B, 3)
   (vi) Pulse oximeter
  (d) Medications
   (i) Phenytoin (Dilantin) prophylaxis (see section V, D, 2)—Dilantin therapy may suppress early seizures (<1 week after injury); therefore patients should be placed on phenytoin in the first 24 hours after severe head injury. After 1 week, it may be discontinued. Controversy exists surrounding prophylaxis against late posttraumatic epilepsy. Some believe that all patients should be discontinued after 1 week, whereas others think that those who are status postcraniotomy, have penetrating injuries, have a prior seizure history, or suffered a posttraumatic seizure should continue treatment for 6 to 12 months (Greenburg, 1994).
   (ii) Ranitidine 50 mg IV q8h
   (iii) Acetaminophen
   (iv) Specific pharmacologic ICP therapy (see section II, B, 3)
   (v) Steroid therapy is not indicated in traumatic brain injury. Outcome is not improved, and the risk of infection and gastric ulcer formation is enhanced.
 (2) Specific ICU issues, including ICP management, seizure prophylaxis, Na management, pulmonary care, DVT prophylaxis, ulcer prophylaxis, and DIC, are discussed elsewhere in this chapter

B. CERVICAL SPINE INJURY

1. General

a. Approximately 10,000 people a year in the United States sustain spinal cord injuries.
b. Etiology includes motor vehicle collision, falls, and diving incidents. There is a clear association with head injury; therefore any patient with a traumatic head injury should be considered to have a cervical cord lesion until proven otherwise.

2. **Neurologic syndromes**
a. Incomplete lesion: This is defined by the presence of any neurologic function below the level of the injury, including sacral sparing (perirectal sensation, voluntary anal contraction, toe flicker). These injuries have a better prognosis for recovery than complete lesions. By itself, the presence of the bulbocavernosus reflex has no prognostic meaning. Incomplete lesions may by grouped into general patterns defined below.
   (1) Central cord syndrome: Upper > lower extremity weakness, varying sensory disturbances below the level of the lesion.
   (2) Brown-Séquard's syndrome: Ipsilateral loss of motor function, proprioception, and vibrioception with contralateral loss of pain and temperature. This has the best recovery prognosis of all defined incomplete syndromes.
   (3) Anterior cord syndrome: Bilateral loss of motor function and pain and temperature below level of lesion with intact proprioception and vibrioception.
b. Complete lesion: Absence of any neurologic function below the involved level. Failure to regain any function by 24 hours has dismal prognosis for any distal neurologic recovery.
3. **Evaluation:** See section I, B, 3.
4. **General principles of management**
a. Surgical: Acute (within 24 hours) surgical treatment is dependent on neurologic function on admission, whether that condition is worsening or improving, the presence of a traumatic spinal hematoma or acutely herniated disk, and the associated vertebral body fracture. The presence of a complete lesion is an exclusion criteria for acute operative intervention. Oftentimes the patient may be taken for vertebral stabilization after days of medical care in the ICU to ultimately assist with rehabilitation.
b. ICU care
   (1) Admission
      (a) General
         (i) Vital signs and neurologic checks q1h
         (ii) Bed rest, hard collar, rotatory bed
         (iii) NPO until abdomen cleared for tube feeding
         (iv) IVF: NS with 20 mEq KCl at 100 to 125 ml/hr
         (v) intakes and outputs, frequent nasotracheal suctioning
      (b) Laboratory tests: routine laboratory evaluation with emphasis on ABGs
      (c) Monitors
         (i) Cardiac monitor
         (ii) Pulse oximeter
         (iii) Foley catheter
         (iv) Arterial line
         (v) PA catheter or CVP via central line if hemodynamically unstable

      (vi) Intubation and ventilation if the patient is unable to adequately ventilate, oxygenate, or maintain airway

  (d) Medications

      (i) Methylprednisolone (Solu-Medrol) protocol for 24 hours: if injury within 8 hours bolus with 30 mg/kg and after 45 minutes begin 5.4 mg/kg/hr for 23 hours

      (ii) Ranitidine 50 mg IV q8h

      (iii) Acetaminophen

      (iv) Pressors (dopamine or phenylephrine) to keep MAP greater than 80

(2) ICU issues

  (a) General: ICU issues, including Na management, general pulmonary care, DVT prophylaxis, ulcer prophylaxis, and DIC, are discussed in section VII.

  (b) Issues specific to the spinal cord–injured patient.

      (i) Cardiovascular: Neurogenic shock is common after cervical cord injury. A generalized loss of sympathetic tone occurs, which dilates the systemic vasculature and produces bradycardia. The combination of these two pathophysiologic responses often drops the MAP, and a common response is to overhydrate the patient. This will result in pulmonary edema as the fluid more easily passes into the interstitial space of the lungs, worsened by the loss of sympathetic tone. Therefore pressors, such as phenylephrine or dopamine, may be used in an effort to keep the MAP greater than or equal to 80 for the first few days after injury.

      (ii) Pulmonary: Cervical spine injuries at or above the C4 level will necessitate mechanical ventilation. Below this, the further down the level of the lesion, the less the chance of initial intubation or prolonged mechanical ventilation. The level of the lesion combined with shrewd medical management determines the success in ventilator weaning. Pulmonary toilet is crucial in these patients, as is medical management to avoid pulmonary edema and pneumonia, both of which can easily tip the scales in the favor of prolonged ventilation.

      (iii) Gastrointestinal: Ileus is common after spinal cord injury, and tube feeding should be slowly advanced as tolerated after the acute injury phase.

      (iv) Autonomic instability: Temperature control, bowel and bladder function, postural hypotension, and other autonomic functions become dysregulated after spinal cord injury. In addition to acute care, these problems continue to be significant in the chronic care of the spinal cord–injured patient.

SUGGESTED READINGS

Greenburg MS: *Handbook of neurosurgery,* ed 3, Lakeland, Fla, 1994, Greenburg Graphics.

Guy J, McGrath BJ, Borel CO, et al: Perioperative management of aneurysmal subarachnoid hemorrhage: part 1. Operative management, *Anesth Analg* 81:1060-1072, 1995.

Haines DE: *Correlative neuroanatomy, the anatomic basis of some common neurologic deficits,* Baltimore, 1985, Urban & Schwarzenberg.

McGrath BJ, Guy J, Borel CO, et al: Perioperative management of aneurysmal subarachnoid hemorrhage: part 2. Postoperative management, *Anesth Analg* 81:1295-1302, 1995.

Osborn AG: *Diagnostic neuroradiology,* St Louis, 1994, Mosby.

Plum F, Posner JB: *The diagnosis of stupor and coma,* ed 3, Philadelphia, 1982, FA Davis.

Ropper AH, editor: *Neurological and neurosurgical intensive care,* ed 3, New York, 1993, Raven Press.

Rowland LP, editor: *Merritt's textbook of neurology,* ed 8, Philadelphia, 1989, Lea & Febiger.

Wilkins RH, Rengachary SS, editors: *Neurosurgery,* vols 1-3, ed 2, New York, 1996, McGraw-Hill.

PART III

Specialized Patient Management

TRAUMA

Scott C. Silvestry

I. INITIAL MANAGEMENT

Admission to the surgical intensive care unit (SICU) should be considered for injured patients with severe or multiple traumatic injuries, airway concerns, significant medical comorbidity, or advanced age. Patients arriving in the SICU from the emergency department or operating room are assumed to have unrecognized injuries. Late recognition of significant injuries is not uncommon in multiple-injury patients. Vigilance must be maintained in seeking undiagnosed injuries on repeat examination to avoid the morbidity associated with a delay in diagnosis. The initial evaluation should be identical to the initial assessment in the emergency department.

14

A. AIRWAY MANAGEMENT

1. **Goals of management** are to secure and protect an adequate airway.
2. **Cervical spine injury is assumed** until radiographic and clinical clearance is confirmed. Semirigid collars are maintained in the SICU until all cervical views or clinical examination can be safely obtained.
3. **As a general principle,** hypothermic patients (patients with core temperatures less than 35.5° C) should remain intubated.

B. VENTILATION AND OXYGENATION

1. **The initial examination** should include an observation of chest expansion and the confirmation of bilateral breath sounds.
2. **The endotracheal tube should be examined** for a properly inflated cuff, and the distance from the tip should be noted (usually 22 to 24 cm). In addition, the CXR will provide confirmatory data.
3. **End-tidal CO_2, pulse-oximetry oxygen saturation, and ABG analysis** provide confirmation of adequacy of oxygenation and ventilation.

C. VASCULAR ACCESS

1. **IV access should be identified by location, size, and current fluid type.** IV location and patency should be confirmed; this step is essential should sudden hemodynamic compromise occur.
2. **Arterial lines should be checked** for proper placement, proper waveform, and secure position.
3. **Special lines,** such as central venous lines and Swan-Ganz catheters, should be examined.

D. LABORATORY STUDIES

Appropriate laboratory studies should be obtained. In particular, a coagulation profile including PT, PTT, platelet count, fibrinogen level, and presence of fibrin split products facilitates rational treatment of bleeding diatheses.

E. FLUID RESUSCITATION

1. **On arrival in the SICU, many patients will not be fully resuscitated.**
2. **Basic indexes,** such as vital signs, assessment of peripheral perfusion via extremity temperature, capillary refill, and urine output, can guide

initial fluid management. Patients with multiple injuries and an unclear fluid status should undergo early invasive monitoring (Swan-Ganz catheterization). The use of Svo$_2$ and continuous cardiac output Swan-Ganz catheters greatly assist fluid management and the determination of need for inotropic support.

3. **Adequate perfusion** by clinical or catheter-based measurements should be confirmed. Assessment of cardiac function and volume status should be completed on admission to the SICU to allow comparison between expected and actual volume requirements.

F. **PHYSICAL EXAMINATION**

1. **Complete head-to-toe trauma survey** should be performed on admission to the SICU.

2. **Defining the precise mechanism of injury** allows consideration of injury complexes and associated diagnoses with attention to level of severity.

3. **The initial physical examination provides a baseline evaluation,** enabling the detection of previously missed injuries and the development of complications. Special attention should be paid to the abdominal examination for any change from initial trauma examination, including the onset or alteration of tenderness, the presence of dullness to percussion, tympany, bowel sounds, and guarding.

G. **RADIOGRAPHS**

1. **An admission-portable CXR** allows confirmation of central line, endotracheal tube, NG tube, and chest tube placements. Careful attention should be directed to mediastinal and pulmonary structures.

2. **All previous studies should be reviewed,** and the final reading by the radiologists should be noted.

II. THORACIC TRAUMA

A. **PNEUMOTHORAX**

1. **Chest pain and shortness of breath** are the most common symptoms.

2. **Physical findings** include decreased breath sounds and decreased chest wall motion. Patients on ventilators will demonstrate significantly higher airway pressures.

3. **CXR demonstrates a hyperlucent area with absent lung markings.** Small pneumothoraxes may only be identified on expiratory films taken with the patient upright. Unilateral deep sulcus on a supine CXR also indicate the presence of pneumothorax, which needs chest tube thoracostomy. Other indications for a chest tube include rib fractures in a patient scheduled for the operating room, subcutaneous emphysema, and emergent decompression of a presumptive tension pneumothorax.

4. **Placement of a 28-F or 32-F chest tube may be diagnostic and therapeutic.**

a. Incomplete reexpansion of the lung after chest tube placement results in persistent air leaks and delay in resolution. Management involves higher suction pressures or placement of an additional chest tube to accommodate higher airflow.

b. Large air leaks should arouse suspicion of a tracheobronchial injury (see section II, F).

c. Continuous air leaks that do not vary with respiration can be associated with esophageal injury (see section II, J).

B. TENSION PNEUMOTHORAX

1. **Tension pneumothorax is an immediately life-threatening problem.** In the SICU, tension pneumothorax most often develops as a complication of mechanical ventilation.

2. **A tension pneumothorax results from a check-valve effect,** which allows accumulation of air under pressure within the pleural space but does not allow egress of air. Positive intrapleural pressures of only 10 to 15 cm H_2O significantly impede venous return to the heart.

3. **The diagnosis is based on clinical findings.** Respiratory compromise and hypotension associated with decreased breath sounds and hyperresonance to percussion on the affected side identify a tension pneumothorax. The trachea may shift away from the affected side. Patients requiring mechanical ventilation will demonstrate elevated airway pressures.

4. **Decompression should be performed immediately,** preceding radiographic confirmation. A 14- or 16-gauge catheter inserted in the second or third intercostal space in the midclavicular line is effective; a rush of air confirms the diagnosis. Placement of a standard chest tube should follow the decompression.

C. PULMONARY CONTUSION

1. **Pulmonary contusion is a direct injury to the lung associated with hemorrhage and subsequent edema.**

2. **Diagnosis** is confirmed by radiographic findings of pulmonary infiltrates and consolidation.

3. **Mild contusions may be treated with the following:**

a. Aggressive pulmonary toilet, including chest physiotherapy and endotracheal suctioning

b. Pain control of associated rib fractures

c. Avoidance of fluid overload

d. Consideration of thoracic epidural analgesia to control splinting

4. **Moderate to severe contusions require intubation and mechanical ventilation** based on standard criteria: Pao_2 less than 60 mm Hg, $Paco_2$ greater than 55 mm Hg, respiratory rate greater than 30.

a. Treatment goals should be to maintain O_2 saturation greater than 90% while maintaining Fio_2 less than 0.5 to prevent O_2 toxicity.

b. PEEP is effective in increasing functional residual capacity and in improving oxygenation. Cardiac output determinations, Svo_2, and pulmonary compliance measurements allow selection of optimal PEEP settings. Optimal PEEP should be obtained through 2- to 5-minute trials with ABG sampling and hemodynamic measurements at graduated PEEP intervals.

   c. Fluid overload should be avoided. Invasive hemodynamic monitoring, including PA catheterization, is indicated to allow optimal fluid management.

   d. The hematocrit should be maintained at levels to optimize Do_2. Oximetric PA catheterization enables precise calculation of Do_2.

5. Complications of pulmonary contusion include the following:

   a. Infection

     (1) The injured lung is susceptible to bacterial colonization.

     (2) Prophylactic antibiotics are not indicated.

     (3) Frequent sputum cultures should be obtained.

     (4) Antibiotic therapy is initiated for the treatment of documented pneumonia.

   b. Barotrauma: most common manifestation is development of a pneumothorax

6. Patients with severe contusions are expected to have a gradual improvement in ABGs and clinical condition, which allows progressive ventilation weaning. Failure to demonstrate improvement should arouse suspicion of superimposed pneumonia or PE.

D. FLAIL CHEST

1. Flail chest results when a segment of chest wall loses continuity with the remainder of the bony thorax.

2. The flail segment will demonstrate paradoxical respiratory movement; however, the primary pathophysiology results from injury to the underlying lung.

3. Therapy is directed toward the underlying lung injury and pain control.

E. HEMOTHORAX

1. The initial treatment of hemothorax in the SICU is the placement of a 36-F chest tube. Only 15% of patients require operation.

2. Indications for operation include the following:

   a. Initial output greater than 1000 ml

   b. Hourly output greater than 300 ml/hr

   c. Total output greater than 2000 ml

3. A hemothorax that is not evacuated by a chest tube predisposes to fibrothorax. Video-assisted thorascopy or formal thoracotomy for evacuation of residual clot may be indicated.

F. TRACHEOBRONCHIAL INJURIES

1. Only 30% of the cases are diagnosed within the first 24 hours.

2. Signs include mediastinal or subcutaneous emphysema and presence of pneumothorax. A large air leak will often be present from chest tubes. Proximity to the path of a penetrating object should arouse suspicion.

3. Diagnosis is made by bronchoscopy.

4. Treatment involves operative repair.

5. The two clinical syndromes seen with delayed diagnosis are the following:

   a. In patients with incomplete injuries, the bronchus will heal with a stricture. Atelectasis and recurrent infection will occur distally, and ultimately tissue destruction will occur.

b. In patients with circumferential lacerations, granulation will occur at each end. The distal bronchial tree will fill with mucus, and radiographic studies will demonstrate complete atelectasis. At this point, management involves pulmonary resection.

G. MYOCARDIAL CONTUSION

1. **This diagnosis should be considered** in patients sustaining blunt trauma to the anterior chest and in patients demonstrating evidence of severe thoracic trauma, such as scapular fracture or high cervical rib fracture. Initial manifestations may include arrhythmia or hypotension.

2. **The diagnosis is based on ECG and cardiac isoenzyme determination.** ECG findings include new ST segment changes, PVCs, conduction system defects, and atrial arrhythmias.

3. **Echocardiography** will identify associated wall motion abnormalities in severe cases and allow identification of a pericardial effusion, if present.

4. **Management of a myocardial contusion includes the following:**
a. Provide ECG monitoring for 24 hours. A lack of ECG findings rules out significant myocardial injury.
b. Measure serial cardiac isoenzymes.
c. Treat ventricular ectopy with lidocaine.

5. **If a new postinjury murmur is found,** it should be evaluated with an echocardiogram.

H. AORTIC TRANSECTION

1. **Injury to the aorta may occur with severe deceleration.** The most common site of aortic transection is immediately distal to the left subclavian artery.

2. **Diagnosis of an aortic transection involves the following:**
a. CXR: Several cardinal features are sought:
   (1) Widened mediastinum
   (2) Fractures of the first and second ribs
   (3) Scapular fractures
   (4) Deviation of the esophagus (NG tube)
   (5) Loss of definition of the aortic knob
   (6) Deviation of the trachea or depression of the left main stem bronchus
   (7) Apical cap
   (8) Left pleural effusion
b. CT scan of the chest: This may demonstrate severe injury to the aorta and may expedite the decision for surgery. However, this study usually serves as a screening: presence of mediastinal hematoma suggests significant thorax trauma and warrants aortography to rule out transection.
c. Transesophageal echocardiography: This is used as a diagnostic addition in patients with suspected blunt thoracic injury, especially the descending thoracic aorta either preoperatively or intraoperatively.
d. Aortography: The definitive test; should maintain a low threshold for obtaining this study.

14

TRAUMA

3. **Therapy** involves left posterolateral thoracotomy with primary or graft repair.

4. **Outcome** after repair of aortic transection often is dictated by severity of other associated injuries (e.g., closed head injury or pulmonary contusion).

5. **Complications of an aortic transection repair include:**
   a. Paraparesis or paraplegia occurs in approximately 5% of patients.
   b. Acute renal failure may occur and is usually reversible.
   c. Postoperative bleeding after the correction of coagulation parameters suggests a mechanical source.

I. DIAPHRAGMATIC INJURY

1. **A diaphragmatic rupture usually requires significant blunt trauma.** The tears are usually radial and more common on the left side.

2. **Diagnosis can be difficult in the early postinjury period.** CXR findings include irregularity or elevation of the diaphragm, a loculated hydro-pneumothorax, or a subpulmonary hematoma.
   a. Contrast studies are used to confirm the diagnosis.
   b. The presence of a NG tube or abdominal viscera in the hemithorax on plain films will establish the diagnosis.

3. **The stomach is the most frequent organ involved in herniation** and may result in gastric volvulus. Injuries to the liver and spleen are frequently associated.

4. **Diaphragmatic tears** should be repaired in one or two layers with a nonabsorbable suture. For acute injuries, repairs should be performed through an abdominal approach. This facilitates reduction of herniated abdominal contents and allows for optimal examination of intraabdominal viscera.

5. **Late repairs** should be performed through a thoracotomy because dense peritoneal adhesions are usually present.

J. ESOPHAGEAL INJURIES

1. **These injuries most commonly occur with penetrating trauma** and should be suspected in all cases of penetrating chest trauma.

2. **Symptoms include dysphagia and hematemesis.**

3. **Findings** include subcutaneous or mediastinal emphysema, fluid levels within the mediastinum, or pleural effusion.
   a. If a chest tube has been placed, finding an air leak that does not vary with respiration suggests an esophageal leak.
   b. Particulate matter in chest tube drainage also indicates an esophageal injury.

4. **Gastrografin swallow** is used in most patients who are suspected to have injury to the esophagus. Esophagoscopy can be used in patients unable to cooperate or in patients taken emergently to the operating room for associated injuries.

5. **Early treatment** involves debridement, primary repair, and drainage with chest tubes.

6. **Complex injuries and those recognized late** (longer than 12 hours postinjury) may require diversion and drainage.

7. **Adequate nutrition** is an absolute priority after repair and can be delivered with TPN or enteral via a jejunostomy feeding tube.
8. **Gastrografin swallow is obtained 5 to 7 days after repair.** Oral feeding is initiated after documentation of no extravasation.

III. GENERAL PRINCIPLES IN ABDOMINAL TRAUMA

A. ACUTE MANAGEMENT

1. **A subset of patients is managed in the SICU** after sustaining abdominal trauma without having undergone abdominal exploration. A high index of suspicion for occult injuries is required, as well as repetitive and thorough physical examinations by the same examiners. Negative peritoneal lavage or CT scans do not exclude significant intraabdominal injury.
2. **A second group of patients will have undergone exploration.** Meticulous attention must be directed toward identifying occult injuries and early recognition of complications. The SICU physician must have a thorough understanding of the injuries identified and the therapeutic procedures performed during the laparotomy.

B. OCCULT INJURIES

Significant injuries may be missed during the diagnostic workup or the laparotomy.

1. **Unrecognized sources of bleeding**
a. Associated signs may include hemodynamic instability, falling hematocrit, peritoneal irritation, or increasing abdominal girth.
b. A CT scan is a sensitive diagnostic test to evaluate the abdomen.
c. Abdominal trauma ultrasonography is increasingly utilized to screen for major abdominal injury in select patients in place of diagnostic peritoneal lavage. A four-quadrant and subxiphoid survey is performed to determine the presence of abnormal fluid collections or hepatic/splenic lacerations.

2. **Hollow viscus perforation**
a. Signs include peritoneal irritation, continued sepsis, and clinical deterioration.
b. Both peritoneal lavage and CT scan can miss this injury. In addition, peritoneal lavage itself may result in intestinal perforation.

C. LATE COMPLICATIONS

1. **Intraabdominal abscess:**
a. Most patients with abscesses will have a persistent fever and an elevated WBC count with a leftward shift.
b. Ileus and abdominal distention are frequently present. In some cases, hyperbilirubinemia or sepsis may increase in severity. Multisystem organ failure may follow any delay in diagnosis and treatment.
c. A CT scan of the abdomen and pelvis is the diagnostic test of choice.
d. Management of an abscess requires either CT-guided catheter drainage or open drainage.

2. **Bowel obstruction** (early, postoperative) is most commonly caused by adhesions.

14

TRAUMA

3. **Stress gastritis** with associated upper GI bleeding is a frequent complication in the trauma patient. Prophylaxis with histamine antagonists,
antacids, or sucralfate should be used in all trauma patients.

IV. SPECIFIC ABDOMINAL INJURIES

A. SPLENIC TRAUMA

1. **The spleen is frequently injured in blunt trauma.**
2. **Symptoms** include LUQ pain and left shoulder pain (Kehr's sign). Physical findings may include LUQ tenderness, tachycardia, and hypotension.
Radiographic findings include left lower rib fractures, an elevated left
hemidiaphragm, and gastric displacement.
3. **Patients in the SICU who do not manifest an overt surgical abdomen
should undergo a CT scan** to establish the diagnosis in the setting of
equivocal physical findings and evidence of ongoing blood loss.
4. **Injuries are classified by the severity** as demonstrated by CT scan
(Table 14-1).
5. **Nonoperative management of splenic injuries** has been used in an
effort to avoid splenectomy and postsplenectomy sepsis. Criteria for nonoperative management are listed:
a. CT scan suggests isolated, low-grade splenic injury (no other significant
intraabdominal injuries).
b. Hemodynamic stability
c. Normal level of consciousness
d. Absence of coagulopathy

TABLE 14-1

SPLENIC INJURY SCALE

Injury Grade*		Description†
I	Hematoma	Subcapsular, nonexpanding, <10% surface area
	Laceration	Capsular tear, nonbleeding, <1 cm parenchymal depth
II	Hematoma	Subcapsular, nonexpanding, 10%-50% surface area; intraparen-chymal, nonexpanding, <2 cm diameter
	Laceration	Capsular tear, active bleeding; 1-3 cm parenchymal depth, does not involve a trabecular vessel
III	Hematoma	Subcapsular >50% surface area or expanding: ruptured subcap-sular hematoma with active bleeding; intraparenchymal hema-toma >2 cm or expanding
	Laceration	>3 cm parenchymal depth or involving the trabecular vessels
IV	Hematoma	Ruptured intraparenchymal hematoma with active bleeding
	Laceration	Laceration involving segmental or hilar vessels, producing major devascularization (>25 % of spleen)
V	Laceration	Completely shattered spleen
	Vascular	Hilar vascular injury that devascularizes spleen

*Advance one grade for multiple injuries.
†Based on most accurate assessment at autopsy, laparotomy, or radiologic study.

6. Nonoperative management of splenic injuries includes the following:

a. Bed rest

b. Serial hematocrit determinations

c. Serial abdominal examinations

7. Operative management of splenic injuries includes both splenic salvage and splenectomy.

a. Splenic salvage is appropriate in patients with hemodynamic stability and no major associated injuries.

b. Splenectomy is still commonly used; usually for class IV or V splenic injuries.

8. Complications of splenectomy or splenorrhaphy for splenic injury include the following:

a. Hemorrhage is the most common complication. Coagulation abnormalities and hypothermia should be corrected. Continued evidence of blood loss mandates reexploration. Approximately 3% of patients treated with splenorrhaphy will require subsequent splenectomy secondary to postoperative bleeding.

b. Subphrenic abscess is treated by drainage.

c. Pancreatitis is managed with bowel rest, NG decompression, and hyperalimentation if required. If pancreatic injury is suspected intraoperatively, drains should be left in the splenic bed.

d. Postsplenectomy sepsis is characterized by an abrupt onset and an aggressive course.

    (1) The incidence is greatest in children.

    (2) Polyvalent pneumococcal vaccine should be given to patients before discharge (protective against 80% of pneumococcal strains).

    (3) Prophylactic penicillin should be given to children after splenectomy.

B. HEPATIC INJURY

1. Recognition of liver injuries has increased since CT scanning is more frequently used. Injuries are classified according to severity on CT scan (Table 14-2).

2. Nonoperative management of hepatic injury is reserved for the hemodynamically stable patients with isolated hepatic injury. Conversion to operative management is indicated with hemodynamic instability, increased intraabdominal pressure that may lead to decreased urine output, or signs of peritoneal irritation suggesting associated perforated viscus.

3. Intraoperative management of hepatic injury includes the following:

a. Temporary control of hemorrhage

    (1) Pringle's maneuver

    (2) Direct manual compression or specialized vascular clamping of the parenchyma

    (3) Packing with gauze

b. Definitive control of hemorrhage

    (1) Direct suture ligation

    (2) Debridement of nonviable tissue

TABLE 14-2		
LIVER INJURY SCALE		
Injury Grade		Description*
I	Hematoma	Subcapsular, nonexpanding, <10% surface area
	Laceration	Capsular tear, nonbleeding, <1 cm parenchymal depth
II	Hematoma	Subcapsular, nonexpanding, 10%-50% surface area; intraparenchymal, nonexpanding, <2 cm diameter
	Laceration	Capsular tear, active bleeding; 1-3 cm parenchymal depth, <10 cm in length
III	Hematoma	Subcapsular >50% surface area or expanding: ruptured subcapsular hematoma with active bleeding; intraparenchymal hematoma >2 cm or expanding
	Laceration	3 cm parenchymal depth
IV	Hematoma	Ruptured intraparenchymal hematoma with active bleeding
	Laceration	Parenchymal distribution involving 25%-50% of hepatic lobe
V	Laceration	Parenchymal distribution involving >50% of hepatic lobe
	Vascular	Juxtahepatic venous injury (retrohepatic vena cava/major hepatic veins)
VI	Vascular	Hepatic avulsion

*Based on most accurate assessment at autopsy, laparotomy, or radiologic study.

    (3) Omental packing
    (4) Dexon mesh hepatorrhaphy
    (5) Hepatic artery ligation
    (6) Hepatic resection

4. Postoperative management of hepatic injury includes the following:
a. Aggressive correction of coagulation abnormalities with platelets and/or FFP
b. Correction of hypothermia
c. Prevention of hypoglycemia with administration of 10% dextrose solutions after hepatic resection

5. Subcapsular hematomas may be managed nonoperatively in stable patients with bed rest, serial physical examination, hematocrit determinations, and repeat CT scanning.
a. One third of these patients requires operation.
b. Signs of rupture or abscess formation require immediate operative intervention.
c. Enlargement of contained hematomas may be initially managed with arteriography and embolization but may also require operative intervention.

6. Complications of hepatic injuries include the following:
a. Ongoing bleeding (despite correction of hypothermia and coagulation parameters) should be treated with early reoperation.
b. Abscesses are common after hepatic trauma (10% to 20%), secondary to retained bile, blood, and necrotic tissue.
    (1) Clinical signs include fever, sepsis, and persistent hyperbilirubinemia.

(2) Diagnosis is established by CT scan.

(3) Treatment is percutaneous or open drainage.

c. Hyperbilirubinemia is a common early finding related to multiple transfusions and transient hepatic dysfunction. A persistent elevation may also indicate infection.

d. Hematobilia:

(1) Clinical findings include abdominal pain and GI bleeding (usually melena) with a history of abdominal trauma.

(2) Diagnosis is established by angiography.

(3) Embolization is usually successful. Several operative strategies have been used, including resection, ligation of hepatic artery branches, and debridement.

C. GASTRIC INJURY

1. **Gastric injuries most commonly occur with penetrating trauma.** Diagnosis may be suspected if a bloody NG aspirate is present.

2. **Most gastric injuries can be repaired primarily.**

3. **NG suction should be maintained postoperatively until peristalsis has returned.**

4. **Complications of gastric injury includes the following:**

a. Significant bleeding occur from a suture line. Management involves reexploration for hemostasis.

b. Subhepatic, subphrenic, or lesser sac abscesses are suspected in patients with persistent fever and elevated WBC counts. Treatment is drainage.

D. DUODENAL INJURY

1. **Delays in the diagnosis of duodenal injuries are common.**

a. Retroperitoneal duodenal injuries may be missed at laparotomy unless meticulous care is given to inspection of the entire duodenum.

b. Mortality rates of 25% to 40% have been reported secondary to delay in diagnosis and severity of associated injuries.

2. **Clinical findings are nonspecific** but include fever; tachycardia; and abdominal, back, or shoulder pain. Testicular pain is associated with retroperitoneal injuries.

3. **Plain films may demonstrate free air, loss of the right psoas margin, air outlining the right kidney or right psoas muscle, or retroperitoneal gas bubbles.**

4. **CT scans** are very helpful in evaluating pancreatic and duodenal injuries.

5. **Gastrografin swallows** will demonstrate duodenal leaks, as well as intramural hematomas.

6. **Intramural hematoma causes partial small bowel obstruction** with nausea, vomiting, and abdominal pain.

a. UGI series is diagnostic, showing a "coiled spring" appearance in the second and third portions of the duodenum.

b. Nonoperative treatment with TPN is usually successful.

7. **Operative management depends on the location and severity of injury.**

a. The most important procedure is to establish effective drainage.

14

TRAUMA

b. Simple lacerations can be closed transversely, and repairs can be buttressed with omental or jejunal patches.

c. Resection of the duodenum and pancreatic head are used rarely for extensive destruction or devascularization. Duodenal diverticularization and pyloric exclusion are two useful techniques for severe injuries that avoid formal resection. Duodenal diverticularization involves antrectomy with Billroth II gastrojejunostomy and vagotomy, closure of the duodenal stump, repair of the duodenal laceration, and decompression with a tube duodenostomy. Pyloric exclusion involves repair of the duodenal laceration followed by closure of the pylorus with absorbable suture through a gastrotomy, which is the site for a gastrojejunostomy

8. Postoperative care for duodenal injuries includes the following:

a. Bowel rest with NG or gastrostomy tube decompression should be maintained for 5 to 7 days.

b. Water-soluble contrast studies can be obtained to evaluate the repair.

c. Drains should be maintained until an oral diet has been resumed.

9. Complications include the following:

a. Duodenal fistula
   (1) Initial management includes bowel rest, gastric decompression, sump drainage of the fistula, and TPN.
   (2) Fistulas that fail to close necessitate reoperation.

b. Intraabdominal abscess

E. PANCREATIC INJURY

1. After upper abdominal trauma, patients with pancreatic injuries often display only mild symptoms. The development of significant pain, tenderness with loss of bowel sounds, and peritoneal signs may be delayed. A common indication for exploration in these patients is associated intraperitoneal injuries.

2. Serum amylase levels are not reliable indicators of pancreatic trauma; only 66% of patients with significant blunt pancreatic trauma have hyperamylasemia. Hyperamylasemia without other signs of injury is not an indication for exploration.

3. CT scan should be obtained. Retroperitoneal injuries may be missed by peritoneal lavage.

4. Operative management is dictated by the extent of injury and is based on the location of the injury, involvement of the pancreatic duct, and associated injury to the duodenum and common bile duct.

a. Isolated injuries not involving the duct should be treated with drainage.

b. Body or tail injuries including the duct can be treated with distal pancreatectomy.

c. Complex injuries involving the duodenum and head of pancreas are associated with a high mortality rate. Surgical options include the following: duodenal diverticularization, pancreaticojejunostomy, and pancreaticoduodenectomy (mortality rate approaches 40%, usually from hemorrhage).

5. Complications of pancreatic injuries include the following:
a. Pancreatic fistulas (occur in approximately 10% of patients)
   (1) These fistulas can usually be managed nonoperatively.
   (2) Management of high-volume fistulas should include TPN.
   (3) Octreotide may be useful in shortening the time to closure.
b. Pancreatitis (occurs in up to 10% of patients)
   (1) Management is nonoperative and includes bowel rest and TPN.
   (2) Recurrent pancreatitis should trigger an evaluation for ductal stricture by ERCP.
c. Pancreatic pseudocysts
   (1) Clinical findings include abdominal pain, nausea, abdominal mass, and a persistently elevated serum amylase.
   (2) Diagnostic tests include ultrasound, CT, and ERCP.
   (3) Treatment consists of internal drainage via cystogastrostomy or Roux-en-Y cystojejunostomy.
d. Pancreatic abscess
   (1) Signs of sepsis are usually evident.
   (2) CT scanning is the diagnostic test of choice.
   (3) Management includes drainage and IV antibiotics.
e. Hemorrhage
   (1) Significant bleeding may occur secondary to erosion of retroperitoneal vessels.
   (2) Immediate reexploration is necessary.

F. SMALL INTESTINE INJURIES

1. Most small bowel injuries are managed by repair or resection with reanastomosis.

2. Complications include:
a. Intraabdominal abscess or generalized peritonitis may result from anastomotic breakdown.
   (1) Signs include fever, abdominal pain, tenderness, and leukocytosis.
   (2) Treatment is usually reexploration with resection and reanastomosis.
b. Enterocutaneous fistulas also result from failure at a repair site or anastomosis.
   (1) Most fistulas close with nonoperative management, including TPN.
   (2) High-output fistulas that fail conservative management require resection with reanastomosis.
c. Obstruction:
   (1) Early obstruction will frequently resolve with NG decompression.
   (2) Criteria for operative intervention include fever, leukocytosis, tachycardia, and peritoneal signs, as well as failure of nonoperative therapy.

G. COLON INJURIES

1. The majority of colon injuries are caused by penetrating trauma.
Injury to the colon is often first identified at laparotomy performed for penetrating trauma. Colon injuries secondary to blunt trauma are difficult to diagnose; both peritoneal lavage and CT scan may miss hol-

low visceral injury. Concerns over rectal injury warrant proctoscopic examination.

2. **Management** is based on location and extent of injury, as well as delay to time of surgery.

a. Primary repair is used in stable patients with minimal contamination and minimal delay.

b. Unstable patients with extensive injuries or established peritonitis are treated with resection with end colostomy.

c. Rectal injuries should be treated with proximal diversion. Drainage of the presacral space is imperative. Adequate debridement of devitalized tissue decreases the incidence of abscess and subsequent sepsis. Distal washout of the rectum with dilute antibiotic solutions may also reduce infection.

3. **Complications** include intraabdominal abscess, which occurs in 5% to 15% of patients and can usually be managed with percutaneous drainage.

H. PELVIC FRACTURE

Many patients with pelvic fractures have high-energy traumatic injuries and present with thoracic and abdominal injuries in addition to pelvic injuries. These other injuries usually take precedence except in the setting of pelvic fracture—related hemorrhage.

1. **Evaluation**

a. Pain or instability on pelvic examination signals the presence of pelvic skeletal injury.

b. The anteroposterior (AP) pelvis, inlet, and outlet tilt x-ray views are usually adequate to diagnose major pelvic disruption.

c. Pelvic CT aids in the evaluation of posterior ring injury, associated acetabular fractures, and evaluation of displacement injuries.

2. **Classification** (Table 14-3) is determined by involvement of the ring and stability of the pelvis in the vertical and rotational planes.

TABLE 14-3	
TILES CLASSIFICATION OF PELVIC RING INJURY	
Type	Description
Type A	Stable
A1	Fractures of the pelvis not involving the ring
A2	Stable, minimally displaced fractures of the ring
Type B	Rotationally unstable, vertically stable
B1	Open book
B2	Lateral compression, ipsilateral
B3	Lateral compression, contralateral (bucket handle)
Type C	Rotationally and vertically unstable
C1	Rotationally and vertically unstable
C2	Bilateral
C3	Associated with an acetabular fracture

3. Treatment

a. Treatment of hemorrhagic shock is the first priority in pelvic injury.
  (1) Control of hemorrhage involves general resuscitation, IV fluids, blood transfusion, and correction of coagulopathy.
  (2) Rule out associated intraabdominal source of bleeding with CT scan or supraumbilical peritoneal lavage. Laparotomy for intraabdominal source of bleeding may take priority to control of pelvic bleeding.
  (3) Application of external fixator.
  (4) Arteriography indicated in the setting of hypotension associated with pelvic injury when external fixator fails to control blood loss. During arteriography, one or both internal iliac arteries are embolized.

b. Need for internal fixation is addressed after hemorrhage is controlled, usually within the first 24 to 48 hours. Need for stabilization relates to classification.
  (1) Type A: Symptomatic treatment only, internal fixation is not required.
  (2) Type B1: Less than 3 cm anterior diastasis, conservative treatment only. More than 3 cm diastasis, closed reduction and anterior stabilization indicated.
  (3) Type B2: Less than 30 degrees rotational stability and less than 1.5 cm leg length discrepancy requires symptomatic treatment and protected weight bearing only. More than 30 degrees rotational stability and more than 1.5 cm leg length discrepancy requires reduction and stabilization.
  (4) Type C1 should be treated with reduction and stabilization

4. Open pelvic fractures

4. Open pelvic fractures are associated with significantly higher mortality than closed fractures, relating to acute hemorrhage and late incidence of sepsis and multisystem organ failure. Treatment involves control of hemorrhage, irrigation and debridement, broad-spectrum antibiotics, and colonic diversion in the setting of associated rectal injuries.

SUGGESTED READINGS

D'Amico TA, Pruitt SK, editors: *Handbook of surgical intensive care: practices of the surgical residents at Duke University Medical Center,* ed 5, St Louis, 1995, Mosby.

Hoyt D, Potenza BM, Cryer HG, et al: Trauma. In Greenfield LJ, et al, editors: *Surgery: scientific principles and practice,* Philadelphia, 1996, JB Lippincott.

Jurkovich GJ, Carrico CJ: Trauma: management of acutely injured patient. In Sabiston DC, editor: *Textbook of surgery: the biological basis of modern surgical practice,* ed 15, Philadelphia, 1996, WB Saunders.

Wilson RE, Walt AJ, editors: *Management of trauma: pitfalls and practice,* ed 2, Baltimore, 1996, Williams & Wilkins.

TRANSPLANTATION

Larkin J. Daniels

I. THE DONOR

A. IDENTIFICATION OF CANDIDATES FOR ORGAN DONATION

1. All deaths should initiate an inquiry for organ and tissue donation.

a. Tissue donation
  (1) Any aged patient without viral disease
    (a) HIV infection
    (b) Rabies
    (c) Active hepatitis
    (d) Jakob-Creutzfeldt disease
  (2) No cardiovascular function necessary
  (3) Tissues for donation
    (a) Cornea
    (b) Skin
    (c) Bone and tendon
    (d) Heart valve

b. Solid organ donation
  (1) Patient criteria
    (a) Nonseptic cadaver with beating heart
    (b) No extracranial malignancy
  (2) Other relative guidelines
    (a) All organs—no IV drug use (check for track marks)
    (b) Renal
      (i) Absence of primary renal disease or urinary tract infection
      (ii) Stable creatinine less than 1.5 or returning to normal in response to hydration
      (iii) Moderate or no pressor requirement (dopamine < 10 mg/kg/min)
      (iv) Less than 65 years of age
    (c) Pancreas
      (i) Absence of diabetes mellitus (not diabetes insipidus)
      (ii) No pancreatitis
    (d) Hepatic
      (i) Absence of primary hepatic disease, fatty infiltration, and alcoholic history
      (ii) Normal hepatic enzymes
    (e) Cardiac
      (i) Absence of primary cardiac disease or traumatic contusion
      (ii) Normal valve and wall motion on echocardiography
      (iii) Normal coronary angiography (over 40 years of age)
      (iv) Less than 55 years of age
    (f) Pulmonary
      (i) Absence of primary pulmonary disease, neurogenic pulmonary edema, chest trauma, or effusion

15

(ii) PEEP less than 10 mm Hg, Po_2 greater than 300 torr on Fio_2 of 1.0, peak airway pressure less than 30 mm Hg

(iii) Less than 55 years of age

2. **Establish a trusting, nonconfrontational relationship with the donor's family.**

a. Emphasize that the patient is dead and not being "kept alive by machines."

b. Take cultural and religious preferences into consideration.

c. Stress that donation does not cost the donor's family anything.

d. Emphasize that donation does not preclude an open-casket funeral.

B. **CRITERIA FOR BRAIN DEATH DECLARATION (Box 15-1)**

1. **Definition of death** as stated by the Uniform Determination of Death Act: irreversible cessation of circulatory and respiratory functions or all brain function, including brain stem

a. Declaration of death must be made in accordance with accepted medical standards.

b. Minor local variations of this act exist.

BOX 15-1

DUKE UNIVERSITY CRITERIA FOR DETERMINATION OF ADULT BRAIN DEATH

I. CLINICAL CRITERIA

A. Known Irreversible Etiology

Exclude CNS depressants (e.g., barbiturates, benzodiazepines), hypothermia (core temperature less than 32.2° C), and neuromuscular blockading medications within 24 hours.

B. Two Examinations*

At least 6 hours apart demonstrating the following:

1. Unresponsive coma
2. Absent brain stem function
(a) No pupillary light response
(b) No corneal response
(c) No oculocephalic response
(d) No response to caloric stimulation (50 ml cold water AU)

C. Apnea

No spontaneous respiration after appropriate testing, i.e., respiratory drive test.

II. CONFIRMATORY TESTS

Confirmatory tests are recommended, especially in the setting of hypoxic-ischemic injury and in periods of observation of less than 12 hours, but remain optional at the discretion of the attending physician.

A. Isoelectric EEG

B. Arteriogram or Nuclear Medicine Study

To demonstrate absence of cerebral circulation.

*The first examination may be performed by senior neurology house staff or by an attending neurologist. The second examination is performed by an attending neurologist.

2. Conditions for the diagnosis of brain death
a. Core temperature less than 32.2° C
b. Absence of pharmacologic sedation or neuromuscular blockade
c. Absence of metabolic causes of coma
   (1) Hyperosmolar coma
   (2) Hepatic encephalopathy
   (3) Preterminal uremia
d. Absence of shock
e. Normal toxin screen

3. Physical examination for the diagnosis of brain death (two examinations required, 6 hours apart)
a. Absence of all cephalic reflexes
   (1) Pupillary
   (2) Corneal
   (3) Gag
   (4) Oculocephalic (doll's eyes)
   (5) Oculovestibular (tympanic membrane caloric response)
b. Absence of decerebrate or decorticate posturing
c. Absence of seizure activity
d. May be presence of spinal reflexes (nonpurposeful response to pain)

4. Clinical studies for confirmation of brain death (to be performed once)
a. Electrocerebral silence on EEG
b. Nonresponsive apnea test
   (1) Ventilate the cadaver for 10 minutes with 100% O_2 and draw baseline ABG
   (2) Stop ventilation and begin CPAP only with 100% O_2.
   (3) Follow the O_2 saturation closely to ensure that hypoxia does not occur.
       (a) Patients in neurogenic pulmonary edema may not tolerate this maneuver.
       (b) P_{CO_2} will rise 3 torr/min in the absence of ventilation.
   (4) After approximately 10 minutes (variable depending on starting P_{CO_2}), observe the cadaver for any respiratory effort for 2 minutes.
       (a) Draw ABG to confirm a P_{CO_2} greater than 60 torr.
       (b) No respiratory effort for 2 minutes with P_{CO_2} greater than 60 torr indicates nonresponsiveness.
   (5) For cadavers with low pulmonary compliance, hypoxia, or neurogenic pulmonary edema, use the following procedures:
       (a) Ventilate with F_{IO_2} of 0.9 and F_{ICO_2} of 0.1.
       (b) Use capnographic monitoring to establish hypercarbia.
       (c) Draw ABG to confirm a P_{CO_2} greater than 60 torr.
       (d) Stop ventilation for 2 minutes to observe for respiratory effort.
c. Cerebral angiogram or nuclear medicine brain scan to demonstrate absence of cerebral blood flow (optional)

5. Logistical concerns for brain death declaration
a. Documentation of brain death
   (1) Entered in official medical record
   (2) Carried out by two competent, independent examiners

15

TRANSPLANTATION

   b. Brain death declaration
      (1) Pronounced by a brain death committee
      (2) Follows predetermined hospital approved guidelines (see Box 15-1)
      (3) Should exercise caution in children less than 5 years of age because
          of their extraordinary ability to recover function after extreme injury

C. STABILIZATION OF HEART-BEATING CADAVERS

1. **Ensure that all care is of therapeutic benefit to the patient until brain
   death is declared.**
   a. Maximization of cerebral O_2 delivery, usually at the expense of O_2 delivery to visceral organs, is mandatory.
   b. At the time of brain death declaration, all care should be redirected
      toward preservation of O_2 delivery to the individual organs for donation.

2. **Maintain core temperature at or around 37° C.**
   a. Pathophysiology
      (1) Loss of cerebral thermoregulation in the hypothalamus and brain
          stem–controlled vasomotor responses
      (2) Rapid loss of heat and eventual hypothermic-induced arrhythmias
   b. Methods to maintain body temperature
      (1) Warm with overhead heaters and warmed blankets.
      (2) Keep the room closed and the room temperature elevated.
      (3) Warm inspired gases to 38° C.
      (4) Warm all intravenous fluids to 38° C.

3. **Reduce cerebral edema by reversing hypovolemia and hyperosmolar
   states if present.**
   a. PA catheter may be necessary to establish volume status.
   b. Transfusion to a hemoglobin greater than 10 mg/dl.
   c. Maintenance of a urine output of 100 ml/hr.

4. **Prevent donor hypoxia.**
   a. Keep Po_2 greater than 100 torr.
      (1) Fio_2 can be increased as needed.
      (2) Hb levels in excess of 15 mg/ml may help provide adequate O_2 delivery in hypoxic donors.
   b. Optimize pulmonary toilet and use bronchodilator therapy for reactive
      airway disease.
   c. Treat correctable injuries (chest tube insertion for pneumothorax or
      hemothorax).
   d. Perform a CXR evaluation for pulmonary edema.
      (1) Neurogenic pulmonary edema
          (a) Low to normal filling pressures
          (b) Nonsegmental infiltrates
          (c) Treated with PEEP and O_2
      (2) Cardiogenic pulmonary edema
          (a) High filling pressures and low cardiac output
          (b) Treated with dopamine or dobutamine
      (3) Aspiration
          (a) Segmental infiltrate
          (b) Treated with pulmonary toilet

e. Judicious use of PEEP.
    (1) Hypoxia requiring PEEP usually contraindicates pulmonary donation.
    (2) Excessive PEEP may contribute to hemodynamic instability.

5. Prevent hemodynamic instability.
a. Hypotension unresponsive to volume or low-dose inotropic support
    (1) Sign of impending complete circulatory collapse
    (2) Mandates expedient removal of viable organs
b. Intervention
    (1) Volume expansion is the most important first step.
    (2) Administer dopamine up to 10 mg/kg/min if inotropic support is needed.
    (3) Phenylephrine less than 2 mg/kg/min may improve Do_2.
        (a) SVR must be measured and followed closely.
        (b) The measurement of Svo_2 is beneficial in this setting.
        (c) Discontinue use if Do_2 does not improve.
    (4) Use of epinephrine, norepinephrine, or high-dose phenylephrine is contraindicated.

6. Treat bradycardia only if systemic perfusion is threatened.
a. Atropine
    (1) Nonresponsiveness to atropine is the rule because cadavers have no vagal tone.
    (2) Trial dose of 1 mg may be used because postsynaptic neural tone may still be in effect.
b. Isoproterenol 1 mg/250 ml, continuous IV infusion
    (1) Titrate to desired heart rate.
    (2) Increased splanchnic blood flow from β-adrenergic effects may require additional volume to prevent paradoxical hypotension.
c. Transvenous pacing occasionally required

7. Normalize ventilation and minimize ventilator-induced barotrauma.
a. Do not compromise oxygenation.
b. Take care to protect the integrity of the alveoli for pulmonary transplantation.
c. Sacrificing the lungs as donor organs to maintain visceral oxygenation is appropriate.

8. Correct electrolyte abnormalities.
a. Measure serum osmolarity and serum levels of Na^+, K^+, Ca^{2+}, Mg^{2+}, and PO_4^{2-}.
    (1) Correct levels to physiologic range.
    (2) Levels may be significantly altered after premorbid aggressive diuresis.
b. Diabetes insipidus has the following considerations:
    (1) Pathophysiology
        (a) Lack of ADH production following loss of CNS function
        (b) Subsequent massive diuresis a frequent occurrence
    (2) Treatment
        (a) Replace urine output ml-for-ml with crystalloid containing the appropriate concentration of Na^+ and K^+ as determined by urine electrolyte measurement.

(b) Exercise caution when K^+ requirements exceed 40 mEq/hr.

(c) Measure serum and urine electrolytes frequently.

(d) Urine losses exceeding 500 ml/hr may require pharmacologic intervention.

    (i) Vasopressin: Initially, administer 1 to 5 U bolus IV. Follow with infusion starting at 1 U/hr. Titrate to keep urine output between 200 and 500 ml/hr—vasopressin is a potent renal and splanchnic vasoconstrictor. Immediately discontinue if urine output drops below 200 ml/hr.

    (ii) DDAVP (alternative): Administer 2 mg as a single bolus. Repeat as needed (generally q12h).

9. Control hyperglycemia.

a. Administer insulin, 100 U in 100 ml NS by IV infusion.

b. Titrate to prevent glucosuria (usually serum glucose < 180).

10. Contact the Organ Procurement Agency.

a. Inform them of the potential donor.

b. Initiate their standard protocol for organ retrieval and tissue typing.

D. CONSIDERATION OF NONHEART-BEATING DONORS

1. Procedure recently instituted in effort to increase donor organ supply.

2. Currently, at Duke, protocol only in place for retrieval of kidneys.

3. Most feasible in settings of patients demonstrating early signs of cardiopulmonary instability or in cases of planned withdrawal of ventilatory support.

4. Procedure requires rapid cooling of abdominal organs after cardiopulmonary arrest.

a. Topical cooling of organs via minilaparotomy

b. Catheter placement into femoral artery and vein to perfuse abdominal organs with preservation solution

5. Patient transfer to operating room for organ harvest should occur within 2 hours of arrest.

6. Kidney transplants from non–heart-beating donors currently suffer from high incidence of ATN.

7. Results have improved with use of pulsatile perfusion to evaluate kidney function before transplantation.

II. THE RECIPIENT

A. PREOPERATIVE ASSESSMENT

1. The preoperative assessment varies widely, depending on institutional protocols.

2. The assessment also depends on the specific organ(s) to be received.

3. The general guidelines for potential recipients upon arrival on the day of transplantation are the following:

a. Obtain a complete history, with emphasis on symptoms suggesting potential infection.

    (1) Recent myalgia or pyrexia

    (2) Oropharyngeal discomfort or dental caries

      (3) Cough

      (4) Dysuria

      (5) Diarrhea, constipation, or rectal disorders

  b. Perform a complete physical examination.

  c. Perform the following laboratory studies.

      (1) CBC with differential

      (2) Serum electrolytes, serum liver function, and PT and PTT

      (3) Urinalysis and urine culture (if not anuric)

      (4) CMV and HSV serologies

      (5) Blood type confirmation

      (6) Posteroanterior and lateral CXR

      (7) ECG (except for heart recipients)

  d. Rule out concomitant malignancy.

      (1) New, suspicious cutaneous or pulmonary lesions, or adenopathy

      (2) Rectal bleeding or other symptoms or signs of potential malignancy

  e. Rule out presensitization.

      (1) Obtain serum for a current crossmatch between recipient serum and donor cells.

         (a) T-cell lymphocytotoxic crossmatch is standard (must be negative before transplant).

         (b) B-cell and monocyte crossmatching are performed at many institutions.

      (2) Rules for ABO and Rh factors in transplantation are the same as in blood transfusions.

      (3) Determine the patient's panel reactive antibody percentage.

         (a) A general measure of the humoral presensitization against all human lymphocyte antibodies (HLAs)

         (b) Graded from 0 (good) to 100 (bad)

         (c) If high (>30%), may warrant the use of enhanced induction therapy

  f. Establish venous and/or arterial access with strict aseptic technique.

4. Organ-specific evaluation procedures include the following:

  a. Renal

      (1) Perform HLA typing before transplantation.

      (2) Determine whether dialysis is required.

         (a) Anticipate intraoperative fluid administration.

         (b) Determine the potential for delayed graft function.

         (c) Obtain the patient's "dry weight."

         (d) Document the daily urine output from native kidneys.

      (3) Culture peritoneal dialysate, if applicable.

      (4) Perform a preoperative transfusion.

         (a) Use sparingly the day of surgery.

         (b) Use only if cardiac comorbidities mandate the need for increased O_2-carrying capacity.

    b. Pancreas
       (1) Usually transplanted with a kidney as a simultaneous kidney pancreas transplantation
       (2) Routine renal evaluation
       (3) Should stabilize glucose levels in the 150 to 200 mg/dl range
    c. Hepatic
       (1) Blood products
          (a) Estimate blood products that will be required.
          (b) Confirm availability with blood bank before beginning the procedure.
       (2) HLA typing: not performed before transplantation
    d. Cardiac and pulmonary
       (1) HLA typing: not performed before transplantation
       (2) No other special evaluations

B. TRANSPLANT UNIT LOGISTICS
1. Assignments should be made to avoid cross-coverage with septic or infected patients.
2. Strict hand washing by all personnel is mandatory.
3. Private rooms are preferred.
    a. Additional isolation procedures are usually not necessary.
    b. When induction therapy is used, masks should be worn.

C. PERIOPERATIVE CARE
1. Daily evaluation for signs of infection
    a. Examination of oropharyngeal region
       (1) Thrush
       (2) Herpetic or CMV lesions
    b. Otic examination for otitis; seen with the following:
       (1) Prolonged NG suction
       (2) Prolonged endotracheal intubation
    c. Skin inspection
       (1) Wounds
       (2) Skin folds and the sacral and perianal regions
    d. Body fluids
       (1) Clarity of urine and other drainage should be noted.
       (2) Prompt culture should be performed if indicated.
    e. Mental status examination (CNS infections)
2. Laboratory studies tailored to address individual organ function
    a. CBC
       (1) Lymphopenia
          (a) May be a sign of overaggressive immunosuppression
          (b) Occurs with use of antilymphocyte preparations
          (c) CMV infection
          (d) Poor nutrition
       (2) Neutrophil proliferation
          (a) Emerging bacterial infections
          (b) Steroid induction therapy

b. Close monitoring of serum glucose during steroid induction

c. Routine electrolytes

d. Serum amylase
   (1) Should be monitored periodically during induction
   (2) Used to rule out steroid-induced pancreatitis

3. Prophylactic antibiotics

a. Same guidelines as for other surgical procedures of similar magnitude and scope

b. Urinary prophylaxis with doxycycline 100 mg PO daily
   (1) Used for renal and simultaneous kidney pancreas recipients
   (2) Continued until the bladder anastomoses are healed (4 weeks)

c. Pneumocystis prophylaxis
   (1) Used for pancreas, cardiac, and pulmonary grafts
   (2) Administration of trimethoprim 160 mg/sulfamethoxazole 800 mg PO 3 times a week

d. Oral fungal prophylaxis
   (1) Nystatin oral suspension 5 ml PO swish and swallow bid, or clotrimazole lozenges 10 mg PO qid
   (2) Appropriate for all immunosuppressed patients until the end of the induction period (usually 4 weeks)

e. Additional organism-specific coverage if cultures from the organ transport medium or the donor return positive

4. CMV prophylaxis

a. Protocols vary in some centers based on organ transplanted

b. Need for prophylaxis based on relative risk for infection

c. All recipients receiving an antilymphocyte antibody preparation require prophylaxis

d. Infection risk dependent on history of infection (serology) of donor and recipient
   (1) Low risk—donor negative/recipient negative
   (2) Moderate risk—donor negative/recipient positive or donor positive/recipient positive
   (3) High risk—donor positive/recipient negative

e. General guidelines for prophylaxis
   (1) Low risk—no prophylaxis
   (2) Moderate risk
      (a) Ganciclovir 5 mg/kg IV q12h for 14 days or until discharge (d/c)
      (b) Acyclovir 800 mg PO tid for 6 weeks total treatment (converted upon d/c)
   (3) High risk
      (a) Ganciclovir 5 mg/kg IV q12h for 14 days, then d/c
      (b) Ganciclovir 1g PO tid for 3 months
      (c) Regimen repeated for active infection or relapse

5. HSV prophylaxis

a. Acyclovir 200 mg PO tid

    b. Should be given postoperatively to all HSV-positive patients for 4 to 12 weeks

6. Peptic ulcer prophylaxis with an H$_2$ antagonist

a. Patients receiving steroids

b. Patients that are NPO

7. Drains

a. Should be closed-suction drains

b. Should be removed early in perioperative course

8. Management of hypertension

a. Appropriate adjustment of intravascular volume status

b. Use of antihypertensives (captopril, clonidine, nifedipine, and propranolol)

    (1) Avoidance of β-blockers and thiazide diuretics in pancreas recipients

    (2) Occasional PRN use of agents to acutely lower BP

        (a) Sublingual nifedipine 10 mg

        (b) Intravenous labetalol 20 mg load, 0.5 to 2 mg/min infusion hydralazine 10 to 20 mg

        (c) Sodium nitroprusside

            (i) Avoid using this agent in recipients of hepatic allografts.

            (ii) Metabolites are hepatotoxic.

9. Maintenance of patient hygiene (oral and cutaneous)

a. Maintenance is critical in preventing infectious complications.

b. Patients should be bathed daily with a bacteriostatic soap.

c. Skin desiccation can be prevented with a moisturizer, such as lanolin.

10. Constipation prevention

a. Use a stool softener (docusate sodium 100 mg PO tid).

b. Above may minimize bacterial translocation during defecation and perirectal injury.

11. Enteral nutrition

a. Reinstate as early as possible.

b. Use vitamin supplementation.

D. ORGAN-SPECIFIC PERIOPERATIVE CARE

1. Renal

a. Hourly assessment of intravascular volume status

    (1) Urine output measured hourly until stable function achieved

    (2) Physical examination

    (3) Measurement of the CVP

b. Posttransplant diuresis

    (1) Common after short ischemic times (e.g., living related donors)

    (2) Can precipitate electrolyte abnormalities, hypovolemia, and shock

    (3) Treatment

        (a) Fluid replacement (Table 15-1)

        (b) Frequent evaluation of serum electrolytes

TABLE 15-1

POSTOPERATIVE FLUID ORDERS AFTER RENAL TRANSPLANTATION

Urine Output (ml/hr)	IV Replacement (ml/hr)*
<75	Output + 50 and reassess volume status
75-100	Output + 50
100-200	Output + 25
200-300	Output
300-400	Output − 50
400-600	Output − 100
600-800	Output − 200
>800	Output − 50 and reassess volume status†

*Use D2.5½NS. For massive output, hyperglycemia may require lower glucose concentrations.
†If severe hypovolemia ensues, additional fluid replacement may be required.

c. Posttransplant oliguria
 (1) Generally secondary to ATN
 (2) Associated with long ischemic times or donor instability
 (3) Evaluation and treatment
  (a) If the patient is hypovolemic, replenish the intravascular volume.
  (b) If the patient is euvolemic, avoid fluid overload and consider dialysis.
  (c) Rule out anastomotic complications (see below).
  (d) If oliguria persists for 5 days, consider the following:
   (i) A biopsy is indicated to rule out superimposed rejection or cyclosporine toxicity.
   (ii) Consider withdrawing cyclosporine (prolonged ATN can be exacerbated by even normal cyclosporine levels).
   (iii) Consider antirejection therapy.
d. Posttransplant anuria
 (1) Managed like oliguria
 (2) Particular emphasis on ruling out technical complications
e. PO intake resumed on the day of surgery
f. Bladder spasm
 (1) A frequent complaint in young transplant patients
 (2) Treated with oxybutynin (Ditropan) 5 mg PO qid
2. Pancreas and simultaneous kidney-pancreas
a. Assessment of the intravascular volume status (same as for solitary renal allografts)
 (1) Excessive hydration
  (a) Increases pancreatic graft edema
  (b) Increases pancreatic complications
 (2) Additional caution in achieving euvolemia
b. Loss of HCO_3^- in patients with bladder drainage of pancreatic graft
 (1) May lead to chronic metabolic acidosis

        (2) Fluid replacement with D2.5½NS supplemented with
           1 to 2 ampules of sodium bicarbonate/L

  c. Generally normal glucose tolerance by the first postoperative day
      (1) An insulin drip is frequently used to avoid stimulating endocrine
         function.
      (2) Hypoglycemia is treated with glucose administration.

  d. Measurement of urinary amylase for patients with bladder drainage of
     pancreatic graft
      (1) High amylase values (10,000 to 100,000 U/L) indicate good pan-
         creatic function.
      (2) Timed measurements to compensate for varied urine volume should
         be 1000 to 8000 U/3 hours. Urinary pH should also be monitored
         and should be greater than 7.

  e. PO intake
      (1) Can resume the day of surgery for bladder drainage of graft
      (2) Delayed for enteric drainage of graft

  f. Bed rest usually extended for 72 hours
      (1) Prevents positional damage to the pancreatic graft
      (2) Should keep graft in a nondependent position

  g. Venous thrombosis
      (1) Early complication
      (2) Prevention
         (a) Enteric-coated aspirin
         (b) Dipyridamole administration

3. Hepatic

  a. Venovenous bypass
      (1) Often used during the operative procedure
      (2) Groin and axillary incision evaluations daily

  b. Management of intravascular volume—hepatic blood flow
     maximization
      (1) Wide portal to central venous gradient
      (2) Reduction of hepatic edema
      (3) Therapeutic intervention
         (a) Maintain a low CVP.
         (b) Use colloids/blood products instead of crystalloid for volume re-
           placement.
         (c) Use diuretics.

  c. Coagulopathy
      (1) Common in the early postoperative period
      (2) Management
         (a) Provide a continuous infusion of FFP (50 to 100+ ml/hr).
         (b) Administer vitamin K (phytonadione 10 to 20 mg/day IV).
         (c) Provide an infusion of cryoprecipitate for fibrinogen less than
           100 mg/dl
         (d) Platelet consumption may require platelet transfusion.
         (e) Failure to correct suggests a primary nonfunction (see below).

   d. Electrolyte abnormalities
     (1) Frequent in those patients with massive transfusion requirements and serum electrolytes
     (2) Monitored and replace electrolytes as necessary
   e. Hypoglycemia
     (1) Results from inability to initiate gluconeogenesis in the newly transplanted liver
     (2) May require infusion of D10W
   f. Hypoalbuminemia: occasionally requires infusion of albumin
   g. Liver function tests
     (1) Measured daily
     (2) Should decrease rapidly in the first 2 postoperative days
       (a) Obstructive LFT elevation suggests technical biliary anastomotic problems
       (b) Hepatocellular enzyme elevation considerations are as follows:
         (i) Vascular complications
         (ii) Rejection
         (iii) Primary nonfunction of the graft
   h. Mental status examination daily to assess improvement in metabolic encephalopathy
   i. Bed rest extended for 48 hours
   j. Primary graft nonfunction
     (1) Occurs in approximately 5% of patients
     (2) Necessitates immediate retransplantation

4. Cardiac
   a. The transplanted heart is denervated and thus insensate.
     (1) There is no angina during ischemia.
     (2) The sinoatrial (SA) node has no direct autonomic control.
       (a) Cardiac output: very preload dependent
       (b) Chronotropic support to maintain a rate of 100 beats/min: direct pacing, or isoproterenol
     (3) Loss of vagal innervation increases sensitivity to catecholamines
   b. Cardiac function should be monitored as with any postoperative cardiac procedure.
   c. Daily ECGs should be performed. (Maintain consistent lead placement.)
   d. Chest tubes and invasive monitors should be removed as early as possible.
   e. Endomyocardial biopsy should be performed.
     (1) At least weekly in the early postoperative period
     (2) Only reliable means of diagnosing rejection early
   f. Enteral nutrition and ambulation should be instituted on the second postoperative day.

5. Pulmonary
   a. Steroids may be withheld during the first postoperative week to aid in bronchial healing.
   b. Transplanted lung should be kept in the nondependent position.

   c. Position should be changed frequently (q1h).

   d. Early extubation is critical for postoperative recovery.

   e. Chest tubes and invasive monitors should be removed as early as possible.

   f. Daily CXRs are performed.

     (1) Aggressively evaluate infiltrates.

     (2) Empirically treat infiltrates with antibiotics.

   g. Indications for bronchoscopy include the following:

     (1) Pulmonary toilet

     (2) Diagnostic lavage and biopsy after deterioration in pulmonary function

   h. Enteral nutrition and ambulation considerations include the following:

     (1) Institute on the second postoperative day.

     (2) Take special care to avoid aspiration.

III. IMMUNOSUPPRESSION

A. INDUCTION THERAPY

1. Methylprednisolone

a. 250 to 2000 mg/day

b. Followed with prednisone taper

   (1) Begin when oral intake resumes.

   (2) Prednisone 5 mg PO is equivalent to methylprednisolone 4 mg IV.

2. Antibody preparations directed against T cells

a. Used in patients at high risk for rejection

   (1) All pancreas, cardiac, and lung recipients

   (2) Highly sensitized renal recipients

   (3) Currently being evaluated for both induction and treatment of rejection in solid organ transplants

b. Available preparations

   (1) CD3–T cell receptor monoclonal antibodies—OKT3

   (2) IL-2 receptor monoclonal antibodies—Basiliximab (CHI, Simulect), daclizumab (Zenapax)

   (3) Polyclonal antibodies—RATG (rat), Atgam (equine), Thymoglobulin (rabbit)

c. Adverse effects

   (1) Fever, rigors, and myalgias are common after the first 2 to 3 doses. Premedicate using acetaminophen 650 mg PO/PR, and diphenhydramine 50 mg IM/PO.

   (2) Pulmonary edema

     (a) Avoid fluid overload.

     (b) Institute dialysis for patients without renal function.

   (3) Development of anti-antibodies

     (a) Occurs with repeated usage of the same preparation

     (b) Inhibits effectiveness in 40% to 60% of patients

     (c) Especially common with older monoclonal preparations (OKT3)

     (d) Skin testing with test doses of polyclonal preparations

(4) Additional side effects of polyclonal preparations
    (a) Thrombocytopenia and neutropenia
    (b) Serum sickness
(5) OKT3: associated with a reversible encephalopathy

d. Dosage
    (1) The dosage is variable for polyclonal preparations.
    (2) OKT3 is given 5 mg/day.
    (3) Treatment lasts for 10 to 14 days.

B. MAINTENANCE THERAPY

1. Glucocorticosteroids

a. Primarily methylprednisolone or prednisone
b. Side effects of steroid use
    (1) Glucose intolerance
    (2) Peptic ulceration
    (3) Delayed wound healing or skin friability
    (4) Psychosis
    (5) Fluid retention
    (6) Adrenal suppression
    (7) Osteoporosis with avascular necrosis
    (8) Increased susceptibility to bacterial, fungal, and viral infections
c. Dosage
    (1) Use high doses (1.25 mg/kg/day of prednisone) for induction.
    (2) Taper to moderate doses (0.5 mg/kg/day) in early perioperative period.

2. Azathioprine (Imuran)

a. Mechanism—inhibitor of de novo purine synthesis
b. Side effects
    (1) Leukopenia
    (2) Hepatotoxicity
    (3) GI intolerance
c. Dosage
    (1) Begin at 2 mg/kg/day rounded to the nearest 50 mg.
    (2) Reduce dose by half if patient is dialysis dependent.
d. Required monitoring of the total leukocyte count
    (1) Reduce dose if this parameter is less than 7000/mm^3.
    (2) Withhold dose if this parameter is less than 3500/mm^3.

3. Cyclosporine (Sandimmune, Neoral)

a. Mechanism—inhibits calcineurin activity in T cells, resulting in blunting of cellular activation.
b. Side effects
    (1) Nephrotoxicity
        (a) Nephrotoxicity can occur regardless of the serum drug level.
        (b) Biopsy may aid in diagnosis.
    (2) Other side effects
        (a) Hypertension
        (b) Hirsutism
        (c) Hypercholesterolemia

15

TRANSPLANTATION

      (d) Hyperkalemia

      (e) B-cell lymphoma

      (f) Acne vulgaris

c. Dosage

    (1) Begin at 1 to 4 mg/kg IV given over 6 to 12 hours.

    (2) Convert to 8 to 15 mg/kg PO when oral intake is feasible (oral dose = 3 × IV dose).

    (3) Taper dose over the first several weeks to approximately 1 to 3 mg/kg daily.

d. Monitoring of serum drug levels

    (1) Desired levels

      (a) Levels are kept between 100 and 250 ng/ml if measured by HPLC.

      (b) Levels are kept in the 500 to 700 ng/ml range if measured by RIA.

    (2) Drugs that lower serum levels

      (a) Rifampin, trimethoprim IV, isoniazid

      (b) Carbamazepine

      (c) Phenobarbital

      (d) Phenytoin

    (3) Drugs that raise serum levels

      (a) Anabolic steroids

      (b) High-dose methylprednisolone

      (c) Ketoconazole

      (d) Calcium channel blockers

4. FK506 (tacrolimus, Prograf)

a. Mechanism of action

    (1) Inhibits calcineurin activity in T cells similar to cyclosporine

    (2) Acts via interaction with FK-binding proteins, resulting in blunting of T-cell activation.

b. Currently being used in place of cyclosporine in some protocols and for cyclosporine-resistant rejection.

c. Side effects

    (1) Nephrotoxicity

    (2) CNS effects—tremor or headache

    (3) Hypertension

    (4) GI—nausea or diarrhea

    (5) Metabolic—hyperglycemia, hyperkalemia, or hypomagnesemia

d. Dosage

    (1) Begin with 0.075 mg/kg PO q12h as soon as NG tube removed.

    (2) Recommended dosing range is 0.075 to 0.015 mg/kg PO q12h.

    (3) Can be given IV if patient is unable to tolerate oral dosing; continuous infusion 0.05 to 0.1 mg/kg/day.

e. Monitoring of serum drug levels

    (1) Desired levels

      (a) 0 to 6 months posttransplant—8 to 12 ng/ml

      (b) 6 to 12 months posttransplant—5 to 8 ng/ml

      (c) Longer than 1 year posttransplant—5 to 7 ng/ml

(2) Levels drawn with morning laboratory tests before AM dose
(3) For patients with renal and hepatic dysfunction, dose at lowest value of recommended ranges
(4) Drugs that raise serum levels
    (a) Nephrotoxic agents—aminoglycosides, amphotericin B, cisplatin, and cyclosporine
    (b) Antibiotics—erythromycin and clarithromycin
    (c) Calcium channel blockers
    (d) Methylprednisolone
    (e) Metoclopramide
(5) Drugs that lower serum levels
    (a) Anticonvulsants—phenobarbital, phenytoin, and carbamazepine
    (b) Rifamycins

5. Mycophenolate mofetil (CellCept)

a. Mechanism of action
  (1) Reversible inhibition of final stages of de novo purine synthesis
  (2) Location of inhibition in pathway provides for high specificity for lymphocytes
  (3) Blocks proliferation of both T and B lymphocytes
b. Currently used in some clinical protocols in lieu of azathioprine
c. Side effects
  (1) Leukopenia
  (2) Sepsis
  (3) GI—diarrhea
  (4) Possible teratogen
d. Dosage
  (1) 1g PO bid, beginning when NG removed.
  (2) No efficacy advantage demonstrated for any dose above 3 g/day.
  (3) Because of renal excretion, in setting of renal insufficiency, avoid doses greater than 1 g PO bid.
e. Monitoring of serum drug levels
  (1) Recommended monitoring of CBC
    (a) Weekly in first month
    (b) Twice monthly for second and third months
    (c) Monthly through first year
  (2) Drug interactions
    (a) Drugs that raise serum levels: acyclovir and probenecid
    (b) Drugs that lower serum levels: antacids and cholestyramine

6. Rapamycin

a. Mechanism of action
  (1) Binds to FK-binding protein similar to FK506
  (2) Target of drug-protein complex is at cell membrane level, resulting in inhibition of growth factor–mediated signaling.
b. Currently being used at some centers in clinical trials in various allograft protocols.

15

TRANSPLANTATION

   c. Because of effects on nonhematopoietic cells, considered to have potential applicability in treatment of other clinical problems.
     (1) Autoimmune diseases
     (2) Arterial restenosis after angioplasty or bypass

IV. REJECTION
A. HYPERACUTE REJECTION
1. Caused by presensitization of the recipient to an antigen expressed by donor
2. Mediated by antibodies binding to the antigen
a. Complement system activated
b. Procoagulant state produced that results in graft thrombosis
3. Occurs within the first minutes to hours after graft reperfusion
4. Treatment
a. There is no treatment.
b. Graft loss results.
5. Prevention
a. Preoperative verification of proper ABO matching and a negative crossmatch
b. Prevented in 99.5% of transplants
B. ACCELERATED ACUTE REJECTION
1. An anamnestic response to a donor antigen (pretransplant exposure to the antigen)
2. Occurs within the first 4 to 8 postoperative days
3. Biopsy to distinguish between two types
a. Vascular rejection
   (1) Primarily mediated by antibody secreted by memory B cells
   (2) Not treatable
b. Accelerated cellular rejection
   (1) Mediated by memory T cells
   (2) Sometimes responds to antilymphocyte immunosuppressants (see above)
C. ACUTE CELLULAR REJECTION
1. Acute cellular rejection is caused primarily by T cells.
2. This type of rejection evolves over a period of days to weeks.
a. Can occur at any time after the first postoperative week
b. Most common in the first 6 months posttransplant
c. Can be precipitated by viral or bacterial infection
3. Treatment leads to successful restoration of graft function in 90% to 95% of cases.
a. Biopsy should precede treatment.
b. Institute methylprednisolone bolus therapy.
   (1) Administer 250 mg to 1 g IV qd for 3 to 5 days.
   (2) Follow with a taper to the patient's baseline prednisone dose.
   (3) If there is a failure to respond, consider the possibility of a steroid-resistant rejection or an error in diagnosis. Use of an antilymphocyte antibody preparation may be indicated (see section III, A, 2).

(4) Depending on organ transplanted, consider empiric CMV treatment with ganciclovir.

D. CHRONIC REJECTION

1. Chronic rejection occurs over a period of months to years.

2. There is no treatment.

3. Biopsy is indicated to rule out a treatable source of graft dysfunction.

4. Acute rejection can be superimposed on chronic rejection.

E. ORGAN-SPECIFIC CONSIDERATIONS

1. Acute renal graft rejection

a. Symptoms

    (1) Graft pain and malaise

    (2) Rarely present in patients receiving cyclosporine

b. Signs

    (1) Fever and graft tenderness (rarely present)

    (2) Rapidly rising creatinine

    (3) Mild leukocytosis

    (4) Decreased urine output

    (5) Fluid retention and edema

c. Diagnosis

    (1) Rule out obstruction.

        (a) Flush Foley with 10 to 30 ml sterile saline.

        (b) Flush stent with 2 ml sterile saline.

    (2) Rule out hypovolemia.

        (a) Challenge with volume if clinically indicated.

        (b) Allografted kidneys are exquisitely sensitive to hypovolemia.

    (3) Rule out vascular and ureteral anastomosis problems in the first 10 postoperative days with a ^{99m}Tc DTPA renal scan.

        (a) Will determine if the graft is perfused

        (b) Will show if urine is being made but is not entering the bladder (ureteral leak)

    (4) Perform a needle core biopsy under ultrasonic guidance.

        (a) Allows for histologic examination of graft

        (b) Will provide evidence either for or against rejection

    (5) Currently there is no gold standard for the diagnosis of acute rejection.

        (a) Empiric therapy may be required.

        (b) If there is no evidence of rejection, reducing the cyclosporine dose may improve function.

    (6) Standard treatment protocol for acute renal graft rejection is the following:

        (a) Methylprednisolone 250 to 1000 mg IV, qd for 3 days, then rapid steroid taper to maintenance doses of prednisone

        (b) Antilymphocyte antibody preparations if no improvement seen after 2 to 3 days

2. Acute pancreas rejection

a. The most sensitive indicator of pancreatic rejection is rejection of the accompanying kidney.

  b. Isolated pancreatic rejection is more difficult to diagnose.
    (1) It is better to make the diagnosis before the onset of hyperglycemia.
    (2) Isolated pancreatic rejection is generally asymptomatic but may be accompanied by malaise or fever.
    (3) Decreased urinary amylase is a sign of acute pancreatic rejection.
      (a) One of the earliest signs
      (b) Occurs before hyperglycemia
  c. Diagnosis of acute pancreatic rejection includes the following considerations:
    (1) The diagnosis is based on changing trends of the biochemical monitors of pancreas function.
    (2) Graft thrombosis should be ruled out in the early postoperative period.
      (a) Clinical signs
        (i) Rapid-onset hyperglycemia
        (ii) Low urine amylase
      (b) May require reexploration or arteriography
  d. Empiric treatment is the standard.
    (1) Biopsy confirmation is less common.
    (2) Cystoscopic transvesical needle biopsy can be performed in bladder drainage patients.
  e. Treatment for acute pancreatic rejection is as follows:
    (1) The treatment is the same as for renal allografts.
    (2) Treatment with methylprednisolone may precipitate hyperglycemia.

3. Acute hepatic rejection
  a. Diagnostic signs
    (1) Elevations in the serum transaminase levels
    (2) Persistent coagulopathy
    (3) Hypoglycemia
    (4) Secretion of watery bile or absence of bile flow from the T tube (if present)
  b. Evaluation
    (1) Treatment is often empiric; coagulopathy may contraindicate percutaneous biopsy.
    (2) Rule out portal or hepatic arterial thrombosis.
      (a) Perform Doppler ultrasound.
      (b) Confirm impaired blood flow by arteriogram.
    (3) Rule out hepatitis.
      (a) Serum viral antibody titers
        (i) Hepatitis A, B, and C
        (ii) Herpes, CMV
        (iii) Adenovirus
      (b) Immunosuppression reduction if positive
    (4) Rule out biliary stricture or leak.
  c. Treatment: same as for renal allograft rejection

4. Acute cardiac rejection

a. Cardiac rejection is asymptomatic and has no ECG changes until it reaches the later stages.

b. The earliest ECG finding is voltage loss, especially in the limb leads.

c. Diagnosis of acute cardiac rejection includes the following considerations:

    (1) Established by examination of routine transvenous endomyocardial biopsies

    (2) Accelerated atherosclerosis

        (a) Considered a form of chronic rejection

        (b) Confirmed by coronary angiography

d. Treatment is generally the same as for renal allografts.

5. Acute pulmonary rejection

a. All pulmonary recipients experience acute rejection in the first 3 postoperative months.

b. Diagnosis of acute pulmonary rejection includes the following considerations:

    (1) Bronchoscopy and biopsy are based on reduced pulmonary function and infiltrates on CXR.

    (2) V/Q scanning is sometimes used.

    (3) Pneumonia must be ruled out.

c. Treatment is generally the same as for renal allografts.

V. COMPLICATIONS

A. TECHNICAL COMPLICATIONS

1. Renal

a. Vascular compromise

    (1) Arterial stenosis and venous outflow obstruction may be related to the following:

        (a) Anastomosis

        (b) Position of transplanted kidney

    (2) Evaluate perfusion with a ^{99m}Tc DTPA renal scan.

    (3) Postoperative bleeding may require evacuation of hematoma to prevent vascular compromise.

b. Ureteral compromise

    (1) Ensure Foley catheter patent by flushing with 30 ml sterile saline q4h.

    (2) Ensure stents are patent by irrigating 2 ml of sterile saline q4h.

    (3) Ultrasound examination of the kidney can reveal perigraft collections suggestive of urinoma.

    (4) Evaluate excretion with a ^{99m}Tc DTPA renal scan.

    (5) Evaluate anatomy with a stentogram if a stent is in place.

2. Pancreas

a. Vascular compromise—presentation

    (1) Rapid rise in serum amylase

    (2) Drop in urine amylase (bladder drainage only)

    (3) Hyperglycemia

   b. Exocrine drainage breakdown
     (1) Bladder leak and/or leak of enteric contents
     (2) Mandates immediate reoperation
   c. Graft pancreatitis
3. Hepatic
   a. Vascular compromise
     (1) Vascular compromise presents as a rapid deterioration in graft function.
     (2) Venous thrombosis leads to rapid accumulation of ascites.
     (3) Arterial thrombosis leads to graft dysfunction or leak from an ischemic bile duct.
     (4) Doppler ultrasound is the diagnostic test of choice.
   b. Management
     (1) Thrombosis usually requires emergent retransplantation.
     (2) Biliary leaks are treated with drainage or reoperation.
     (3) Strictures can usually be stented nonoperatively.
4. Cardiac transplant complications related to CPB (see Chapter 16)
5. Pulmonary—early technical problems
   a. Most often related to bronchial anastomosis
   b. Require reoperation
B. INFECTIOUS COMPLICATIONS
Infectious complications are common and diverse.
1. Infections in the early perioperative period
   a. Preexisting infections in the recipient
     (1) Urinary tract infections
     (2) Pneumonia
     (3) Contaminated vascular access
     (4) Reactivated hepatitis B or herpes simplex
     (5) Infection with *Strongyloides stercoralis*, an intestinal nematode
       (a) Can present as overwhelming gram-negative sepsis related to *Escherichia coli*
       (b) Treatment: oral thiabendazole and IV antibiotics for the gram-negative sepsis
       (c) 50% mortality rate
   b. Infections arising from the donor
     (1) Check cultures from the transport media.
       (a) Institute appropriate prophylaxis if *Pseudomonas* or *Candida* organisms cultured
       (b) Treat other organisms based on clinical indications
     (2) Treat the CMV-seropositive donor with ganciclovir 5 mg/kg IV q12h.
     (3) Other blood-borne diseases can be transmitted via the graft.
   c. Wound infections (usually related to technical problems)
   d. Intraabdominal infection
     (1) All transplant patients with unexplained fever should be evaluated by abdominal CT.
     (2) Symptoms will be muted or absent as a result of immunosuppression.

     (3) Differential diagnosis includes the following:
       (a) Diverticulitis
       (b) Cholecystitis
       (c) Peptic perforation
       (d) Appendicitis
  e. Pneumonia (common)

2. Infections beyond the first month

a. Bacterial superinfection
    (1) Prolonged intubation
    (2) Drains in place for long periods of time

b. Viral infections
    (1) CMV infection considerations include the following:
      (a) Presentation
        (i) Pneumonia
        (ii) Esophagitis, colitis, and gastritis
        (iii) Retinitis
        (iv) Hepatitis
        (v) Unexplained fever
        (vi) Falling leukocyte count
      (b) Immunosuppressive effects of CMV can lead to opportunistic infection
      (c) Treat with ganciclovir as above
    (2) EBV, HSV, VZV, and adenoviral infection
    (3) Late presentation of hepatitis C

c. Fungal infections
    (1) Primarily pneumonia or nasopharyngeal infection
    (2) Superinfection of transcutaneous catheters
    (3) Metastatic infection (common)
      (a) Cutaneous infections should be excised.
      (b) CT scan of the chest and brain to evaluate metastatic spread.
    (4) Treatment with amphotericin or fluconazole (required)
    (5) Fungal CNS infections
      (a) Alterations in neurologic examination
      (b) Lumbar puncture and CT investigations
    (6) Specific fungal pathogens
      (a) *Pneumocystis carinii*
        (i) Presents as life-threatening pneumonia.
        (ii) Prophylaxis with trimethoprim/sulfamethoxazole for most patients.
        (iii) Pentamidine therapy added if infection develops.
      (b) *Listeria monocytogenes*
        (i) CNS infection is empirically assumed if bacteremia is present.
        (ii) Treat with ampicillin and gentamicin.
      (c) Mycobacterial infection
        (i) Presentation same as in non–immunosuppressed patients
        (ii) Standard treatment regimen

15

TRANSPLANTATION

SUGGESTED READINGS

Austen KF, Burakoff SJ, Rosen FS, et al, editors: *Therapeutic immunology,* Cambridge, UK, 1996, Blackwell Science.

Flye MW, editor: *Principles of organ transplantation,* Philadelphia, 1989, WB Saunders.

Rubin RH, Young LS, editors: *Clinical approach to infection in the compromised host,* ed 3, New York, 1994, Plenum.

Starzl TE, Demetris AJ, editors: *Liver transplantation,* St Louis, 1990, Mosby.

Thomson AW, Starzl TE, editors: *Immunosuppressive drugs: developments in antirejection therapy,* London, 1994, Edward Arnold.

Tilney NL, Strom TB, Paul LC, editors: *Transplantation biology: cellular and molecular aspects,* Philadelphia, 1996, Lippincott-Raven.

CARDIAC SURGERY

Hartmuth Bruno Bittner

I. POSTOPERATIVE ASSESSMENT

A. INITIAL ASSESSMENT

Destabilization may occur during transport from the operating room to the ICU. A brief examination should be performed, and a report of the intraoperative course communicated.

1. Airway and ventilation

a. Check the endotracheal tube position and cuff pressure, and listen for air leaks.

b. Auscultate to ensure bilateral breath sounds; check the end-tidal CO_2.

c. Examine the chest for symmetric respiratory motion.

d. Initial ventilator settings: mode SIMV/PS, TV 10 to 12 ml/kg, Fio_2 60%, PEEP 5 cm H_2O, pressure support 10 cm H_2O, and rate 10 to 14 breaths/min.

2. Circulation

a. Palpate bilateral femoral and pedal pulses, and assess capillary refill.

b. Auscultate the heart. Rubs are often present when mediastinal chest tubes are used and are of no significance.

3. Report

a. Inquire about the operative procedure, intraoperative complications, hemodynamic course, weaning off cardiopulmonary bypass, and arrhythmias.

b. General postoperative plan should be discussed, including for fluid management; weaning from drips; dosages of inotropic, antiarrhythmic, and vasoactive drugs; extubation goals; and fast track or standard care protocol options.

B. EXPANDED ASSESSMENT

1. Hemodynamics and monitoring

a. Note vital signs, including HR, BP, PA pressure, PCWP, temperature, O_2 saturation, respiratory rate, and airway pressure.

b. Compare immediate ICU recordings with intraoperative hemodynamic assessment.

c. Abrupt changes in BP may occur immediately on arrival in the ICU, often as a result of the short-lived pressors administered by the transporting physician en route from the operating room.

(1) Correlate arterial line with cuff pressure.

(2) Check the quality of carotid and femoral artery pulses.

(3) If bradycardic, initiate pacing.

(4) Trendelenburg's position for severe SBP decrease (<90 mm Hg) and volume bolus of 250 ml.

2. Specific devices

a. Intraaortic balloon pump

(1) Set trigger mode (ECG or arterial BP) and timing of balloon inflation/deflation. Inflation must occur just after aortic valve closure for dia-

stolic augmentation; deflation should be complete before ventricular ejection for optimal afterload reduction.

(2) Note BP with the IABP turned off.

b. Chest tubes and suction devices

(1) Note the number and location of each mediastinal and pleural chest tube and/or drain.

(2) Ensure that suction tubing is attached and that bubbling is present in the proper chambers. Check for tubing kinks and obstructive blood clots. Chest tubes to 20 cm H_2O suction.

(3) Note amount of collected blood at the time of arrival in the ICU.

(4) Check for the presence of air leaks. These may be a result of intraoperative injury to the lung or, more commonly, to air leaking around the chest tube insertion site or a tubing connector.

c. External pacemaker settings

(1) External pacemakers are typically DVI devices (dual chamber pace, ventricular sense, inhibit pacing in response to native beat).

(2) Ventricular and atrial pacing capture thresholds should be determined by initiating pacing at a higher rate than the heart's intrinsic rate, then gradually reducing the output current until loss of pacing occurs. These numbers should be recorded for both atrial and ventricular wires.

(3) If external pacing is required, the output current of the pacemaker should be set to twice the threshold level.

(4) For capture failure, increase output, check connections, exchange polarity and/or cable. If pacing is not required, the pacemaker should be set to the demand mode at a "backup" rate of 60 beats/min.

3. Laboratory studies

a. ABG, CBC, PT, PTT, electrolytes, glucose, BUN, creatinine, ionized calcium, and magnesium.

b. If chest tube output greater than 200 ml/hr or suspicious for coagulopathy: repeat ACT (to assess reversal of heparin) and send for DIC screen (PT, PTT, fibrinogen, and fibrin split products).

c. Stat portable CXR.

4. Patient history

a. Review cardiac history, risk factors, previous MI, arrhythmias, cardiac catheterization, PTCA failure, thrombolytic therapy, and emergency operation

b. Previous medications

c. Pertinent comorbidity that may affect immediate postoperative course: history of previous surgery, tobacco use, asthma, COPD, pulmonary vascular disease (PVD), renal function, neurologic disorders, especially history of CVA

5. Postoperative orders

a. Vital signs: usually q15min for 1 hour, then q30min for 4 hours, then hourly thereafter

b. Activity: bed rest until extubated and/or removal of PA catheter

c. NPO; NG tube to continuous low-wall suction until extubation
d. Chest tubes to 20 cm H_2O suction
e. Foley catheter to straight drain
f. Ventilator settings (check initial postoperative ABG analysis and make appropriate changes)
g. External warming devices for hypothermia ($\leq 36.0°$ C)
h. Medications:
   (1) Antibiotics
   (2) Analgesics and sedatives: morphine 1 to 4 mg IV q30min PRN pain, midazolam 2 mg q1-2h PRN agitation
   (3) Inotropic, antiarrhythmic, and vasoactive drugs
   (4) Ulcer prophylaxis to keep gastric pH greater than 6
   (5) Acetaminophen: 650 to 1300 mg suppository PR q4h PRN for temperature greater than 38.2° C
   (6) Albuterol nebulizers: 0.5 ml in 2.5 ml 0.9% NaCl q4h for wheezing
   (7) Diabetic management: SSI therapy SQ with blood glucose checks q6h, or continuous insulin infusion with hourly blood glucose measurements to keep blood glucose below 200 mg/dl

II. EARLY POSTOPERATIVE COURSE (FIRST SEVERAL HOURS IN ICU)

A. HEMODYNAMICS AND MONITORING

1. **Hypothermia-induced vasoconstriction** characterizes this period.
2. **Treat the resultant hypertension with titratable sodium nitroprusside.** Specify mean or SBP range. Sudden episodes of hypotension may be encountered, resulting from rewarming vasodilation and instability of vascular tone.
3. **Ensure optimum O_2 delivery:** arterial oxygenation saturation greater than 90%, Hgb greater than 8.5 mmol/L, and cardiac index greater than 2 L/min/m^2.
4. **Weaning of inotropes is typically delayed** until several hours of stability have been achieved and the patient is fully rewarmed.
5. **In rare cases, patients manifest a hyperdynamic state,** characterized by tachycardia, hypertension, and elevated cardiac index. These patients may be treated judiciously with labetalol 2.5 mg IV bolus. Repeated administration q10min at higher doses may be performed until the desired effect is achieved.
6. **Shivering is commonly seen** and may not only be related to hypothermia. Mild shivering requires no treatment. Excessive shivering causes increased Vo_2, acidosis, and CO_2 production and may be treated with meperidine 25 to 50 mg IV qh.

B. RESPIRATORY

1. **Delay weaning from the ventilator** for several hours after arrival to ensure hemodynamic stability. Note that narcotics or sedatives given as patients emerge from anesthesia may compromise spontaneous breathing.

16

CARDIAC SURGERY

2. **In patients with stable blood gases and low chest tube output,** rapid extubation may be accomplished by reducing the rate in a SIMV mode.

C. RENAL

1. **Urine output** should be maintained above 0.5 ml/kg in all patients. Depending on the length of the procedure, the skill of the perfusionist, and the effectiveness of ultrafiltration during CPB, the patient may arrive in the ICU several kilograms over preoperative weight because of intraoperative fluid administration and CPB priming.

2. **Furosemide** 10 to 20 mg IV/PO bid over 3 days is usually effective in inducing diuresis in patients with adequate cardiac output. Ethacrynic acid 25 to 50 mg IV qd can be used in patients who are unresponsive to furosemide.

3. **Serum creatinine may be lower than baseline** as a result of CPB-induced hemodilution, even in patients with renal insufficiency. Over a period of hours it can be expected to rise to baseline and as a result of mild renal injury and ATN from CPB often exceeds baseline by a small degree.

4. **Patients with baseline renal insufficiency may be treated with dopamine** 2.5 to 3.0 μg/kg/min to increase renal blood flow.

D. WOUNDS AND CHEST TUBES:

Pleural drainage may be greater than 200 ml/hr for the first 1 to 6 hours. Ideally, drainage should taper off gradually to 20 to 30 ml/hr. Abrupt decrease in output may result from obstructing thrombus within the chest tube. Obstructing thrombus may be removed by gently milking or "stripping" the chest tube using devices designed for this purpose or with lubricated fingers.

E. NEUROLOGIC STATUS

1. **Assess pupillary responses and gag reflex.**

2. **All patients should be able to follow simple commands and move all four extremities.**

III. INTERMEDIATE POSTOPERATIVE COURSE (6 TO 12 HOURS AFTER ARRIVAL)

A. HEMODYNAMICS

1. **Hypothermia-induced vasoconstriction should resolve,** and patients no longer require vasodilator drugs. Patients who are hypertensive despite normothermia may be treated with prazosin, hydralazine, or ACE inhibitors.

2. **Cardiac output should continue to improve,** and inotropic drugs should be slowly weaned with the goal of discontinuance 12 to 18 hours postoperatively.

3. **Remove PA catheter from patients who are off inotropes** and continue to be hemodynamically stable. Note that many patients can be managed without a PA catheter.

B. RESPIRATORY

The patient should be extubated, oversedation with narcotics and CO_2 retention should be avoided, pulmonary toilet is emphasized.

C. RENAL

1. **Urine output may diminish** despite adequate cardiac output and BP. Furosemide should be given to maintain a urine output greater than 0.5 ml/kg/hr.
2. **Significant kaliuresis is common,** especially when diuretics are used, and necessitates frequent (q4-6h) measurements of serum potassium with IV supplementation as needed. Many ICUs apply potassium supplementation protocols.

IV. LATE POSTOPERATIVE COURSE (12 TO 24 HOURS AFTER ARRIVAL)

A. HEMODYNAMICS

1. **Inotropes should no longer be required.**
2. **In stable patients not needing inotropes,** PA catheters are pulled after extubation.
3. **Oral β-blockers** (atenolol 12.5 to 25 mg bid or propranolol 10 mg qid) may be administered to patients with preoperative ejection fraction of greater than 35% as prophylaxis against atrial arrhythmias.

B. RESPIRATORY

1. **More than 90% of patients** should be extubated by 24 hours postoperatively.
2. **Supplemental oxygen** (2 to 4 L/min by nasal prongs) is often needed for 48 to 72 hours postoperatively until patients are ambulatory and excess fluid is removed.

C. RENAL

1. **Continued diuresis with furosemide** is maintained until patients achieve their preoperative weight and room air O_2 saturation greater than 90%. Patients who display significant renal injury with elevated serum Cr should not be over diuresed because this may impair renal perfusion and result in further injury.
2. **Hypokalemia** (serum K < 4.5 mEq/L) is treated with oral potassium supplementation.

D. WOUNDS AND CHEST TUBES

1. **Chest tubes may be pulled** when output is less than 20 ml/hr for 3 to 4 hours, no air leak is present, and the CXR demonstrates no undrained fluid.
2. **Chest tubes should always be pulled after extubation.**

V. POSTOPERATIVE COMPLICATIONS

A. LOW CARDIAC OUTPUT

The factors determining CO are heart rate, preload (filling pressures), after-load (vascular resistance), and contractility. Low cardiac output is a syndrome consisting of inadequate tissue perfusion, defined as a CI less than 2 L/min/m². A management algorithm is given below.

1. **Bradycardia and arrhythmias**
a. Cardiac output increases with increasing HR. In general, a HR less than 60 beats/min should be treated by atrial pacing to a rate of 100 to

16

CARDIAC SURGERY

110 using temporary epicardial wires. Increasing HR above 110 seldom provides further increases in cardiac output and may be detrimental in terms of increased myocardial oxygen demand and decreased ventricular filling.

b. AV pacing may be used in patients with complete AV block. Ventricular pacing alone may be associated with a 10% to 20% decrement in cardiac output.

c. Patients with no epicardial pacing wires may be paced using a PA catheter equipped with pacing electrodes or a temporary transvenous pacing lead. β-Agonist infusions may also provide positive chronotropy.

2. Low preload (CVP < 10 mm Hg, pulmonary artery diastolic pressure [PAD] or PAWP < 12 to 15 mm Hg)

a. Between 250 and 500 ml colloid bolus or transfuse blood products if low hematocrit (<25%).

b. Higher filling pressures may be required to obtain adequate ventricular filling because ventricular compliance may decrease after cardiac surgery.

c. LV preload is generally limited by the development of pulmonary edema at filling pressures greater than 20 mm Hg.

3. Increased afterload

a. The normal systemic afterload is 900 to 1400 dyne/sec/cm^{-5}.

b. Sodium nitroprusside 1 to 10 μg/kg/min is the vasodilator of choice because of its short half-life and relative specificity as an arterial vasodilator. Cyanide toxicity can occur as a result of high doses for several days and is manifested as an elevation of mixed venous O_2, metabolic acidosis, convulsions, disorientation, muscle spasms, and anorexia. Treatment for cyanide intoxication is IV infusion of 25% sodium thiosulfate, 150 mg/kg over 15 minutes.

c. Nitroglycerin is primarily a venous vasodilator but does have limited arterial vasoactivity, as well. It also has the added benefit of being a coronary arterial dilator. Dosage is 0.5 to 3 μg/kg/min.

4. Contractility and myocardial dysfunction

a. Mild diastolic dysfunction (decreased ventricular compliance) is common after cardiac arrest. Therefore it is imperative that preload be maximized before attributing poor cardiac output to lack of myocardial contractility.

b. Systolic dysfunction may be a result of inadequate revascularization, acute graft occlusion, or prolonged cross-clamp time (ischemia).

c. Systolic function may be enhanced with inotropic drugs. Inotropic drugs should be started at low doses, then titrated to desired effect. Similarly, once started, these drugs should be weaned gradually (as tolerated). Abrupt cessation may result in hemodynamic decompensation.

d. Common choices of inotropic support: dopamine, dobutamine, and epinephrine. Consider phosphodiesterase inhibitors (milrinone, amrinone) for low CO states associated with elevated PA pressure and increased PVR, and for patients with right ventricular dysfunction.

e. Patients on higher doses of inotropes in need of central line change require overlapping drip change to avoid hemodynamic decompensation.

B. TAMPONADE

1. **Pericardial fluid** can develop in more than 80% of postoperative patients, but only 1% develop clinically significant tamponade.

2. **The classical Beck's triad** (increased CVP with distended neck veins, hypotension, and muffled heart tones) is infrequently found in postoperative open heart surgery patients. Important signs are low CO, decrease in urine output, CVP exceeding mean PA pressure, and rapid increase in left and right atrial pressures tending to equalize.

3. **Tamponade** is almost invariably associated with progressive widening of the mediastinal shadow on follow-up CXR, often occurring after abrupt cessation of mediastinal chest tube output.

4. **The diagnosis is usually made on clinical indexes and high level of suspicion.** It may be confirmed by bedside cardiac ultrasound showing poor RV filling resulting from free wall compression.

5. **The primary treatment, however, is volume expansion and immediate decompression of the pericardium.** Inotropes may transiently improve hemodynamics. Vigorous stripping of mediastinal chest tubes may be effective, but patients are usually returned to the operating room for direct evacuation of pericardial clot. Acute, life-threatening tamponade with rapid onset of hemodynamic instability demands immediate opening of the sternotomy with evacuation of clot in the ICU.

C. MECHANICAL SUPPORT OF THE FAILING HEART

Indicated for failure to wean from CPB, low CO state unresponsive to inotropic agents, and as a bridge to cardiac transplantation.

1. **Counterpulsation—intraaortic balloon pump:** Most commonly used mechanical device, usually duration of support 3 to 10 days. Also used for unstable angina and malignant arrhythmias.

a. Physiologic effects are reduction of left ventricular afterload, increase in aortic root and coronary perfusion pressure, and reduction of left ventricular wall tension and Vo_2.

b. Inflation must occur after the aortic valve is closed for diastolic augmentation, and deflation must be completed before aortic valve opening for afterload reduction.

c. Trigger modes include ECG (most frequently used) and pressure.

d. Position is just distal to the origin of the left subclavian artery, and above renal and mesenteric arteries.

e. Complications, such as limb ischemia and thromboembolic events, balloon rupture, and aortic dissection, require immediate removal.

f. Before removal of the balloon, normalize platelet count and coagulation status. During the removal, allow femoral artery to bleed antegrade and retrograde to prevent thromboembolization.

g. Transthoracic and transaortic insertion is done in patients with severe PVD and aortobiiliac disease that precludes common femoral or external iliac artery insertion.

16

CARDIAC SURGERY

h. Contraindications to IABP include aortic insufficiency, aortic dissection, severe atherosclerotic disease, and recent thoracic aortic grafts.

2. **Temporary external ventricular assist devices**

a. Duration of support usually up to 10 days.

b. The most commonly used nonpulsatile temporary assist devices are the BioMedicus centrifugal pump (Medtronic-BioMedicus, Eden Prairie, Minn.) and the Archimedes screw axial flow hemopump. A temporary pulsatile pump is the Abiomed BVS 5000 (Abiomed, Danvers, Mass.), which is pneumatically actuated by an external drive console with gravity filling. The insertion of these devices is similar to cannulation for CPB. For left ventricular assist device (LVAD) insertion, a cannula is placed into the left atrium (through right superior pulmonary vein) and outflow is to the ascending aorta. In RVAD, the right atrium and pulmonary artery are cannulated. Patients are sedated, heparinized (ACT 180 seconds to 200 seconds), and flow is maintained at 2 to 4 L/min. Cardiac echo is frequently used to assess ventricular function and recovery potential.

c. Major complications include bleeding, right ventricular failure, renal failure, infection, neurologic deficits, thromboembolization, and blood cell degradation.

D. ARRHYTHMIAS

1. **Atrial fibrillation**

a. Early atrial fibrillation is diagnosed in up to one third of patients and usually occurs in the first 3 postoperative days.

b. Prevention is preferable and is usually achieved by prompt treatment of hypokalemia and hypomagnesemia, maintenance of Sao_2 greater than 90%, prevention of acidosis, and prophylaxis with β-adrenergic blockers.

c. Treatment: see Chapter 6.

2. **Atrial flutter**

a. Diagnosis: a regular atrial rate of 250 to 350 beats/min (typically 300 beats/min) on an atrial ECG using the external atrial pacing wires.

b. In patients with external atrial pacing wires, rapid atrial pacing may restore sinus rhythm.

3. **Ventricular arrhythmias**

a. PVCs are common after cardiac surgery. Unifocal PVCs raise the possibility of endocardial stimulation by a misplaced PA catheter tip. Treatment is relocation of the catheter; lidocaine is ineffective in suppressing mechanically induced PVCs. Multifocal PVCs are more likely a result of global metabolic insult and should prompt a thorough search for electrolyte imbalances, hypoxia, or myocardial ischemia. PVCs that occur greater than 10 to 12/min may be treated with a test dose of lidocaine 100 mg IV. Successful suppression of PVCs with the test dose may be followed by lidocaine 1 to 2 mg/kg IV continuous infusion.

b. Ventricular tachycardia/fibrillation is treated with immediate cardioversion and lidocaine 100 mg IV followed by lidocaine 1 to 2 mg/kg IV infusion.

E. HEMORRHAGE

1. **High chest tube output** (greater than 200 ml/hr) is either a result of a coagulopathy or focal mechanical bleeding site.

2. **Hemodynamically stable patients who are bleeding** should undergo thorough reversal of any coagulopathy. The order of treatment of coagulopathy is (a) reversal of heparin, (b) correction of hypocalcemia and hypothermia, (c) replacement of clotting factors, and (d) correction of thrombocytopenia. Apply the "five P rule": *P*EEP (increase to 8 cm H_2O column), *p*rotamine (if ACT remains abnormal), *p*lasma (transfuse FFP), *p*ressure (lower SBP and MAP with sodium nitroprusside [Nipride] as tolerated; elevating the head of the bed 45 degrees is helpful in decreasing venous pressure in the thorax and controlling persistent venous oozing), and *p*latelet transfusion.

a. Heparin reversal is guided by the ACT. Prolonged ACT is treated by repeated administration of protamine and measurement of ACT until a normal value is achieved. Heparin "wash-out" may cause delayed prolongation of the ACT after initially normal values and is treated with protamine. Excessive protamine (protamine-to-heparin ratio greater than 1.3:1.0) can produce significant prolongation of the ACT and may further increase clotting time and reduce platelet aggregation and function.

b. Prolongation of the PT/PTT indicates the need for FFP; hypofibrinogenemia requires cryoprecipitate.

c. Thrombocytopenia (platelet count < 50,000/mm^3) is treated with pooled platelets. Patients who receive aspirin preoperatively and bleed postoperatively should receive one pooled unit of platelets regardless of absolute platelet count. Acetaminophen 650 mg PR and diphenhydramine 25 mg IV may ameliorate transfusion-related fever.

d. Aprotinin (preferred for redo sternotomies) and aminocaproic acid 5 g IV bolus followed by 1g IV q1h bolus × 5 hours inhibits clot lysis and is sometimes helpful.

3. **Patients who have chest tube output** greater than 500 ml/hr or who display hemodynamic instability should be reexplored. After coagulopathy has been reversed, output greater than 100 ml/hr for 4 or more hours should also warrant reexploration.

F. RENAL FAILURE

1. **Mild elevation of the serum creatinine** is not an uncommon occurrence 24 to 48 hours postoperatively and requires no treatment.

2. **Hemodilution while on CPB may lower the serum creatinine** below the preoperative value, and a return to the preoperative value is expected with postoperative diuresis.

3. **Low-dose dopamine** (2.5 to 3.5 µg/kg/min) administered postoperatively has not been shown to ameliorate the renal dysfunction caused by intraoperative ischemia. However, in some patients with postoperative oliguria (despite adequate cardiac output), low-dose dopamine may potentiate the effect of diuretic drugs.

16

CARDIAC SURGERY

4. **Oliguria** (<30 ml/hr) warrants assessment of renal perfusion, SBP should be greater than 100, and Swan-Ganz catheter should be placed to ensure CI greater than 2 L/min/m². Bladder obstruction should also be ruled out. If renal perfusion is adequate and bladder obstruction is not present, loop diuretics should be used. Initially, furosemide 20 mg IV and increase by 20-mg increments until adequate urinary output is achieved. If furosemide fails to stimulate a response, ethacrynic acid 50 mg or metolazone 2.5 to 20 mg should be attempted.

5. **In patients requiring dialysis,** peritoneal dialysis is preferred because of its minimal effect on hemodynamics.

G. NEUROLOGIC COMPLICATIONS

1. Cerebrovascular accident

a. One of the most devastating complications following cardiac surgery is CVA. Incidence is 2% to 4%. The cause of stroke after cardiac surgery is usually embolic.

b. CVA is associated with an in-hospital mortality of 15% to 30%.

c. Evaluation of neurologic deficits includes a thorough neurologic examination, head CT, and consultation of the neurology service.

d. Treatment of focal neurologic deficit includes nonspecific measures, such as preventing hypoxia, hypoglycemia, and maintaining a higher blood pressure of systolic values between 150 to 180 mm Hg using intravascular volume expansion or dopamine infusion. The question of whether treatment should include anticoagulation is largely unresolved. The decision of anticoagulation has to be weighed between possible cardiac complications associated with postoperative anticoagulation and the chance to reduce recurrent events. Supportive services and rehabilitative care is initiated, such as occupational and physical therapy.

2. Peripheral nerve injuries

a. Peripheral nerve injury is quite common, and most deficits resolve within several months after surgery. These injuries include brachial plexus injury, unilateral vocal cord paralysis, and phrenic nerve damage.

b. Numbness in the last 2 to 3 digits is a frequent brachial plexus injury from stretching and compression of nerves during chest retraction. Also, the exposure of the femoral vessels, harvest of saphenous vein, and improper positioning may cause nerve injury. Treatment consists of physical therapy and counseling.

3. Neuropsychiatric changes

a. Frank postoperative psychosis may follow an initially lucid postoperative interval. Contributing factors include advanced age, presence of preoperative psychiatric illness, hypoxia, electrolyte disturbance, narcotic/benzodiazepine use, sleep deprivation, and ICU environment. Reorientation of the patient to time, date, and place is usually helpful. Contributing medications should be discontinued and hypoxia and electrolyte disorders corrected.

b. In severely agitated patients, haloperidol should be administered. In more difficult scenarios, psychiatric consultation is warranted.

4. Seizures

a. Systemic events that lower seizure threshold need to be considered to initiate treatment. Typically, these are hypoxemia, severe hyperglycemia, hypomagnesemia, hypocalcemia, hypoglycemia, hyponatremia, low levels of anticonvulsants, chronic meperidine treatment, and lidocaine antiarrhythmic therapy.

b. Management of postoperative seizures include close monitoring of vital signs, provision of a safe airway, and maximization of oxygen. Venous blood should be obtained for glucose, electrolytes (especially sodium and potassium), calcium, magnesium, CBC, ABGs, anticonvulsant level, if indicated, and 25 to 50 ml of 50% dextrose.

c. Parenteral anticonvulsants: lorazepam 2 to 4 mg IV or diazepam 5 to 30 mg IV push until seizure stops. Phenytoin is then loaded with 15 mg/kg IV and continued to achieve therapeutic serum levels. If seizures continue, consider general anesthesia with neuromuscular blockade. Phenobarbital 1 mg/kg IV every 5 to 10 minutes until seizure stops, up to 10 to 15 mg/kg (700 to 1000 mg over 30 minutes).

H. GASTROINTESTINAL COMPLICATIONS

1. Cholecystitis, calculous or acalculous.

2. Bowel perforation most commonly occurs as a result of a duodenal ulcer and is manifested as free air on the upright abdominal x-ray in association with abdominal pain and peritoneal signs. Duodenal perforation is rare in patients receiving adequate prophylaxis with H_2-blockers and/or buffering agents.

3. Bowel ischemia may occur intraoperatively because of insufficient flow during CPB or postoperatively because of low CO or embolus. Intraoperative ischemia may not manifest symptoms for the first 2 to 3 postoperative days, even with frank bowel necrosis. The cecum is the most commonly involved bowel segment.

4. Pancreatitis can be diagnosed with serum amylase and lipase. Treatment is usually bowel rest and supportive care.

I. INFECTIONS

1. Infections are rarely apparent before the patient leaves the ICU.

2. Mediastinitis is suspected in all patients with an unstable sternum. Sternal stability is assessed by gently rocking the sternum with hands placed to either side of the sternotomy. An alternative method is to place a hand on the upper third of the sternal incision while the patient coughs. In either case, a "clicking" sensation is indicative of an unstable sternum.

3. Sternal instability in association with an unexplained fever and leukocytosis is sufficient for the diagnosis of mediastinitis, even in the absence of purulent drainage.

4. Preferred treatment of mediastinitis is immediate reopening of the sternal wound, thorough irrigation of the mediastinum, IV antibiotics,

16

CARDIAC SURGERY

and q12h dressing changes. Delayed closure with appropriate muscle or omental flaps is accomplished in 4 to 5 days.

VI. FEATURES OF SPECIFIC CARDIAC OPERATIONS

A. CORONARY ARTERY BYPASS GRAFTING

1. **Graft occlusion:** Early graft occlusion occurs in 5% to 10% of patients. Presentation varies with the extent of ischemic myocardium and collateral flow. Signs of graft occlusion include sudden hypotension, ventricular arrhythmias, abrupt loss of contractility (not explainable by other mechanisms), and typical ECG changes (ST segment elevation). Emergent cardiac catheterization is diagnostic. Therapy for patients with severe ischemia consists of immediate reoperation.

2. **Mammary artery spasm:** Presentation similar to graft occlusion. Diagnosis is confirmed by cardiac catheterization. Initial therapy should consist of nifedipine 10 mg SL followed by Nipride and nitroglycerin infusions in an attempt to abort the spasm. Refractory spasm that results in hemodynamic instability is treated with reoperation and replacement of the mammary artery with a vein graft.

B. VALVULAR OPERATIONS

1. **Anticoagulation:** Therapeutic anticoagulation should be delayed for at least 48 hours postoperatively to ensure hemostasis. For mechanical prostheses, IV heparin is then started while warfarin (Coumadin) anticoagulation is achieved. Bioprosthetic valves require either aspirin or short-term warfarin anticoagulation (3 months).

2. **Arrhythmias:** Operations on both the mitral and aortic valves may result in injury to the cardiac conduction system and result in AV conduction delays or complete AV dissociation. The injury may be apparent immediately postoperatively or 24 to 48 hours later as a result of progressive inflammation and/or myocardial edema. Digoxin, β-adrenergic blockers, and calcium-channel blockers are stopped. Temporary pacing is continued, and if complete block persists for greater than 1 week, a permanent pacemaker is placed.

3. **Excessive preload:** Patients undergoing mitral valve replacement for mitral stenosis require special attention with respect to blood volume expansion because these patients exhibit a pronounced descending limb of the Starling curve. Acute fluid overload may initiate a downward spiral of reduced myocardial contractility.

4. **Hypertension:** Close vigilance is required to maintain a mean BP near 70 mm Hg because even transient hypertensive episodes may disrupt an aortotomy incision after aortic valve replacement (AVR).

C. VENTRICULAR ANEURYSMECTOMY

1. **Resection of a ventricular aneurysm should increase ejection.**

2. **Excessive resection of aneurysmal tissue** may result in a small ventricular chamber and poor diastolic performance. Cardiac output in these patients is especially dependent upon heart rate.

3. **Avoid hypertension:** keep MAP at 70 mm Hg.

D. LONG-TERM LVAD

1. **Types:** Thoratec (LVAD or BiVAD, pump external; Thoratec, Pleasanton, Calif.), Novacor (LVAD only, pump internal; Baxter Corp., Deerfield, Ill.), HeartMate (LVAD only, pump internal; Thermedics, Woburn, Mass.).
2. **Indications:** bridge to cardiac transplantation. Cardiogenic shock, PAWP greater than 20 mm Hg, CI less than 2.0 L/min/m^2, and failure of inotropes and IABP.
3. **Contraindications:** CVA, renal or hepatic failure, coagulopathy, and active infection.
4. **Acute complications:** right ventricular failure and hemorrhage.
5. **Goal:** recondition patient in preparation for heart transplant, and try to achieve physical rehabilitation and ambulation as soon as possible.
6. **Late complications:** drive line and pocket infections, thromboembolism.
7. **Chronic anticoagulation:** Novacor—warfarin, HeartMate—aspirin or low-dose warfarin.

E. CARDIAC TRANSPLANTATION

1. **Accepted treatment option** for end-stage heart disease not amenable to medical or other surgical therapy. A Vo_2 value between 10 and 15 ml/kg/min may be an objective indication if a steady decline has been noted. A fixed pulmonary vascular resistance (PVR) greater than 6 Wood units or a transpulmonary gradient greater than 15 mm Hg are contraindications. Severe dysfunction of other organ systems and malignancy are also contraindications.
2. **Postoperative course is dominated by denervated recipient heart physiology.** The cardiovascular system is circulating catecholamine dependent. Stress responses to hypovolemia, hypoxia, and anemia are delayed. This can lead to orthostatic hypotension secondary to lack of compensatory tachycardia. Myocardial ischemia can be silent resulting from lack of ascending nerve fibers. The transplanted heart relies on Frank-Starling mechanisms to increase CO. Pacing and isoproterenol are most effective ways to increase heart rate and therefore CO.

SUGGESTED READINGS

Cohn LH: The role of mechanical devices, *J Cardiovasc Surg* 5:278-281, 1990.

DiSesa VJ: Pharmacologic support for postoperative low cardiac output, *Semin Thorac Cardiovasc Surg* 3:13-23, 1991.

Hendren WG, Higgins TL: Immediate postoperative care of the cardiac surgical patient, *Semin Thorac Cardiovasc Surg* 3:3-12, 1991.

Inada E: Blood coagulation and autologous blood transfusion in cardiac surgery, *J Clin Anesth* 2:393-406, 1990.

Kirklin JW, Barratt-Boyes BG: *Postoperative care in cardiac surgery*, ed 2, New York, 1993, Churchill Livingstone.

Mangano DT: Myocardial ischemia following surgery: preliminary findings. Study of perioperative ischemia research group, *J Cardiovasc Surg* 5:288-293, 1990.

Scott WJ, Kessler R, Wernly JA: Blood conservation in cardiac surgery, *Ann Thorac Surg* 50:843-851, 1990.

PEDIATRIC SURGERY

Bryan C. Weidner

A. NEONATAL TRANSITIONAL PHYSIOLOGY

1. Respiratory

a. Fetal respiratory gas exchange occurs across the placenta.
   (1) O_2 uptake is enhanced by left-shifted dissociation curve of fetal Hgb.
   (2) Carrying capacity is improved by high Hgb concentration (14 to 20 g/dl).
b. Bronchial tree differentiation occurs between 24 and 28 weeks of gestation.
   (1) Cells lining the bronchial tree differentiate into type I lining cells or type II pneumocytes.
   (2) There is subsequent development of alveoli through 36 weeks of gestation.
c. Pulmonary surfactant is a combination of surface-active phospholipids and proteins.
   (1) Produced by type II pneumocytes
   (2) Lines terminal lung air spaces
   (3) Essential for maintaining alveolar stability
      (a) A change in pattern of amniotic fluid phospholipids (ratio of lecithin to sphingomyelin) reflects lung maturity.
      (b) L/S greater than 2 predicts less than 5% risk of developing hyaline membrane disease.
      (c) L/S greater than 3.5 predicts pulmonary maturity in infants of diabetic mothers.
      (d) Pulmonary maturity in infants at less than 34 weeks' gestation may be accelerated by maternal treatment with glucocorticoids (betamethasone or dexamethasone administered over 48 hours).
      (e) Exogenous surfactant may be administered to deficient infants (beractant [Survanta] 4 ml/kg via endotracheal tube q6h × 4 or colfosceril [Exosurf] 5 ml/kg via endotracheal tube q12h × 2-4).
         (i) Can decrease severity of hyaline membrane disease
         (ii) Can decrease incidence of pneumothorax
         (iii) Improves survival rates
d. Chest wall compliance decreases with increasing gestation.
   (1) Premature infants with pliable, compliant chest walls may be inefficient in generating effective negative intrathoracic pressure for inspiration.
   (2) The work of breathing is great for newborns with lung disease and high chest wall compliance.
   (3) Fetal fluid disappearance from the airways and alveoli occurs in conjunction with increased lung lymphatic flow after birth to permit gas exchange.

17

309

2. **Cardiovascular**
   a. Anatomic differences in fetal/postnatal circulation
   b. Fetal circulation
      (1) High fetal pulmonary vascular resistance
      (2) Low systemic resistance associated with placental circulation
      (3) Results in right-to-left flow across the ductus arteriosus
   c. Changes at birth
      (1) Lung expansion with increased alveolar Po_2
      (2) Resultant PA vasodilatation and decreased pulmonary vascular resistance
      (3) Increased arterial and mixed venous O_2 tension, which mediates umbilical artery and ductus arteriosus constriction
         (a) Ductus arteriosus and PA smooth muscle remain sensitive to changes in O_2 tension postnatally.
         (b) Hypoxemia from lung disease may lead to:
            (i) PA vasoconstriction
            (ii) Ductus dilatation with worsening shunt
            (iii) Worsening hypoxemia
      (4) Increased pulmonary venous return and systemic venous resistance
         (a) Increase in LAP to level above that of RA
         (b) Functional closure of right-to-left shunt through the foramen ovale

3. **Nutritional**
   a. All fetal nutrients are supplied by mother.
   b. Glucose is most important energy substrate for the fetus.
      (1) Diffusion across the placenta maintains a fetal blood glucose at 75% of the maternal level.
      (2) Fetal gluconeogenesis and glycogen stores are low.
         (a) Low glucagon levels
         (b) High insulin levels
      (3) Maintenance of postnatal glucose levels includes the following:
         (a) Oral intake
         (b) Increased glucagon levels
         (c) Decreased insulin levels
      (4) Newborns have limited ability to utilize fat or protein to synthesize glucose.
      (5) Hypoglycemia (<30 mg/dl) considerations include the following:
         (a) Manifestations
            (i) Apathy, weak cry
            (ii) Cyanosis
            (iii) Seizures
            (iv) Asymptomatic
         (b) Risk inversely related to gestational age
      (6) Hyperglycemia considerations include the following:
         (a) Result of reduced insulin response

(b) Most frequently seen in immature infants receiving parenteral nutrition

(c) May result in intraventricular hemorrhage and fluid/electrolyte derangements

c. Calcium is also important in fetal development.

(1) Necessary for normal fetal bone mineralization

(2) Delivered to fetus by active transport across the placenta (especially third trimester)

(3) Postnatal transient hypocalcemia

(a) Loss of maternal source

(b) Renal immaturity

(c) Parathyroid suppression from high fetal calcium

(d) Usually resolves by second day of life

(4) Persistent hypocalcemia

(a) Infants at risk

(i) Preterm or surgical infants

(ii) Infants requiring transfusions

(iii) Infants of diabetic mothers

(b) Symptoms

(i) Jitteriness

(ii) Seizures

(iii) Increased muscle tone

(c) Treatment

(i) 10% calcium gluconate 1 ml/kg IV over 10 minutes

(ii) Continuous ECG monitoring

(5) Hypomagnesemia

(a) May accompany hypocalcemia

(b) Treated with 50% magnesium sulfate 0.2 mg/kg IM

B. PEDIATRIC VITAL SIGNS AND MONITORING

1. Heart rate and rhythm

a. Monitor with continuous ECG.

b. Normal values vary with age (Table 17-1).

c. Increase in cardiac output is achieved by increase in HR.

d. Bradycardia frequently results from hypoxia and may be seen in patients in shock.

2. Blood pressure

a. Normal values vary with age (see Table 17-1).

b. Doppler ultrasound is the most accurate noninvasive method.

TABLE 17-1

NORMAL VITAL SIGNS OF CHILDREN

Age (years)	Pulse (bpm)	Blood Pressure (mm Hg)	Respirations (breaths/min)
0-1	120	80/40	40
1-5	100	100/60	30
5-10	80	120/80	20

17

PEDIATRIC SURGERY

   c. Intraarterial monitoring can be used for critically ill patients.
     (1) Radial, dorsalis pedis, and temporal arteries are common sites.
     (2) Umbilical artery may be used in newborns.
   d. Hypotension usually occurs very late in profound shock.

3. Central venous catheters
   a. CVP reflects volume status in the absence of cardiopulmonary disease.
     (1) Catheter tip should be in superior vena cava or RA.
     (2) Conditions that elevate CVP include the following:
       (a) Positive-pressure ventilation
       (b) Pneumothorax
       (c) Pericardial tamponade
       (d) Abdominal distention
     (3) The CVP trend is more useful than absolute numbers.
   b. Preferred sites for placement include the following:
     (1) Older infants and children—subclavian vein
     (2) Younger infants—facial vein
     (3) External or internal jugular or basilic veins acceptable
     (4) Femoral catheter placement less preferable because of contamination of groin

4. PA catheters
   a. Allow measurement of PA and pulmonary artery wedge pressures.
   b. Allow calculation of cardiac index (normal: 3.5-4.5 $L/min/m^2$) and Vo_2.

5. Oxygenation and ventilation
   a. Variance of normal respiratory rate with age (see Table 17-1)
   b. Apnea monitor
     (1) The tendency for apnea is greater with premature infants.
     (2) Many other pathologic conditions increase the frequency and severity of apneic events.
   c. Pulse oximetry
     (1) Measures Sao_2 by absorption spectrophotometry
     (2) Benefits
       (a) Rapid response time
       (b) Continuous monitoring
       (c) No calibration required
     (3) Limitations
       (a) Patients with poor arterial pulsations
       (b) Anemia
       (c) Jaundice, dark skin
   d. End-tidal carbon dioxide
     (1) Noninvasive, continuous monitor of alveolar, and therefore arteriolar, CO_2
     (2) Based on absorption of infrared light by carbon dioxide gas
   e. ABG
     (1) May use umbilical artery in newborn
     (2) Useful for monitoring adequacy of oxygenation, ventilation, and perfusion

6. **Urinary output**
a. Useful parameter in monitoring fluid management
b. Continuous monitoring
   (1) Foley catheter
   (2) Bag placed over urethral opening in smaller infants
c. Appropriate urinary output is 1 to 2 ml/kg/hr

7. **Body weight**
a. Acute changes reflect changes in total body water.
b. Serial measurements are useful guides in fluid replacement.
c. Newborns undergo significant diuresis on the first day of life with normal loss of total body water and weight.

8. **Temperature**
a. Skin probes continuously monitor body temperature in neonates and infants
b. Heat production in newborn
   (1) Newborns cannot shiver
   (2) Heat production through reflexive increase in nonshivering thermogenesis (mobilization of brown fat deposits) with capacity proportional to body weight.
c. Heat loss in newborn
   (1) Loss of amniotic fluid insulation at birth can result in significant heat loss.
   (2) Heat loss is proportional to body surface area.
      (a) Newborns at disadvantage because body surface area is quite large in proportion to body weight.
      (b) Rate of heat loss may overwhelm heat-producing capacity in newborn.
   (3) Heat loss may necessitate use of thermally controlled environment (overhead radiant heaters or warming lamps).

C. **FLUIDS AND ELECTROLYTES**
1. **Renal function**
a. GFR in a newborn is 25% that of an adult.
   (1) GFR reaches adult levels by 18 to 24 months.
   (2) GFR in a preterm infant is slightly lower than in a full-term infant.
b. Concentrating ability in infants is lower than in adults.
   (1) Preterm infant—400 mOsm/kg
   (2) Full-term infant—600 mOsm/kg
   (3) Adults—1200 mOsm/kg
c. Premature neonates must diurese significant extracellular and postnatal total body water in a short period after birth.
   (1) Total body water
      (a) 80% of body weight at 32 weeks' gestation
      (b) 75% by the end of the first postnatal week
      (c) Adult levels (60%) by 18 months
   (2) Extracellular fluid volume
      (a) 45% body weight at birth
      (b) 20% by 24 months

17

PEDIATRIC SURGERY

2. **Fluid and electrolyte requirements include the following:**
a. Insensible water loss
   (1) Loss from the respiratory tract (one third of total loss)
       (a) Loss is 12 ml/kg/day for full-term infants in a thermoneutral environment and 50% humidity.
       (b) Loss increases (up to 10 times) with increasing prematurity.
   (2) Loss from skin
       (a) Stratum corneum
           (i) Major barrier component of the skin
           (ii) Less well developed in premature infants
       (b) Warmers, phototherapy
           (i) May increase skin loss by up to 50% in full-term infants
           (ii) May increase skin loss by up to 100% in premature infants
       (c) Perspiration
           (i) Full-term infants sweat if body temperature is greater than 37.5° C.
           (ii) Premature infants do not sweat at birth.
b. Renal water requirements
   (1) Depend on solute load and concentrating ability of the kidneys.
   (2) Concentrating ability of kidneys depends on gestational age.
   (3) Solute loads are the following:
       (a) At birth—15 mOsm/kg/day
       (b) After the second week of life—30 mOsm/kg/day
       (c) Increased solute load results from oral diet, catabolic state, and postsurgery/trauma
c. Gastrointestinal water loss
   (1) Normal stool water loss is relatively inconsequential.
   (2) Vomiting, diarrhea, and fistula output should be measured and replaced.
d. Sodium
   (1) Two mEq/kg/day for full-term newborns
   (2) Between 4 and 5 mEq/kg/day for critically ill premature infants
   (3) Newborns able to retain sodium but cannot excrete excess well
e. Potassium
   (1) Two mEq/kg/day, required
   (2) Significant catabolic state with protein and potassium loss may require more
f. Bicarbonate
   (1) Metabolic acidosis from underperfusion
       (a) Treat underlying cause.
       (b) Manage temporarily with dilute bicarbonate solutions (1 mEq/kg).
   (2) Metabolic alkalosis accompanying vomiting or orogastric suctioning
       (a) Result of dehydration and loss of gastric HCl
       (b) Correction with appropriate fluid/electrolyte replacement

D. VENTILATORY SUPPORT

1. **Monitoring:** See section I, B, 5.
2. **Mechanical ventilation**
a. Indications
   (1) Severe respiratory acidosis (pH < 7.2)
   (2) Severe hypoxemia (Pao_2 < 60 mm Hg, Fio_2 > 70%)
   (3) Neonatal apnea
   (4) Pulmonary toilet
   (5) Airway obstruction
   (6) Patient fatigue
b. Endotracheal tubes
   (1) Size
      (a) Premature infants: 3 mm
      (b) Full-term newborns through 6 months: 3.5 mm
      (c) Age greater than 6 months: (16 + age)/4 mm
   (2) Uncuffed tube for infants and young children
   (3) May remain in place for weeks before tracheostomy needs to be considered
c. Ventilatory mode (see Chapter 21)
   (1) Children heavier than 10 kg can be managed with volume-cycled ventilators
   (2) Infants lighter than 10 kg are best managed with pressure-cycled ventilators
   (3) PIP
      (a) Increasing PIP increases tidal volume, improves CO_2 elimination
      (b) From 12 to 18 cm H_2O (normal lungs), 20 to 25 cm H_2O (respiratory distress syndrome)
   (4) PEEP
      (a) Prevents alveolar collapse
      (b) Increasing PEEP may increase oxygenation but decrease ventilation
      (c) From 2 to 3 cm H_2O (normal lungs), 4 to 5 cm H_2O (respiratory distress syndrome)
   (5) Frequency: Between 10 and 20/min (normal lungs), 20 to 40 (respiratory distress syndrome)
   (6) I:E ratio
      (a) Normally 1:2
      (b) Reversal of I:E ratio may improve oxygenation but increase mean airway pressure
   (7) Fio_2
      (a) Initial setting 100%
      (b) Titrate to keep Pao_2 60 to 80 mm Hg
      (c) Complications—atelectasis, bronchopulmonary dysplasia, retrolental fibroplasia in premature infants

17

PEDIATRIC SURGERY

(8) High-frequency ventilation (jet or oscillating)
   (a) Infants who have failed mechanical ventilation
   (b) Frequency 15 to 600
   (c) Fio_2 100% (titrate to Pao_2 60 to 80 mm Hg)
   (d) Theoretically improves oxygenation at lower peak airway pressures
   (e) Less barotrauma
   (f) May decrease output from bronchopleural fistula
   (g) Jet
      (i) Passive exhalation
      (ii) Frequency 150 to 600
   (h) Oscillating
      (i) Active exhalation
      (ii) Frequency 200 to 1000
(9) ECMO: For patients with reversible cardiopulmonary disease who fail conventional ventilatory methods (see Chapter 19)

E. HEMODYNAMIC SUPPORT
1. Shock
a. Sepsis
   (1) Most common cause of shock in infants and children
   (2) Insufficient Do_2
      (a) Severe decrease in SVR with maldistribution of blood flow
      (b) Cardiac output generally elevated but can be depressed
   (3) Usually caused by gram-negative bacteria
   (4) Associated conditions
      (a) Intestinal perforation
      (b) Urinary tract infection
      (c) Respiratory tract infection
      (d) Contaminated IV catheters
   (5) Neonates—particularly susceptible because of immature host defenses
      (a) Decreased storage pool of poorly functioning neutrophils
      (b) Reduced immunoglobulin levels
   (6) Treatment
      (a) Fluid resuscitation
      (b) Broad-spectrum antibiotic administration
      (c) Vasoactive support
      (d) Correctable surgical conditions ruled out
      (e) Experimental treatments
         (i) Granulocyte transfusions
         (ii) Granulocyte colony-stimulating factors
         (iii) Intravenous immunoglobulin
         (iv) Antibodies to endotoxin or TNF
b. Hypovolemic shock
   (1) Dehydration
      (a) Causes
         (i) Sensible losses (e.g., vomiting, diarrhea)
         (ii) Insensible losses (e.g., evaporative, third-spacing)

        (b) Fluid lost usually hypotonic
           (i) More water lost than electrolytes
           (ii) Results in a hypertonic dehydration
        (c) Emergency treatment with hypotonic solutions of NaCl
     (2) Hemorrhage
        (a) May be due to trauma, coagulation abnormality
        (b) Resuscitation with blood/blood products
        (c) Must control hemorrhage
           (i) Operative control if indicated
           (ii) Coagulation factors replaced
  c. Diagnosis
     (1) Clinical evidence of impaired tissue perfusion
        (a) Slow capillary refill (>3 seconds), weak pulses, cool
           extremities
        (b) Tachypnea, tachycardia, hypoxemia, acidosis
        (c) Oliguria
        (d) Altered mental status
        (e) Thrombocytopenia
     (2) Data from invasive monitoring

2. Resuscitation
  a. Fluids
     (1) Lactated Ringer's 20 ml/kg, by rapid IV infusion
        (a) Some prefer colloid (e.g., 5% albumin solution).
        (b) Blood may be used if the hemorrhage is the cause for shock.
        (c) If there is no response, administer second bolus.
     (2) Metabolic acidosis should be treated with $NaHCO_3$
     (3) Consider placing a central venous catheter
     (4) Search for sites of ongoing fluid loss
  b. Pharmacologic support
     (1) May be necessary to optimize cardiac output and Do_2.
     (2) See discussion in Chapter 2.
  c. Progress closely monitored
  d. Underlying cause of hemodynamic instability treated

F. NUTRITION (see Chapter 22)
1. Assessment
  a. Physical variables (weight, length, head circumference, triceps
    skin fold)
  b. Laboratory assessment
     (1) Serum albumin
        (a) From 2.8 to 3.5 g/dl suggests moderate malnutrition.
        (b) Less than 2.8 g/dl indicates severe malnutrition.
        (c) Normal newborns may have low levels.
     (2) Serum transferrin
        (a) More sensitive than albumin
        (b) Shorter half-life (9 vs. 20 days) than albumin
     (3) Lymphocyte count

2. Fluid/electrolyte requirements

a. The volume requirement calculation is based on the infant's weight.
   (1) First 10 kg—100 ml/kg/day (4 ml/kg/hr)
   (2) Next 10 kg—50 ml/kg/day (+100 ml/day for first 10 kg)
   (3) Every kilogram thereafter—20 ml/kg/day (+1500 ml/day for first 20 kg)
b. The volume requirement may increase because of increased insensible losses.

3. Caloric/protein requirement

a. Typical age-dependent requirements are listed in Table 17-2.
b. Ideal diet (percent in calories)
   (1) Carbohydrate 50%
   (2) Fat 35%
   (3) Protein 15% (230 nonprotein kcal/g nitrogen)
c. Requirements increased during certain periods
   (1) Fever increases caloric requirements 12%/° C greater than 37° C.
   (2) Major surgery increases caloric requirements 20% to 30%.
   (3) Severe sepsis increases caloric requirements 40% to 50%.
   (4) Long-term growth failure increases caloric requirements up to 100%.
d. The metabolic rate can be calculated from oxygen consumption (see Chapter 1)
e. A positive nitrogen balance is achieved in an anabolic state

4. Enteral nutrition

a. Always preferable to use GI tract for feedings
   (1) Breast milk is the preferred source of nutrition for infants.
   (2) Commonly used formulas are listed in Table 17-3.
   (3) Enteral nutrition may be most efficient if it is delivered through a feeding tube.
b. Typical protocol for enteral feeding of neonates
   (1) Begin with 15 ml Pedialyte every 3 hours.
   (2) Increase volume 5 ml with each feed for a day.
   (3) Advance to half-strength formula for a day.
   (4) Advance to full-strength formula.
c. Special considerations
   (1) Hyperosmolar feeds may produce diarrhea.

TABLE 17-2

AGE-DEPENDENT CALORIE AND PROTEIN REQUIREMENTS

Age (years)	Kilocalories (kcal/kg/day)	Protein (g/kg/day)
Low-birth-weight infant	130-150	3-4
Neonate	110-120	3.0-3.5
<1year	90-120	2-3
1-7	75-90	2-2.5
12-18	30-60	1.5
18	25-30	1

17

PEDIATRIC SURGERY

TABLE 17-3

COMMONLY USED INFANT FORMULAS

Formula	Calories (kcal/ml)	Na (mEq/L)	K (mEq/L)	Ca (mEq/L)	P (mEq/L)	Fe (mEq/L)	Osmolarity (mOsm/L)
Breast milk	0.67	7	14	340	162	1.5	100
Cow's milk	0.67	25	35	1240	950	1	270
Enfamil	0.67	11	19	546	462	<1	285
Nutramigen	0.67	14	17	630	473	13	450
Portagen	0.67	14	21	630	473	13	210
Pregestimil	0.67	14	17	630	473	13	311
ProSobee	0.67	18	19	788	525	13	250
Similac	0.67	11	19	580	430	<1	285

(2) Non—lactose-containing formulas (e.g., Isomil, ProSobee) may be better tolerated in the early postoperative period.

(3) Predigested formulas may be better tolerated in patients with short gut syndrome.

(4) Increases in volume are usually better tolerated than increases in osmolarity.

5. Parenteral nutrition

a. Route of delivery

   (1) Central venous catheterization

     (a) Permits administration of hypertonic solutions

     (b) Carries the risks of central line placement

   (2) Peripheral route

     (a) Short-term parenteral alimentation

     (b) Partial nutritional support

b. Indications

   (1) Newborns expected to be without enteral nutrition for more than 5 days

   (2) Gastrointestinal disease

     (a) Short bowel syndrome

     (b) Necrotizing enterocolitis

     (c) Inflammatory bowel disease

     (d) Gastroschisis

     (e) Omphalocele

     (f) Intestinal atresia

c. Initiation (Figure 17-1)

   (1) Protein

     (a) Begin at 1 g/kg/day.

     (b) Increase to 2 to 3 g/kg/day.

   (2) Glucose

     (a) Begin at 7 g/kg/day.

     (b) Increase to about 20 g/kg/day.

   (3) Fat (lipid): 1 to 4 g/kg/day as a 10% to 20% emulsion

d. Monitoring

   (1) Daily weight

   (2) Serum electrolytes twice per week

   (3) Serum triglycerides, albumin, liver enzymes, calcium, phosphorous, and magnesium each week

   (4) Vitamins A, D, B_{12}, folate, and zinc each month

   (5) More frequent laboratory assessment at initiation of TPN

e. Complications

   (1) Electrolyte abnormalities, hyperlipidemia, trace element deficiencies

   (2) Fluid overload

   (3) Catheter sepsis

   (4) Hepatic dysfunction, cholestatic jaundice, hyperammonemia

DUKE UNIVERSITY MEDICAL CENTER

DOCTORS' ORDERS

DAILY PARENTERAL ALIMENTATION ORDER SHEET—PEDIATRICS

TECH _____   PHARMACIST _____

DATE	TIME	DOCTORS' ORDERS		HUC ACTION DATE/TIME INITIALS	NURSE ACTION DATE/TIME INITIALS
		PATIENT WEIGHT =	kg		
		TOTAL VOLUME/24 hours=	mls		
		RATE =	ml/hr		
		Containing:			
		Dextrose %	g		
		Crystalline amino acids			
		(AMINOSYN)	g		
		Sodium	mEq		
		Chloride	mEq		
		Potassium	mEq		
		Phosphate	MM		
		Calcium	g		
		(100 mg. calcium gluconate = 0.5 mEq)			
		Magnesium	mEq		
		Multivitamin (PEDIATRIC,TPN)	ml		
		(Circle one desired)			
		Copper	µg		
		Zinc	µg		
		Heparin	units		
		Fat emulsion cc/ hours			
		Physician signature			

FIGURE 17-1

Duke University Medical Center parenteral nutrition doctors' orders sheet.

17

PEDIATRIC SURGERY

II. RESPIRATORY DISTRESS IN INFANTS AND CHILDREN

A. PRESENTATION

1. Assessment

a. Early signs of respiratory distress
   (1) Restlessness, feeding difficulties
   (2) Tachypnea, retractions and stridor
b. Later signs
   (1) Bradycardia, cyanosis
   (2) Unresponsiveness and cardiopulmonary arrest

2. Initial management

a. Chest radiograph
   (1) Obtain on all patients with signs of respiratory distress.
   (2) Help differentiate surgical from nonsurgical conditions.
   (3) Place radio-opaque orogastric tube for assessment of TE anomalies in newborns.
   (4) Lateral soft-tissue films of neck are useful in children with upper airway obstruction.
   (5) Inspiratory/expiratory x-rays or fluoroscopy may demonstrate air-trapping resulting from bronchial obstruction with a radiolucent object.
b. Monitoring
   (1) Observation in an intensive care setting
   (2) Continuous pulse-oximetry
   (3) Serial ABG determinations to assess adequacy of oxygenation, ventilation
c. Maintenance of patent airway
   (1) Endotracheal intubation, tracheostomy if indicated
   (2) Removal of oral, pharyngeal, and tracheal secretions with suctioning
   (3) Use of humidified supplemental O_2

B. SPECIFIC CONDITIONS

1. Congenital diaphragmatic (Bochdalek's) hernia

a. Failure of closure of the posterior pleuroperitoneal canal
b. Permits herniation of abdominal contents into the chest
c. Pathophysiologic consequences
   (1) Inhibition of ipsilateral lung growth
   (2) May also retard contralateral lung growth with mediastinal shift
   (3) Pulmonary vascular immaturity
   (4) May develop pulmonary hypertension and persistent fetal circulation
d. Presentation
   (1) May be diagnosed in utero (maternal referral to tertiary care center indicated)
   (2) May be asymptomatic or have cardiopulmonary collapse
   (3) Physical examination
      (a) Respiratory distress
      (b) Decreased breath sounds in one chest, usually the left (90%)

      (c) Cyanosis

      (d) Scaphoid abdomen

    (4) Bowel gas and nasogastric tube in the chest shown by CXR

    (5) Differential diagnosis

      (a) Diaphragmatic eventration

      (b) Congenital cystic adenomatoid malformation

e. Management

    (1) Orogastric tube for GI decompression

    (2) Endotracheal intubation and mechanical ventilation

      (a) Low Pco_2, high pH maintained

      (b) Tube thoracostomy as needed

    (3) Additional therapies

      (a) ECMO considered for patients not adequately oxygenated with conventional or high-frequency jet ventilation

      (b) Pulmonary vasodilators

    (4) Operative repair of diaphragmatic defect once patient stabilized

2. Congenital cystic adenomatoid malformation

a. Multicystic mass of pulmonary tissue with a proliferation of bronchial structures

b. May be symptomatic in the early neonatal period

c. Treatment

    (1) Surgical excision, usually lobectomy

    (2) Indicated even if the patient is asymptomatic

3. Congenital lobar emphysema

a. Hyperinflated, poorly ventilated lobe (usually upper)

b. Pathophysiology

    (1) A cartilaginous deficiency is in the tracheobronchial tree.

    (2) Bronchial obstruction develops.

    (3) Progressive distress results from compression of surrounding normal parenchyma.

c. High incidence of associated cardiac anomalies

d. Diagnosis

    (1) CXR does not always demonstrate hyperaeration.

    (2) Diagnosis can be made by V/Q or CT scan.

e. Lobectomy—curative; may require emergent surgery

4. Pneumothorax

a. Frequent complication of mechanical ventilation, especially in premature infants

b. Treatment

    (1) May resolve spontaneously in otherwise healthy infants (may hasten resolution by high, inspired Fio_2 improving the gradient for poorly diffusing nitrogen)

    (2) Indications for tube thoracostomy (see Chapter 5)

      (a) Symptomatic pneumothoraxes

      (b) Pneumothoraxes in patients requiring positive-pressure ventilation

17

PEDIATRIC SURGERY

(3) Should perform needle aspiration of chest for immediate decompression of suspected tension pneumothorax

5. Airway obstruction

a. Potentially fatal, necessitating thorough, early, rapid evaluation

b. Relationship of stridor to site of obstruction

    (1) Inspiratory—vocal cord, cervical trachea

    (2) Expiratory—intrathoracic trachea

    (3) Biphasic—subglottic

c. Evaluation

    (1) Awake laryngoscopy in the stable patient can identify the following:

        (a) Palatal defects

        (b) Hypopharyngeal tumors, subglottic masses

        (c) Laryngomalacia

    (2) Lateral airway film may demonstrate the following:

        (a) Epiglottitis

        (b) Supraglottic obstruction

    (3) Unstable patients should be taken to the operating room.

        (a) Intubation or tracheostomy

        (b) Bronchoscopy for complete evaluation from oropharynx to proximal tracheobronchial tree

d. Causes of airway obstruction

    (1) Congenital

        (a) Choanal atresia

        (b) Macroglossia/mandibular hypoplasia

        (c) Laryngomalacia

        (d) Laryngeal web, cyst

        (e) Hemangioma

    (2) Acquired

        (a) Adenoid hypertrophy

        (b) Vocal cord paralysis

        (c) Subglottic stenosis

    (3) Inflammatory

        (a) Epiglottitis

        (b) Croup

        (c) Bacterial tracheitis

        (d) Tonsillar hypertrophy

        (e) Peritonsillar/retropharyngeal abscess

        (f) Foreign body

    (4) Tumor

III. GASTROINTESTINAL EMERGENCIES IN THE NEONATE

A. GENERAL STRATEGY FOR EVALUATION

1. Rule out mechanical obstruction (congenital atresias).

2. Evaluate other causes.

B. INITIAL ASSESSMENT

1. History

a. Maternal hydramnios
  (1) Normal amniotic fluid dynamics
    (a) Swallowed by the fetus
    (b) Resorbed by the intestine
    (c) Excreted by the kidney
  (2) Fetal GI obstruction
    (a) Fetal GI obstruction interrupts the amniotic fluid cycle, causing hydramnios (>2 L amniotic fluid).
    (b) 15% to 20% of these newborns will have GI obstruction.
  (3) Decreased amniotic fluid (oligohydramnios) associated with renal disorders
b. Bilious emesis
  (1) Suggests obstruction distal to the ampulla of Vater
    (a) This is a surgical emergency.
    (b) Consider mechanical obstruction, specifically malrotation with midgut volvulus.
  (2) Non—bile-stained vomitus
    (a) Possible prepyloric obstruction (pyloric atresia/stenosis)
    (b) May be due to nonsurgical, nonobstructing conditions (e.g., GE reflux)
c. Delay of postnatal events
  (1) Normal bowel gas pattern
    (a) Air to the cecum by sixth hour of life
    (b) May take another 20 hours for air to reach rectum
  (2) Failure to pass meconium within 24 hours suggests obstruction

2. Physical examination
a. Abdomen
  (1) Scaphoid: suggests proximal GI obstruction
  (2) Distended
    (a) Suggests distal GI obstruction
    (b) Rapid distention: possible esophageal atresia with distal TE fistula
b. Obvious anomalies
  (1) Incarcerated hernia
  (2) Gastroschisis
  (3) Omphalocele
  (4) Imperforate anus

3. Evaluation
a. Place orogastric tube.
  (1) Aspirate contents; obstruction is suggested if aspirate is greater than 10 ml or fluid is bile-stained.
  (2) Insufflate 25 ml air and clamp tube.
b. Obtain chest/abdominal radiograph.
  (1) Tube coiled in the neck—esophageal atresia (with distal TE fistula if air present in GI tract)
  (2) Free air seen under diaphragm on upright radiograph—hollow viscus perforation

17

PEDIATRIC SURGERY

    (3) Intraabdominal calcifications associated with prenatal perforation

    (4) Failure of air to pass through to the distal bowel

       (a) Suggests intestinal obstruction

       (b) May be difficult to distinguish small from large bowel in a neonate

  c. Obtain contrast study to further evaluate possible intestinal obstruction.

    (1) Proximal bowel obstruction

       (a) Cecum is in the right upper quadrant by barium enema in malrotation.

       (b) Follow a normal barium enema by an upper GI series.

          (i) A barium enema may only be suggestive of malrotation.

          (ii) A barium enema will not demonstrate other causes of proximal obstruction.

       (c) Proceed directly to upper GI series without barium enema.

          (i) If KUB suggests obstruction

          (ii) If suspicion for malrotation is high

       (d) Performing upper GI first may preclude immediate subsequent barium enema because of the residual contrast.

    (2) Distal obstruction

       (a) Contrast enema performed with a high-osmolar, water-soluble agent

       (b) May be therapeutic and diagnostic

C. SPECIFIC CONDITIONS

1. Esophageal atresia (with TE fistula)

  a. Presenting symptoms/radiograph dependent on anatomic configuration

    (1) Pure atresia (5%) or atresia with a proximal fistula (<1%)

       (a) Inability to swallow, excess secretions, tachypnea with aspiration of saliva

       (b) Orogastric tube coiled in mediastinum, no GI air

    (2) Atresia with distal fistula (85%)

       (a) Respiratory distress as a result of reflux of gastric contents in the lungs

       (b) Orogastric tube coiled in mediastinum, normal GI gas pattern

    (3) Fistula alone (5%) has more subtle symptoms

       (a) Intermittent choking

       (b) Cyanosis with feeding

       (c) Recurrent pneumonia

       (d) Plain film usually normal

  b. Preoperative management

    (1) Patient should be placed in a partly upright position with head elevated and with repeated suction of the upper esophageal pouch.

    (2) Assess for associated anomalies (occur in 30% to 40% of cases).

    (3) Preoperative bronchoscopy may be helpful in defining fistula(s).

    (4) Gastrostomy may be placed as a temporizing measure in patients not ready for operative repair.

    (5) "Wide-gap" atresia may benefit from gradual stretching with metal sounds.

c. Postoperative considerations
   (1) Maintain an upright position with neck flexed and orogastric tube securely in place.
   (2) Use nebulized air and intermittent endotracheal suctioning.
   (3) Obtain an esophagram on the fifth postoperative day.
       (a) Remove orogastric tube and initiate feeds if no leak present.
       (b) Remove extrapleural chest tube once feeds have been tolerated for 24 hours.

2. Malrotation

a. Anatomy
   (1) Small bowel primarily on the right side of abdomen
   (2) Colon on the left
   (3) Partial distal duodenal obstruction and failure of the duodenal loop to cross back to the left upper quadrant
b. Clinical presentation
   (1) Acute midgut volvulus
       (a) Sudden onset of bilious vomiting
       (b) With or without abdominal distention and pain
       (c) Results from ischemia caused by occlusion of the superior mesenteric artery by twisted mesentery
   (2) Duodenal obstruction
       (a) May have acute or chronic symptoms
       (b) Results from complete/partial obstruction by peritoneal bands and/or midgut volvulus
c. Management
   (1) Vigorous fluid resuscitation
   (2) Broad-spectrum antibiotics
   (3) Radiographic evaluation
   (4) Emergent operative intervention
       (a) Neonates with bilious emesis in whom malrotation cannot definitively be excluded
       (b) Immediate exploration because acute midgut volvulus is a potentially catastrophic event

3. Abdominal wall defects

a. Gastroschisis
   (1) Intestinal herniation through a perforation in the umbilical ring
       (a) Probably result of atrophy of the right (usually) embryonic umbilical vein
       (b) Not associated with other anatomic anomalies
   (2) Pathophysiologic consequences
       (a) No peritoneal covering over eviscerated bowel
       (b) Inflammation of this bowel a result of irritating effect of amniotic fluid in utero
       (c) Significant fluid loss from the exposed inflamed bowel after birth

        (3) Immediate therapy
            (a) Vigorous fluid resuscitation
            (b) Bowel supported and wrapped in moistened gauze
            (c) Neonate placed in a plastic bag with only head outside
            (d) Operative repair

b. Omphalocele
    (1) Arrest in development of the anterior abdominal wall
    (2) Associated anomalies in 35% of patients
    (3) Immediate treatment
        (a) Fluid losses not excessive if peritoneal lining or sac is intact
        (b) Peritoneal sac protected from rupture preoperatively with petroleum gauze
        (c) Operative repair

c. Perioperative considerations
    (1) Prolonged ventilatory support and TPN are likely to be required.
    (2) Use of a Silastic silo may be necessary.
        (a) Required if the bowel cannot be safely returned to the abdominal cavity because of respiratory compromise
        (b) Permits gradual return of intestines into abdomen over 1 week

4. Necrotizing enterocolitis

a. Most common acquired GI emergency in neonates

b. 50% overall mortality rate

c. Pathophysiology
    (1) Acute inflammatory process involving the intestine
        (a) Gut ischemia/hypoxia
        (b) Bacterial overgrowth or abnormal flora in the presence of enteral feeding
    (2) Associated conditions
        (a) Prematurity with average birthweight of 1.5 g and average gestational age of 31 weeks
        (b) Hypoxia, shock
        (c) Cytopenia
        (d) Umbilical artery catheterization
        (e) Polycythemia
        (f) Congenital heart disease
        (g) Early rapid feedings or hyperosmolar feedings
        (h) Blood transfusions

d. Presentation
    (1) Symptoms
        (a) Lethargy
        (b) Abdominal distention with edema/erythema of the abdominal wall
        (c) Feeding intolerance, bilious emesis
        (d) Bloody diarrhea
    (2) Radiographic findings
        (a) Dilated loops of the intestine may be the only abnormality.
        (b) Characteristic pneumatosis intestinalis may be present.

(c) Portal venous gas suggests advanced disease.

(d) Contrast enema is contraindicated.

e. Management

(1) Nonoperative interventions

(a) Fluid resuscitation and cardiopulmonary support

(b) Bowel rest/decompression and parenteral nutrition

(c) Broad-spectrum antibiotics

(d) Blood cultures

(e) Correction of anemia and coagulopathy

(f) Frequent abdominal examinations (premature infants may not exhibit classic signs of intestinal gangrene, such as fever, leukocytosis, and abdominal tenderness)

(g) Serial abdominal radiographs

(h) Serial lactates may be helpful

(2) Indications for surgical intervention (ideal timing of surgery is after advent of intestinal gangrene but before perforation; negative exploratory laparotomy carries high risk to these extremely ill patients)

(a) Intestinal perforation and pneumoperitoneum

(b) Portal venous gas

(c) Positive paracentesis

(d) Erythema/edema of the abdominal wall

(e) Fixed/tender abdominal mass

(f) Fixed loop on radiograph

(g) Clinical deterioration

(3) Goals of operative intervention

(a) Excision of gangrenous bowel

(b) Exteriorization of marginally viable ends (may require multiple ostomies)

(c) Preservation of as much intestine as possible

IV. PEDIATRIC TRAUMA

A. GENERAL PRINCIPLES

1. Leading cause of death in children (ages 1 to 15)

a. Over 20,000 deaths annually

b. More than 100,000 cases of permanent disability per year (mostly neurologic)

2. Differences from the management of adult trauma

a. Accident patterns

(1) Most accidents result from blunt trauma (80%).

(2) Head trauma is very common.

(a) Results in most morbidity and mortality

(b) Orthopedic injuries responsible for almost all remaining morbidity

b. Physiologic

(1) Small amounts of blood loss represent a significant percentage of total body blood volume.

(2) Water and heat loss can be much greater than in adult trauma.

(3) Gastric dilatation is common in children.
    (a) Vomiting
    (b) Aspiration
(4) Basal metabolic rate/nutritional requirements are higher.
c. Psychologic
    (1) Patients may have difficulty in expressing complaints and assessing pain.
    (2) Fear and stress may result in misleading signs and physical findings.
3. Trauma score (Table 17-4)
a. Reflects severity of injury
b. Patient transferred to pediatric trauma center if score is less than 9
B. EMERGENCY MANAGEMENT
1. Standard ABCs of CPR
2. Vascular access
a. Place a large-bore peripheral intravenous line.
    (1) If not possible, use the following:
        (a) Subclavian line in larger patients
        (b) Distal saphenous vein cutdown in smaller patients
    (2) Groin lines are less favored.
b. Intraosseous catheters may be placed in children 5 years and younger.
    (1) Equipment (any of the following may be used)
        (a) An 18- to 20-gauge spinal needle
        (b) Bone marrow needle
        (c) Commercial intraosseous line kit

TABLE 17-4

PEDIATRIC TRAUMA SCORE

Criteria		Score
Size (kg)	>20	+2
	10-20	+1
	<10	−1
Airway	Normal	+2
	Maintainable	+1
	Not maintainable	−1
Systolic blood pressure	>90 mm Hg (palpable radial)	+2
	50-90 mm Hg (groin pulse only)	+1
	<50 mm Hg (pulse not palpable)	−1
CNS status	Awake	+2
	Partially conscious or unconscious	+1
	Decerebrate	−1
Open wounds	None	+2
	Minor	+1
	Major	−1
Skeletal injury	None	+2
	Closed fracture	+1
	Open/multiple fractures	−1

(2) Placement
(a) Common site is one to two fingerbreadths below tibial tubercle on anteromedial aspect of tibia
(b) Direct needle inferiorly to avoid growth plate
(c) Penetrate bone with continuous pressure and screwing motion
(d) Marrow entry signified by loss of resistance—confirm with aspiration

3. Shock
a. Almost always caused by hemorrhage
b. Treat with vigorous fluid resuscitation

C. ABDOMINOPELVIC TRAUMA
1. Penetrating trauma (20%) is managed in a similar manner as adults.
2. Abdominal trauma in children is usually blunt.
3. Evaluation includes the following:
a. Abdomen assessed through serial examinations
b. Serial laboratory studies (hematocrit, urinalysis, amylase, liver enzymes)
c. CT scanning
(1) Indications
(a) Stable patients with history (e.g., high-energy blunt trauma) or examination suggestive of intraabdominal injury
(b) Multiple system injury, especially head trauma
(c) Significant volume requirement without obvious source of fluid loss
(d) Planned general anesthesia for other injuries making serial abdominal examinations impossible
(e) Gross hematuria
(f) Elevated transaminase levels (SGOT > 200 IU, SGPT > 100 IU)
(2) Can be useful for subsequent follow-up

4. Management
a. Nonoperative
(1) Safe for patients with stable liver or spleen injuries (80% of abdominal visceral bleeding).
(a) Patients are admitted to ICU for monitoring, serial examinations, and serial hematocrits (stable hemoglobin of 7 g/dl considered acceptable).
(b) If patient remains stable and abdominal tenderness resolves, may be transferred out of ICU after 1 to 2 days but is maintained on bed rest.
(c) Patients allowed out of bed by days 4 to 5.
(d) May be discharged by day 7 if no other injury necessitates hospitalization.
(e) Delayed hepatic or splenic hemorrhage requiring laparotomy rare more than 2 days after injury.
(f) No contact sports for 3 months.
(2) Splenic preservation avoids potential complication of postsplenectomy sepsis.

17

PEDIATRIC SURGERY

  b. Indications for laparotomy
     (1) Ongoing hemorrhage and instability
     (2) Peritonitis
     (3) Acute deterioration
     (4) GI perforation
     (5) Transfusion requirement of greater than 50% blood volume in
         24 hours
D. BURNS
See Chapter 18.
E. CHILD ABUSE
1. Incidence is probably over 50,000 cases per year
a. Includes physical injury, emotional abuse, neglect, and sexual
   abuse
b. Demographics
   (1) Children are usually younger (<2 years old)
   (2) Low socioeconomic background
   (3) Young parents
   (4) Average age for sexual abuse is older (10 years of age)
2. Clues to the possibility of child abuse
a. Parents with flat affect or depressed mood
b. Delay in seeking medical attention by parents for child
c. Inconsistent physical history, one that does not fit with physical findings
   in case of injury
d. Injuries are often burns, fractures, soft-tissue injuries, or head
   trauma
e. Radiographic clues
   (1) Multiple healing fractures of different ages
   (2) Liver, splenic, or pancreatic fractures or duodenal
       hematoma
3. Required by state law to report suspected child abuse
F. BIRTH TRAUMA
Incidence is about 0.5% of all births.
1. Larger infants and those with significant congenital anomalies are at greater risk.
2. Typical injuries include the following:
a. Fractures (e.g., clavicle—in cases of shoulder dystocia)
b. Nerve injuries (especially the brachial plexus)
c. Visceral injuries
3. Treatment usually conservative, most resolve with time
4. Hemoperitoneum
a. May result from compression and fracture of liver, spleen, or
   adrenals
b. May necessitate blood transfusion

V. PEDIATRIC EMERGENCY DRUGS AND DOSAGES
See Table 17-5.

TABLE 17-5	
PEDIATRIC EMERGENCY DRUGS AND DOSES	
Drug	Dose
Epinephrine (1:10,000)	0.01 mg/kg (0.1 ml/kg)
Atropine (0.1 mg/ml)	0.01 mg/kg (0.1 ml/kg)
Lidocaine 1% (10 mg/ml)	1 mg/kg (0.1 ml/kg)
Sodium bicarbonate (1 mEq/ml)	1 mEq/kg (1 ml/kg)
Calcium chloride 10% (100 mg/ml)	30 mg/kg (0.3 ml/kg)
Dextrose 50%	0.5 g/kg (1 ml/kg)
Naloxone (0.4 mg/ml)	0.01 mg/kg (0.025 ml/kg)
Dilantin	10 mg/kg
Phenobarbitol	10 mg/kg
Lorazepam (Ativan)	0.05 mg/kg
Valium	0.05 mg/kg
Defibrillation	2 J/kg
Transfusion (ml PRBC)	(Blood volume) $\times$ (desired Hb − present Hb)/23

SUGGESTED READINGS

Foglia RP, Winthrop AL: Abdominal trauma. In Oldham KT, Colombani PM, Foglia RP, et al, editors: Surgery of infants and children: scientific principles and practice, Philadelphia, 1997, Lippincott-Raven.

Kosloske AM: Indications for operation in necrotizing enterocolitis revisited, J Pediatr Surg 29:663, 1994.

Mahaffey SM: Neonatal and pediatric physiology. In Greenfield LJ, Mulholland MW, Oldham KT, et al, editors: Surgery: scientific principles and practice, ed 2, Philadelphia, 1997, Lippincott-Raven.

BURNS

Andrew J. Lodge

I. EPIDEMIOLOGY

A. INCIDENCE
Approximately 2 million per year in United States.
B. HOSPITALIZATION
From 70,000 to 80,000 require hospitalization.
C. MORTALITY RATE
The mortality rate is 4% to 60%, depending on size and depth of burn and presence of inhalation injury.

18

II. INITIAL MANAGEMENT

A. STOPPING THE BURNING PROCESS
1. **Extinguish flames** and remove all involved clothing.
2. **Flush chemical burns** with copious amounts of water.
B. STANDARD ABCS OF ATLS
C. ESTABLISHMENT OF VENOUS ACCESS
1. **Insert a 14- or 16-gauge IV catheter;** place through unburned skin, if possible.
2. **Peripheral veins** are almost always adequate.
D. HISTORY
E. PHYSICAL EXAMINATION
1. **Examine for associated injuries.**
a. Examine for evidence of inhalation injury.
b. Examine for evidence of musculoskeletal and thoracoabdominal trauma.
2. **Monitor vital signs hourly** or more frequently as appropriate.
3. **Obtain baseline body weight.**
F. LABORATORY EVALUATION
1. **ABG with carboxyhemoglobin level**
2. **CBC**—note that RBC loss is proportional to extent of full-thickness burn injury
3. **Electrolytes, BUN, and creatinine**
4. **Urinalysis**
5. **Type and crossmatch**
G. TETANUS PROPHYLAXIS
1. **Known recent tetanus vaccine or booster:** 0.5 ml tetanus toxoid IM
2. **Unknown history of tetanus immunization**
a. Between 250 and 500 U of tetanus-immune globulin IM
b. Active immunization with tetanus toxoid
H. ESTIMATE EXTENT OF BURN
1. **Use the rule of nines** for approximation of BSA burned (Figure 18-1).
2. **The patient's palm is approximately 1% BSA.**
3. **Children have an increased percentage of BSA in the head and neck** compared with adults.

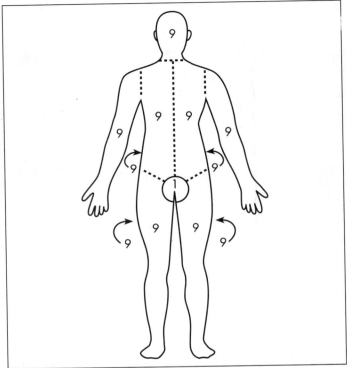

The rule of nines. Each of the above regions represent approximately 9% of BSA.

I. ESTIMATION OF BURN DEPTH

1. Partial-thickness burn
a. Pink or mottled red color
b. Wet appearance
c. Covered with vesicles or bullae
d. Often severely painful

2. Full-thickness burns—all epithelial elements destroyed
a. Charred—may appear translucent
b. Dry appearance
c. May have thrombosed superficial veins
d. Insensate—nerve endings destroyed
e. Often requires excision
f. Always requires cutaneous autografting for wound closure

J. INDICATIONS FOR ICU OR BURN CENTER ADMISSION
1. Adults with greater than or equal to 25% BSA burn
2. Children with greater than or equal to 20% BSA burn
3. Full-thickness burns greater than or equal to 10% of BSA
4. Burns of face, hands, feet, eyes, ears, or perineum
5. High-voltage electric injury
6. Inhalation injury or associated trauma
7. Other medical conditions that increase medical risk

III. FLUID RESUSCITATION

A. MANDATORY IV HYDRATION FOR ALL BURNS 15% BSA
B. PHYSIOLOGIC CONSIDERATIONS
1. **Blood volume decreases** and edema forms most rapidly during the first 8 hours postburn; these processes decrease over the first postburn day
2. **Capillary permeability** begins to return to normal on postburn day 2; edema resorption also begins
3. **Pulmonary edema**
   a. Uncommon during initial resuscitation
   b. Most often occurs during the resorptive phase (commonly 3 to 6 days postburn)
C. IV FLUID THERAPY
1. **Parkland formula for initial resuscitation**
   a. Lactated Ringer's for fluid resuscitation during the first 24 hours postburn
      (1) Infuse 4 ml/kg/% BSA burn.
      (2) Administer half of the calculated volume over the first 8 hours postburn.
      (3) Administer the remaining half of the calculated volume over the next 16 hours.
   b. Second 24 hours postburn
      (1) Administer D5W in sufficient quantities to replace evaporative water loss and maintain serum sodium concentration 140 mEq/L
      (2) Infusion of colloid-containing fluid equivalent to plasma to replace plasma volume deficit
         (a) Approximately 20% to 60% of calculated plasma volume
         (b) Roughly equals 250 ml per each 10% BSA burn over 20%
2. **Modified Brooke formula for initial resuscitation**
   a. Lactated Ringer's for fluid resuscitation during the first 24 hours
      (1) Infuse 2 ml/kg/% BSA burn in adults (3 ml/kg/% BSA burn in children).
      (2) Administer half of the calculated volume over the first 8 hours postburn.
      (3) Administer the remaining half of the calculated volume over the next 16 hours.
   b. Colloid-containing fluid for fluid resuscitation during the second 24 postburn hours

18

BURNS

(1) Add 25 g albumin (1 ampule) to 500 ml NS to yield a concentration of 5 g/dl.
(2) Estimate the plasma volume deficit (based on BSA burn) and replace it with colloid-containing fluid over 24 hours.
    (a) From 30% to 50% BSA burn, infusion of 0.3 ml/kg/% BSA burn
    (b) From 50% to 70% BSA burn, infusion of 0.4 ml/kg/% BSA burn
    (c) Greater than 70% BSA burn, infusion of 0.5 ml/kg/% BSA burn
(3) Use an electrolyte-free water infusion to maintain adequate urine output.
    (a) IV D5W in the adult
    (b) Children
        (i) Children tend to develop hyponatremia with D5W infusion.
        (ii) Infuse D5¼NS or D5½NS.

3. Estimation of insensible fluid losses (important after initial resuscitation)
a. Insensible water loss (ml/hr) = (25 + % BSA burn) × total BSA (m^2).
b. Replace insensible losses with D5W.
c. Inadequate free water replacement may lead to hypernatremia.
d. Anticipate a decreased evaporative loss when open wounds are grafted or covered with biologic dressings.

4. Transfusion of PRBC to maintain hematocrit between 30% and 35%

5. In children, may require maintenance fluid in addition to calculated resuscitation volume

D. EVALUATION OF THE ADEQUACY OF FLUID RESUSCITATION

1. Monitor hourly urine output.
a. Most readily available index of adequate volume resuscitation
b. Insertion of Foley catheter and hourly urine output measurements
c. Adequate urine output—30 to 50 ml/hr in an adult; 1 ml/kg/hr in children less than 30 kg
    (1) Low urine output
        (a) Usually prerenal oliguria
        (b) Acute renal failure extremely uncommon in burn patients
        (c) Administration of additional IV fluid as a fluid challenge
        (d) Maintenance adjustments and fluid infusion replacement based on urine response
    (2) High urine output—greater than 75 ml/hr in adult; greater than 2 ml/kg/hr in children
        (a) Indicates overhydration, unless secondary to glucosuria
        (b) Decrease in fluid administration

2. PA catheterization indications include the following:
a. Poor response to adequate volume resuscitation
b. Underlying cardiac disease
c. Age extremes

3. Body weight should be measured upon admission and every day after.
a. First 48 hours postburn—weight gain of 10% to 20% with adequate resuscitation

b. After 48 hours—1% to 2% weight loss occurs every day
c. From 7 to 10 days postburn—return to preburn weight
4. **Hematocrit is not an accurate indicator** of the adequacy of volume resuscitation.

IV. VASCULAR CONSIDERATIONS
A. VASCULAR COMPROMISE
1. **May occur in full-thickness encircling burns of the extremities** because seared tissue will not expand as edema develops
2. **Signs and symptoms**
a. Progressive paresthesia and deep tissue pain
b. Cyanosis
c. Impaired capillary refill
3. **Doppler ultrasonic flow meter**
a. Useful in evaluation because tissue edema may make palpation of pulses difficult
b. Examination of palmar arch pulses in the upper extremity
4. **Prevention**
a. Elevation of the circumferentially burned limb above heart level
b. Active exercise and muscular contraction
   (1) Periods of 2 to 3 minutes q2h during first 24 to 48 hours postburn
   (2) May enhance venous return and reduce edema
5. **Indications for escharotomy to release compressing eschar**
a. Absence of pulsatile arterial flow
b. Progressive decrease in pulse on serial examination
6. **Escharotomy technique**
a. Sterile bedside procedure
b. No anesthesia necessary (no sensation in areas of full-thickness burn)
c. Scalpel or electrocautery
d. Midmedial and/or midlateral incision through nonviable eschar
   (1) Make incisions only through full-thickness burns.
   (2) Proceed from proximal to distal and always incise eschar across involved joints.
   (3) Stay anterior to the medial epicondyle of the upper extremity to avoid the ulnar nerve.
   (4) Incise through the superficial fascia.
      (a) Incise down to, but not through, underlying subcutaneous tissue.
      (b) Cut eschar edges should separate.
e. Return of distal pulses within a few minutes
   (1) Facilitate venous return by extremity elevation and exercise.
   (2) Failure of pulses to return may have several causes, including the following:
      (a) Hypovolemia
      (b) Subfascial edema secondary to electrical or deep thermal burn, prolonged ischemia, or trauma; may need fasciotomy
f. Topical antimicrobial agent applied to all escharotomy (and fasciotomy) incisions until fully healed (see section V, B)

18

BURNS

B. FASCIOTOMY:
See section VIII, A, 7.

V. PULMONARY CONSIDERATIONS

A. CARBON MONOXIDE INTOXICATION

1. Signs and symptoms

a. Mild intoxication

(1) Palpitations

(2) Mild muscular weakness

(3) Mild headache

(4) Dizziness

(5) Confusion

b. Severe intoxication

(1) Loss of consciousness

(2) Seizures

(3) Neurologic deficit

(4) Pulmonary edema

(5) Myocardial ischemia

(6) Severe metabolic acidosis

2. Carboxyhemoglobin level

a. The carboxyhemoglobin level is determined with ABG.

b. Hgb with bound carbon monoxide cannot transport O_2, so tissue hypoxia may occur.

c. If the carbon monoxide level is greater than 40%, the patient may experience progressive collapse, coma, or death.

3. Treatment

a. 100% O_2

b. Hyperbaric O_2

(1) Indicated in the presence of any of the above signs of severe CO intoxication

(2) If CO-Hb levels are greater than 25%

(3) More liberal use in pregnant patients and children

(4) Use of multiple sessions indicated if neurologic symptoms persist

(5) Logistics may be difficult in the severely burned patient requiring significant resuscitation

B. INHALATION INJURY

1. Present in 3% to 25% of burn victims

2. Presence of inhalation injury substantially increases mortality (6 to 15 times)

3. Rarely a cause of immediate hypoxia (onset often delayed more than 24 hours postburn; 10% of patients will develop ARDS in first week)

4. Risk factors

a. Impaired mental status (ethanol or other drug intoxication, neurologic disease)

b. Head trauma

c. Burns from petroleum products

d. Burns sustained in a closed space

5. Signs and symptoms of inhalation injury

a. Inflammation of oropharyngeal mucosa

b. Facial burns and singed nasal hair

c. Hoarseness, stridor, wheezing, and rales

d. Unexplained hypoxemia

e. Carbonaceous sputum production (most specific sign)

6. Evaluation of possible inhalation injury

a. CXR—notoriously insensitive

b. Flexible fiber-optic bronchoscopy

(1) Perform this procedure when the patient is hemodynamically stable.

(2) Must be performed early if signs of inhalation injury are present.

(3) Anesthetize the nasal mucosa with topical agents.

(4) Administer 100% O_2 to patient for 3 minutes before examination.

(5) Place an appropriately sized endotracheal tube over the scope before examination.

(6) If intubation is necessary, the tube can easily be passed into the trachea over the scope.

(7) Signs of inhalation injury include the following:

(a) Mucosal erythema, edema, blisters, ulcers, or hemorrhage

(b) Carbon particles in major airways

c. Xenon-133 perfusion lung scan—significant inhalation injury suggested by a delay of more than 90 seconds in xenon clearance

d. ABG—for evidence of hypoxia and carboxyhemoglobinemia

7. Treatment of inhalation injury

a. Administer warm, humidified O_2

b. Pulmonary toilet—postural drainage, chest percussion, incentive spirometry, IPPB

c. Bronchospasm treatment

d. Therapeutic bronchoscopy to clear debris

e. Intubation indications

(1) Progressive hypoxia

(2) Pharyngeal, supraglottic, and/or vocal cord edema threatening airway occlusion (on bronchoscopic examination)

(3) Early prophylactic intubation in seriously injured patients with any signs of associated inhalation injury

f. Prophylactic steroids

(1) Not beneficial

(2) May increase the risk of infection

g. Prophylactic antibiotics

(1) Not beneficial

(2) May lead to the emergence of resistant strains of bacteria

h. Positive-pressure ventilation

(1) Initially PEEP at 5 cm H_2O

(2) If Sao_2 is less than 90%, increase Fio_2 to 50% to 60%

18

BURNS

(3) If Sao$_2$ still less than 90%, increase PEEP
(4) If PEEP is greater than 15 or arterial BP falls with increasing PEEP, place pulmonary artery catheter

C. CIRCUMFERENTIAL BURNS OF THE THORAX

1. May mechanically impair ventilation

2. Signs and symptoms

a. Progressive use of accessory muscles of respiration

b. Increase in inspiratory pressures in mechanically ventilated patients (most common indication for thoracic escharotomy)

c. Tachypnea

3. Thoracic escharotomy

a. Use the technique described in section IV, A, 6.

b. Incisions are made bilaterally in anterior axillary lines.

c. Extend incisions from the clavicle to the costal margin.

d. Connect these escharotomies with a costal margin escharotomy if the full-thickness burn involves the anterior abdominal wall.

D. UNEXPECTED RESPIRATORY DEPRESSION IN A PATIENT ACCEPTED IN TRANSFER FROM ANOTHER HOSPITAL

1. The patient may have been given IM or subcutaneous narcotics.

2. These drugs will be systemically absorbed because resuscitation increases tissue perfusion.

3. Treat with IV naloxone (Narcan).

VI. WOUND CARE

A. GENERAL CARE

1. Daily examination of wound until totally healed

2. Daily gentle cleansing with a non–alcohol-containing surgical detergent

3. Gentle debridement of nonviable tissue after cleansing

a. Continue debridement to the point of pain or bleeding.

b. Administer IV analgesia as needed.

c. Wash in a shower or Hubbard tank, but do not immerse.

4. Wound and adjacent margin shaved of approximately 1 inch (do not shave eyebrows)

5. Wound allowed to air dry

B. TOPICAL ANTIMICROBIAL AGENT APPLICATION

See Table 18-1 for list of commonly used topical antimicrobial agents and their characteristics.

1. Should be applied as early as possible to burn to limit bacterial proliferation

2. Application every 12 hours

3. Silver sulfadiazine, mafenide acetate, and silver nitrate are most commonly used and the only agents proven efficacious for major burns

C. BURN WOUND EXCISION

1. Performed only after resuscitation is complete

2. Indications

a. Full-thickness burns

b. Patients requiring debridement of high-voltage electric injury

TABLE 18-1

COMMONLY USED TOPICAL ANTIMICROBIAL AGENTS

Agent	Application	Characteristics	Systemic Effects	Antimicrobial Spectrum	Specific Uses
Silver sulfadiazine (1%) (Silvadene)*	To open wound; painless	Antimicrobial cream; fair to poor eschar penetration	Transient leukopenia (resolves spontaneously)	Broad antibacterial; Candida albicans	Deep partial-thickness burns; full-thickness burns
Mafenide acetate (11.1%) (Sulfamylon)*	To open wound; painful	Antimicrobial cream; excellent eschar penetration	Carbonic anhydrase inhibitor	Broad antibacterial	Burns of external ear; invasive wound infections
Silver nitrate (0.5%)*	With layered dressing; slightly painful	Antimicrobial solution; poor eschar penetration; stains skin, clothes, linens	Electrolyte leeching; methemoglobinemia	Broad antibacterial; antifungal	Partial-thickness burns; burns to face
Bacitracin ointment	To open wound; painless	Polymyxin antibiotic ointment	None	Broad antibacterial	Partial-thickness burns; burns to face
Polymyxin B sulfate	To open wound; painless	Peptide antibiotic ointment	None	Gram-negative bacteria	Partial-thickness burns; burns to face
Neomycin	To open wound; painless	Antibiotic ointment; more prone to resistance and hypersensitivity than bacitracin and polymyxin B	Rare ototoxicity; rare nephrotoxicity	Broad antibacterial	Partial-thickness wounds
Polysporin	To open wound; painless	Combination antibiotic ointment	None	Broad antibacterial	Partial-thickness wounds
Neosporin	To open wound; painless	Combination antibiotic ointment; painless application; rare hypersensitivity	None	Broad antibacterial	Partial-thickness wounds
Acetic acid (0.5%)	With layered dressing	Weak acid	Acidosis with protracted use on large wounds	Broad antibacterial; antipseudomonal	Wounds infected with Pseudomonas aeruginosa

*Only agents proven efficacious for major burns.

3. Contraindications

a. Hemodynamic instability

   (1) Burn excision is accompanied by large-volume blood loss.

   (2) Limit excision to 20% BSA or 2 hours operative time.

b. Pulmonary complications

c. Superficial partial-thickness injury

4. Technique

a. Adequate levels of systemic antibiotics should be present before excision

b. Method of excision

   (1) Tangential "shaving" method

   (2) Excision to fascia

c. Control of hemorrhage

   (1) Thrombin- and/or epinephrine-moistened gauze dressings

   (2) Tourniquet for excision on extremity

   (3) IV or subeschar infiltration with vasopressin

d. May graft immediately or delay

D. BIOLOGIC DRESSINGS

1. Indications and uses

a. Coverage of freshly excised wounds

b. Decreases bacterial proliferation and promotes granulation tissue formation

c. May be used to determine readiness of a site for grafting

d. Decreases the pain of partial-thickness burns and maintains joint mobility

e. Decreases evaporative water loss; prevents wound dessication

2. Types of biologic dressings

a. Human cutaneous allografts

   (1) Dressing of choice

   (2) Donor must be minimal risk, documented HIV seronegative

b. Porcine xenografts

   (1) Readily available

   (2) Less effective than allografts in decreasing bacterial proliferation

c. Bilaminate synthetic dressing

   (1) Only when allografts or xenografts are not available

   (2) Ineffective in decreasing bacterial proliferation

3. Technique

a. Reapply new dressings every 3 to 5 days.

b. Remove and replace dressings more frequently if suppuration occurs between the wound and dressing.

E. BURN WOUND INFECTION

1. Signs of burn wound infection

a. Intraeschar hemorrhage (black or dark hemorrhagic discoloration)

   (1) Most common sign

   (2) May be secondary to minor trauma

b. Conversion of a partial-thickness burn to full-thickness injury— pathognomonic of burn wound infection

c. Erythema and edema at wound edges
d. Degeneration of granulation tissue
e. Marked subeschar suppuration
f. Premature or unexpected eschar separation
g. Hemorrhagic fat necrosis
h. Metastatic abscesses in unburned skin (ecthyma gangrenosum)
i. Vesicular lesions on healing partial-thickness burns—suggest viral infection

2. Diagnosis of burn wound infection

a. A surface culture is unreliable.
b. Wound biopsy is the method of choice.
  (1) Should be performed if any signs of infection are present
  (2) Biopsy viable tissue subjacent or adjacent to the burn wound
  (3) Excision of a 500-mg portion of tissue—tissue sample divided in half
    (a) Send one half of the sample for culture and sensitivity.
      (i) Greater than or equal to 10^5 organisms/g of tissue suggestive but not diagnostic of infection
      (ii) May be due to surface colonization
    (b) Send one half of the sample for histologic examination.
      (i) Place the sample in 10% formalin for rapid processing or examine by frozen section.
      (ii) Invasive infection is present if bacteria are detected in unburned tissue that is adjacent to the wound.

3. Treatment of documented bacterial wound infection

a. Change topical antimicrobial agent to mafenide (Sulfamylon).
b. Administer systemic antibiotics based on the sensitivities of the offending organisms.
c. Use a subeschar injection of antibiotics into the infected burn wound.
  (1) Especially useful in treatment of focal pseudomonal infections
  (2) Before excision of infected wound to reduce bacteremia
  (3) Technique
    (a) One-half daily dose of semisynthetic penicillin (Piperacillin) in 150 to 1000 ml NS q12h
    (b) Injected beneath eschar using a #20 spinal needle to minimize the number of injection sites
d. Excise all infected tissue.
  (1) Adequate blood levels of antibiotics should be present before excision.
  (2) Debride any infected tissue (may be necessary to amputate).
  (3) Cover immediately with a biologic dressing.

4. Nonbacterial burn wound infection

a. *Candida* organisms
  (1) Frequently colonize but rarely cause invasive infection
  (2) Systemic therapy if fungemia occurs
    (a) Amphotericin-B
    (b) With or without 5-fluorocytosine
b. HSV: systemic adenosine arabinoside (Ara-A) or acyclovir

VII. COMPLICATIONS
A. GI COMPLICATIONS
1. Curling's ulcer
a. Acute ulceration of the upper GI tract
b. May progress to hemorrhage or perforation and can be life-threatening
c. Preventive therapy—gastric pH greater than 5 maintained
   (1) H_2 blockers
   (2) Early feeding and antacids (30 ml q1-2h PRN pH < 5)
   (3) Sucralfate may increase risk of pneumonia in ventilated burn patient
2. Ileus
a. Almost always present in burns greater than or equal to 20% BSA
b. Usually resolves spontaneously 2 to 3 days postinjury
c. Treat with NG suction, IV fluids
3. Acalculous cholecystitis
a. Usually causes right upper quadrant pain and jaundice
b. Diagnosis confirmed using abdominal ultrasound
c. Cholecystectomy if distended gallbladder is detected by ultra-sonography
d. Percutaneous cholecystostomy tube placement in critically ill patient
B. RESPIRATORY COMPLICATIONS:
Pneumonia is the most common infectious complication in burn patients.
1. Most commonly resulting from *Staphylococcus aureus* and gram-negative bacteria
2. Can result from hematogenous spread from other sources of infection
C. SUPPURATIVE THROMBOPHLEBITIS
1. Local signs in less than half of the patients
a. Maintain a high index of suspicion in a septic patient with no identifiable source of infection.
b. Every previously cannulated vein is a potential site for infection.
2. Exploration of vein
a. Recovery of normal-appearing blood from the vein is a negative result.
b. Intraluminal pus confirms the diagnosis.
c. Excise veins that contain intraluminal clots.
   (1) Send one segment for histologic examination.
   (2) Send another segment for culture and sensitivity.
3. Treatment
a. IV antibiotics
b. Complete surgical removal of infected vein
4. Prevention—all IV catheters, including central lines, changed at least every 72 hours
D. ACUTE BACTERIAL ENDOCARDITIS
1. Right heart involvement is the most common.
2. All valves can potentially be affected.

VIII. NUTRITION

An enteric tube feeding is usually necessary initially. Early enteral nutrition has been shown to be metabolically favorable and to decrease hospital stay. Avoid TPN if possible (high risk of catheter-related sepsis).

A. CONTROL OF METABOLIC REQUIREMENTS

1. Adequate pain control

2. Warm environment

3. Timely treatment of infection

B. CONTROL OF DIARRHEA

1. Reduced caloric density of feedings

2. Paregoric

C. CALORIC AND PROTEIN REQUIREMENTS

1. Based on percent BSA burn and preburn weight

2. Requirements for patients with more than 40% total BSA burn

a. Some 2000 to 2200 calories/total BSA(m^2)/day

b. From 12 to 18 g nitrogen/total BSA(m^2)/day

IX. SPECIAL CONSIDERATIONS

A. ELECTRICAL INJURY

1. Arrhythmias are common, especially asystole and ventricular fibrillation.

a. ACLS as needed

b. Indications for continuous cardiac monitoring (for a minimum of 48 hours)

    (1) Loss of consciousness

    (2) Abnormal ECG

2. Associated skeletal fractures are common.

a. Falls often associated with the electrical injury (falls from high-voltage towers)

b. Current-induced muscle contractions

    (1) May cause vertebral fractures

    (2) Must exclude cervical spine injury with appropriate radiographs

3. Vascular damage must be excluded.

a. The electrical current may damage the intima, producing thrombosis and/or hemorrhage.

b. Arteriography may be useful.

    (1) Identification of extent of tissue damage

    (2) Determination of level for amputation

4. There may be renal damage secondary to hemochromogens (hemoglobin and myoglobin).

a. Common after electric injury

b. May also occur with burn-associated crush injuries

c. Prevention

    (1) Increase infusion of IV fluids.

        (a) Maintain a urine output of 1 ml/kg/hr.

        (b) Continue until no hemochromogens are present in the urine.

18

BURNS

(2) If excretion of hemochromogens continues or there is a risk of hypervolemia, consider the following:

    (a) Mannitol 25 g IV bolus

        (i) Administer up to 300 g every 24 hours.

        (ii) Mannitol prevents tubular deposition of pigment.

    (b) IV sodium bicarbonate

        (i) Keep the urine pH greater than 6.

        (ii) Alkalinization of urine facilitates hemochromogen excretion.

5. Neurologic damage includes spinal cord deficits.

a. Deficits that appear early may be transient.

b. Deficits that appear late are generally permanent.

6. Cataract formation occurs days to months after head or neck electric injury.

7. Wound care includes the following:

a. Fasciotomy

    (1) Indications

        (a) Cyanosis and impaired distal capillary refill

        (b) Hard, stony muscle by palpation

        (c) Progressively diminishing or absent pulses by Doppler ultrasound examination

        (d) Compartment pressure by wick catheter greater than 30 mm Hg

    (2) Technique

        (a) Perform in the operating room.

        (b) Incise the fascia of each involved muscle compartment.

        (c) If distal pulses do not return after compartment release, amputation may be indicated.

b. Operative debridement

    (1) Delay until resuscitation is complete.

    (2) Debride all necrotic tissue; amputate if necessary.

    (3) Pack the wound open.

    (4) Reexplore the wound 24 to 72 hours later.

        (a) Carry out further debridement, if necessary.

        (b) If all necrotic tissue has been removed, close the wound by skin approximation or grafting.

c. Daily wound inspection with further debridement as necessary

B. CHEMICAL BURNS

1. Initial treatment

a. Remove all involved clothing.

b. Flush with large amounts of water.

    (1) Do not waste time searching for specific neutralizing agents.

    (2) Chemicals burn continuously until washed off.

c. Use IV fluid resuscitation as with other burns.

2. Agents for which specific therapy is indicated

a. Hydrofluoric acid

    (1) Prolonged irrigation with benzalkonium chloride

    (2) Topical application of calcium gluconate gel

      (3) Local injection of 10% calcium gluconate into damaged tissue for treatment of severe pain

      (4) Treatment of hypocalcemia as necessary

b. Phenol

      (1) Initial water lavage

      (2) Lipophilic solvent wash (polyethylene glycol, propylene glycol, or glycerol) to remove residual phenol

c. White phosphorus

      (1) Irrigate wound with saline.

      (2) Cover with moist gauze dressing to prevent ignition.

      (3) A 0.5% to 1% copper sulfate wash followed by copious irrigation will turn retained particles blue-gray.

        (a) Facilitates identification of particles

        (b) Impedes ignition

d. Tar and bitumen burns

      (1) Hot material cooled with cold water

      (2) Wound care

        (a) Do not remove material with a petroleum-based solvent.

        (b) Cover with a petroleum-based ointment and dress daily.

3. Treatment of chemical eye injury

a. Continuous irrigation with water for at least 30 minutes

b. Topical antimicrobial agent

c. Cycloplegic eye drops to decrease synechia formation

d. Lubricant ointments without eye patches

e. Daily monitoring of intraocular pressure

f. Early consultation with an ophthalmologist

18

BURNS

SUGGESTED READINGS

McManus WF, Pruitt BA Jr: Thermal injuries. In Mattox KL, Moore EV, Feliciano DV, editors: *Trauma,* Norwalk, Conn, 1988, Appleton & Lange.

Monafo WW: Initial management of burns [see comments], *N Engl J Med* 335:1581-1586, 1996.

Moylan JA: Burn injury. In Moylan JA, editor: *Trauma surgery,* ed 2, Philadelphia, 1991, JB Lippincott.

Pruitt BA Jr: The burn patient. I. Initial care. II. Later care and complications of thermal injury, *Curr Probl Surg* 16(4-5), 1979.

Pruitt BA Jr, Goodwin CW Jr: Thermal injuries. In Davis JH, editor: *Clinical surgery,* vols 1-2, St Louis, 1987, Mosby.

Pruitt BA Jr, Goodwin CW Jr, Pruitt SK: Burns: including cold, chemical and electrical injuries. In Sabiston DC Jr, editor: *Textbook of surgery,* ed 14, Philadelphia, 1991, WB Saunders.

Rose JK, Herndon DN: Advances in the treatment of burn patients, *Burns* 23(suppl 1):S19-S26, 1997.

Shirani KZ, Vaughan GM, Mason AD Jr, et al: Update on current therapeutic approaches in burns, *Shock* 5:4-16, 1996.

Waymack J, Pruitt BA Jr: Burn wound care, *Adv Surg* 23:261, 1990.

EXTRACORPOREAL MEMBRANE OXYGENATION

Joseph M. Forbess

I. INTRODUCTION

Extracorporeal membrane oxygenation (ECMO) is a mechanical support technique applied for extended periods in patients with severe but potentially reversible pulmonary and/or cardiac disease. ECMO sustains the patient's oxygenation and, if necessary, hemodynamic requirements while allowing the basic disease to resolve under optimal conditions. It is most successfully applied to neonates with acute respiratory failure but has also been used in children and adults.

II. ECMO FOR NEONATES AND INFANTS

A. INDICATIONS AND PATIENT SELECTION

ECMO is indicated for newborns with acute respiratory failure that is refractory to conventional management. It is also used for cardiopulmonary failure in infants after cardiac surgery.

B. GENERAL INCLUSION/EXCLUSION CRITERIA

Because of the increased risk of intracranial hemorrhage, infants less than *34 weeks gestational age* are usually excluded; *2000 grams* is generally considered the minimum suitable birth weight, although low weight alone should not exclude a patient from therapy. Patients with a *significant coagulopathy* or preexisting bleeding complications are at extreme risk while heparinized on ECMO. Most deaths on ECMO result from bleeding complications. Any disorders of coagulation should be corrected before institution of ECMO. *Major intracranial hemorrhage* also precludes systemic heparinization, although most centers would not exclude a patient from ECMO because of a grade I intraventricular hemorrhage (IVH). There should be *no evidence of irreversible brain damage* from IVH or any other cause. Because ECMO is planned as a temporizing measure while the lungs recover from some reversible process, *prolonged mechanical ventilation* (10 to 14 days) and *irreversible lung disease* are considered relative contraindications. An *echocardiogram* should be performed to rule out the presence of *correctable cardiac lesions,* which would require repair and not ECMO. In addition, the presence of *uncorrectable cardiac lesions,* which would not respond to ECMO support, should contraindicate the use of this therapy. Finally, *other lethal congenital anomalies* should be considered contraindications to the institution of ECMO.

The above inclusion/exclusion criteria are derived from the Extracorporeal Life Support Organization's (ELSO) "Guidelines for Neonatal ECMO Consultation." If these above criteria are met, and the patient continues to fail with more conventional support, ECMO should be considered. Rough estimates of this failure include a Pao_2 less than 50 to 60 mm Hg (Fio_2 1.0), PIP of greater than 35 cm H_2O on conventional ventilation, and no improvement after the institution of high-frequency ventilation and/or nitric oxide therapy for approximately 6 hours.

C. NEONATAL DIAGNOSES REQUIRING ECMO

The most common diagnoses of neonates placed on ECMO are as follows:

1. **Meconium aspiration syndrome (MAS):** During delivery, meconium-stained amniotic fluid indicates fetal distress and results from sustained hypoxemia that causes hyperperistalsis and sphincter relaxation. At birth, the neonate may aspirate meconium into the distal airways, causing airway obstruction, inflammation, and chemical pneumonitis. Infants who aspirate meconium may have mild, moderate, or severe respiratory distress at birth. Patients with MAS and severe respiratory distress refractory to conventional therapy are candidates for ECMO.

2. **Persistent pulmonary hypertension of the newborn (PPHN):** In the newborn lung, severe pulmonary vasoconstriction often occurs in response to factors such as hypoxia, hypercapnia, acidosis, and sepsis. The resultant elevation in pulmonary vascular resistance can cause right-to-left shunting of blood flow away from the lungs and through the ductus arteriosus and foramen ovale. As this negative cycle perpetuates, the neonate becomes severely hypoxemic and acidotic. Standard therapy for PPHN consists of mechanical ventilation, induced respiratory alkalosis, and use of various pharmacologic agents. However, approximately 2% to 5% of neonates fail to respond to this therapy and are considered for ECMO.

3. **Congenital diaphragmatic hernia (CDH):** During the embryonic formation of the diaphragm, a defect may result from incomplete closure of the posterolateral communication between the abdominal and thoracic cavities. With incomplete development of the posterior diaphragm, abdominal contents herniate into the chest cavity and interfere with lung development and prevent inflation after delivery. Severe respiratory distress presents as PPHN, and surgical repair is required. Postoperatively, neonates experience a "honeymoon period" of improved pulmonary function, often followed by intractable respiratory failure. ECMO is indicated in patients failing conventional treatment after a honeymoon period. The absence of this honeymoon period is considered evidence of pulmonary hypoplasia and is therefore a contraindication to ECMO.

4. **After cardiac surgery:** Venoarterial ECMO can also serve as a form of mechanical assist in patients with severe cardiac failure. This may be applied preoperatively or postoperatively in patients with correctable cardiac anomalies who experience reversible mechanical failure resulting from severe pulmonary hypertension or depressed myocardial function.

D. ECMO PROTOCOL FOR NEONATES AND INFANTS

After obtaining informed consent to administer ECMO support to a patient, the ECMO team is mobilized. This team usually consists of a select group of respiratory therapists, perfusionists, nurses, and physicians who have combined to establish a safe and reliable protocol for initiating, maintaining, and concluding extracorporeal life support.

1. **Techniques of extracorporeal support:** ECMO is performed by draining venous (deoxygenated) blood, pumping it through an artificial lung where carbon dioxide is removed and oxygen is added, and returning the blood to the circulation via an artery (venoarterial ECMO) or a vein (venovenous ECMO). The features of venoarterial and venovenous ECMO are listed in Table 19-1.

a. The ECMO circuit

(1) The components of a standard ECMO circuit are illustrated in Figure 19-1.

(2) Deoxygenated blood drains passively into a silicone bladder, which operates as the control point of a servoregulated roller pump that draws blood from the bladder. If the pump flow exceeds the passive venous return, the bladder will collapse and the roller pump will automatically slow down or shut off until it reexpands. Blood is then pumped through a silicone membrane lung that is designed for extended periods of ECMO. After passing through a countercurrent heat exchanger, the warmed, oxygenated blood is then returned to the patient via the arterial or venous infusion cannula. A tubing bridge is created between the drainage and perfusion catheters to allow recirculation of the ECMO circuit during priming and weaning. Heparin and fluids are infused into the circuit immediately proximal to the bladder.

b. Cannulation

(1) Venoarterial (VA) ECMO: The functions of both the heart and the lungs are partially or totally replaced. Deoxygenated blood is drained from the RA via a cannula inserted into the right internal jugular or femoral vein while oxygenated blood is pumped through a cannula placed into the right common carotid artery. VA ECMO is the standard for neonates.

(2) Venovenous (VV) ECMO: This type provides gas exchange but no cardiac support. Venous drainage and infusion cannulas are placed into the RA or vena cavae via the right internal jugular or femoral veins. Alternatively, a double-lumen catheter may be positioned in

TABLE 19-1		
COMPARISON OF VENOARTERIAL AND VENOVENOUS ECMO		
Parameter	VA ECMO	VV ECMO
Organ support	Gas exchange and cardiac output	Gas exchange only
Pulse contour	Reduced pulsatility	Normal pulsatility
CVP	Unreliable	Reliable
PA pressure	Unreliable	Reliable
Circuit Svo_2	Reliable	Unreliable
Circuit recirculation	None	15%-50%
Arterial O_2 saturation	95%	80%-95%
Ventilator settings	Minimal	Moderate

19

EXTRACORPOREAL MEMBRANE OXYGENATION

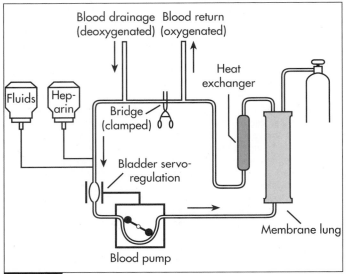

FIGURE 19-1

ECMO circuit schematic. Deoxygenated blood drains passively to a sealed bladder. If negative pressure occurs within the bladder, the roller pump is automatically shut off. After passing through the membrane lung, oxygenated blood is circulated through a countercurrent heat exchanger and back to the patient. Heparin and other infusions are delivered into the circuit immediately before the bladder.

the RA through the right internal jugular vein for both drainage and infusion. In either case, blood is drained from and returned to the venous circulation at the same rate. Therefore ECMO candidates who are hemodynamically unstable and require cardiovascular support should be placed on VA ECMO. In addition, a portion of newly oxygenated blood is removed by the drainage catheter in VV ECMO, and this recirculation fraction increases with the circuit blood flow.

2. **Initiation and management of ECMO:** Cannulation is performed by cutdown and ligation of vessels with strict sterile technique at the ICU bedside, with an operating room team and a complete set of instruments. In the neonate, a 12-Fr or 14-Fr venous cannula and 10-Fr or 12-Fr arterial cannula (for VA ECMO) are inserted into the right internal jugular vein and right common carotid artery, respectively, after receiving a heparin loading dose of 100 U/kg. Because circuit blood flow is limited by the available venous drainage, the venous drainage cannula should be as large as possible.

3. Circuit management

a. Blood flow: The blood flow setting of the ECMO circuit is determined by the oxygen delivery (Do_2) requirements of the patient. Typical blood flow rates are 100 to 150 ml/kg/min in neonates and 80 to 120 ml/kg/min in children.

   (1) VA ECMO: Blood flow during VA ECMO is usually 80% of the total cardiac output, resulting in a diminished but observable pulse pressure. The exact flow rate is best managed by continuous, inline monitoring of the mixed-venous oxygen saturation (Svo_2). An Svo_2 of 75% or greater generally indicates adequate Do_2. Inadequate Do_2, indicated by a falling Svo_2, is initially treated by increasing the circuit blood flow.

   (2) VV ECMO: Blood is drained and returned to the venous circulation at the same rate and thus has no influence on cardiac output or hemodynamics. As a result of recirculation of oxygenated blood, the circuit flow for total respiratory support with VV ECMO is 20% to 50% higher than VA ECMO for the same patient. In addition, the Svo_2 will be falsely elevated and a less reliable source for assessing the adequacy of Do_2. Continuous pulse oximetry provides better information for monitoring Do_2 during VV ECMO.

b. Oxygenation: Oxygenation is controlled by the Fio_2 of the gas connected to the membrane lung. In both VA ECMO and VV ECMO, a postoxygenator Po_2 of 200 to 300 mm Hg is maintained.

   (1) VA ECMO: The systemic Po_2 during VA ECMO results from the combined bypass and nonbypass Do_2. In most cases, the patient's arterial blood will be fully saturated with a Po_2 of 150 to 250 mm Hg.

   (2) VV ECMO: Because of the recirculation of VV ECMO, the patient's Sao_2 will range from 85% to 95%, with a Po_2 of 60 to 80 mm Hg. Patients undergoing VV ECMO may appear slightly cyanotic, although Do_2 is usually adequate if the cardiac output and Hgb are maintained in their normal ranges. If Do_2 is inadequate during maximal settings on VV ECMO, extracorporeal support should be converted to the VA mode.

c. Ventilation: Pco_2 is maintained at a value of 35 to 50 mm Hg by adjusting the "sweep" flow of gas. This is the flow of gas through the oxygenator. Carbon dioxide may need to be added to the sweep gas mixture because of the efficiency with which modern oxygenators remove CO_2.

d. Anticoagulation: Continuous heparin infusion is required throughout the ECMO course. To monitor heparinization, the ACT is measured frequently. The ACT, which is a measure of whole blood-clotting ability, is normally about 100 seconds. During ECMO, the heparin infusion is titrated to maintain an ACT of 150 to 200 seconds.

4. Patient care during ECMO:
Upon initiation of ECMO support, there is usually immediate improvement of the patient's condition and several aspects of care are modified.

a. Pulmonary care

   (1) Ventilator management should be adjusted to minimal settings to provide lung rest and optimum conditions for pulmonary recovery.

19

EXTRACORPOREAL MEMBRANE OXYGENATION

(2) With VA ECMO, ventilator settings should be reduced to an Fio_2 of 0.21, peak airway pressure of 20 cm H_2O, and a respiratory rate of 5 to 10 breaths/min.

(3) With VV ECMO, the ventilator is usually maintained at moderate settings with an Fio_2 of 0.4, peak airway pressure of 30 cm H_2O, and a respiratory rate of 10 to 20 breaths/min. A PEEP of at least 8 cm H_2O should be maintained to prevent atelectasis.

(4) Aggressive pulmonary toilet should be performed several times per day, and a chest film should be ordered daily to assess the lungs, as well as cannula positions.

b. Medications and fluids

(1) An accurate record of fluid balance and daily weights is essential.

(2) Blood is transfused to maintain a hematocrit between 35% and 40%.

(3) Platelets are routinely administered at the initiation of ECMO and daily thereafter to maintain a count between 120,000 and 150,000/mm^3.

(4) Fibrinogen levels are monitored at least daily and maintained at or above 100 mg/dl.

(5) Prophylactic antibiotics are usually given while on ECMO.

(6) Full nutrition should be administered throughout the duration of ECMO support.

(7) Patients requiring ECMO are usually hypervolemic upon initiation of support. In these cases, pharmacologic diuresis is instituted to remove excess fluid and return patients to their dry weights. If diuretics are insufficient, a small, hollow-fiber hemofilter may be placed in the ECMO circuit to supplement urine output and provide hemoconcentration.

(8) Minimal pharmacologic sedation should be applied during ECMO. Seizure activity must be treated promptly.

c. Laboratory studies

(1) Before initiation of ECMO, baseline determinations of CBC, electrolytes, LFTs, and coagulation parameters must be obtained.

(2) During ECMO, the CBC, electrolytes, and coagulation parameters are measured every 8 hours.

(3) ABG is obtained every 8 to 12 hours, and continuous pulse oximeter monitoring is used.

(4) A head ultrasound is performed on neonates to rule out intracranial hemorrhage.

5. **Weaning and decannulation from ECMO:** ECMO support is usually maintained for 4 to 5 days. Indications of lung recovery include an increasing Svo_2 and systemic Po_2, or decreasing Pco_2 while ECMO flow and ventilator settings are constant. Other signs of improvement are noted by increased pulmonary compliance and a normalizing CXR. Cardiac recovery is noted by increased pulse pressure, cardiac output, and Svo_2, in addition to improved contractility as monitored by serial echocardiography.

a. Weaning from VA ECMO
   (1) When significant improvement is documented in native cardiopulmonary function, VA ECMO blood flow is gradually reduced over a period of hours. When the native lungs and heart can provide adequate Do_2 and gas exchange at 20% of the baseline VA ECMO flow, a brief trial off bypass (cannulas clamped, bridge open) is attempted on moderate ventilator settings.
   (2) If this is successful, VA ECMO is started again and the patient is prepared for the sterile decannulation procedure. Anticoagulation of the circuit should be maintained until decannulation is initiated.
b. Weaning from VV ECMO
   (1) A trial wean from VV ECMO consists of decreasing and capping the gas flow to the membrane lung while continuing extracorporeal flow.
   (2) If the native lungs provide adequate gas exchange, ECMO can be discontinued and the cannulas removed. Anticoagulation of the circuit should be maintained until decannulation is initiated.
6. Emergencies during ECMO: Infrequently, an emergency situation, such as circuit disruption or air embolism, may occur and require immediate exclusion from the ECMO circuit. If this situation develops, the following steps must be followed sequentially:
a. Clamp the venous drainage line.
b. Open the tubing bridge.
c. Clamp the infusion line.
d. Increase patient ventilator settings to full support.
e. Disconnect the gas line to the membrane lung.
f. Repair or replace the source of emergency.
g. Evaluate the need for starting ECMO again.
7. Complications
a. Mechanical complications occur in approximately 10% of ECMO applications. These range from frequent minor events, such as cracks in connectors and kinking of tubing, to rare major problems, such as oxygenator failure or circuit rupture. Physiologic instability may be significant until the source has been corrected. It is paramount to recognize nature of the problem *after* the above emergency algorithm for discontinuing ECMO has been followed in an orderly fashion.
b. Medical complications include the following:
   (1) Bleeding is the most common complication during ECMO. Intracranial hemorrhage is the most significant bleeding complication and occurs in 10% to 15% of ECMO cases. Other locations of bleeding include the GI tract and the vascular access sites. Bleeding complications are best managed by titrating heparin to a lower ACT target of 150 seconds and aggressively maintaining a platelet count greater than $150,000/mm^3$. ECMO is usually discontinued in response to confirmed intracranial hemorrhage or uncontrollable bleeding.

19

EXTRACORPOREAL MEMBRANE OXYGENATION

(2) Neurologic: During cannulation for VA ECMO, the right common carotid artery is ligated, with only rare attempts to repair it after ECMO. As a result of collateral blood flow to the brain, acute neurologic sequelae directly related to this ligation are rare, although seizures have been reported in 5% of patients while on ECMO.

(3) Other complications encountered during ECMO include hemolysis, hyperbilirubinemia, renal insufficiency, cardiac arrhythmias, pulmonary hypertension, and sepsis.

8. **Outcome:** As part of its charter, the ELSO maintains an international registry of all patients treated with ECMO. As of July 1997, the registry for neonatal ECMO has recorded 12,016 cases. By diagnosis, babies suffering MAS or PPHN had survival rates of 94% and 84%, respectively, whereas the survival rate of patients with CDH was 59%. Patients with pneumonia or sepsis had a survival of 76%. Combined pediatric/neonatal survival after cardiac surgery was 42%. Several reports of long-term follow-up, including prospective, randomized trials using neurodevelopmental testing, describe approximately 75% of ECMO survivors as normal children.

III. ECMO FOR ADULTS

Although ECMO is standard treatment for newborn infants, it is utilized much less frequently in adult patients. This is largely because of the 90% mortality associated with ECMO in a 1970s NIH-funded prospective randomized trial. A more recent evaluation of adult ECMO in both European and North American centers, with similar inclusion criteria, has demonstrated a survival of 40% to 50%. Patients with cardiac and or respiratory failure may be candidates for ECMO if they are not responding to conventional therapy, have a transpulmonary shunt greater than or equal to 30% on an Fio_2 of 0.6 or greater, or have a static pulmonary compliance of less than 0.5 ml/cm H_2O/kg. Exclusion criteria are age over 60 years, duration of ventilation longer than 7 days, bleeding diathesis, or the presence of some other life-threatening, incurable process.

Although ECMO is used with some success for infants with postcardiotomy cardiac failure, this has not been the general experience in adults, where intraaortic balloon pumps or ventricular assist devices are preferable to VA ECMO. Results have also been disappointing when ECMO has been utilized for early graft failure after lung or heart/lung transplantation. Graft function may return, but patient survival is rare.

As is the case with infants, VV ECMO is utilized if hemodynamic support is not necessary. Venous access may be obtained percutaneously in most adults. Arterial access is usually obtained via sterile cutdown on the common carotid or common femoral artery. Perfusion protocols for adults are similar to those discussed above for infants and neonates. Bleeding is again the most frequent complication, although adults are not as prone to intracranial hemorrhage.

SUGGESTED READINGS

Anderson HL III, Snedecor SM, Otsu T, et al: Multicenter comparison of conventional venoarterial access versus venovenous double-lumen catheter access in newborn infants undergoing extracorporeal membrane oxygenation, *J Pediatr Surg* 28:530, 1993.

Anderson HL III, Steinle C, Shapiro M, et al: Extracorporeal life support for adult cardiorespiratory failure, *Surgery* 114:161, 1993.

Kolla S, Awad SS, Rich PB, et al: Extracorporeal life support for 100 adult patients with severe respiratory failure, *Ann Surg* 226:544, 1997.

Shanley CJ, Hirschl RB, Schumacher RE, et al: Extracorporeal life support for neonatal respiratory failure: a 20-year experience, *Ann Surg* 220:269, 1994.

The University of Michigan Extracorporeal Life Support Home Page: www.med.umich.edu/ecmo/index.html.

The Extracorporeal Life Support Organization Home Page: www.elso.med.umich.edu.

19

EXTRACORPOREAL MEMBRANE OXYGENATION

PART IV

Selected Problems in Patient Management

INFECTION AND SEPSIS

Charles W. Hoopes

I. FEVER AND DISORDERS OF TEMPERATURE HOMEOSTASIS

A. NORMAL TEMPERATURE HOMEOSTASIS

1. **Normal range** for core temperature 36.7° C to 37.6° C. Superimposed normal diurnal variation of 1° C (usually peaking in the evening) and 0.5° C with menstruation

2. **Normal homeostatic mechanisms**

a. Thermal control originates from the preoptic nucleus of the anterior hypothalamus, which directs the autonomic nervous system to regulate cutaneous vasomotor tone, perspiration, cutaneous muscular tone, and endocrinologic effectors of metabolic activity.

b. Nonshivering thermogenesis, the exaggerated metabolic activity of brown fat (significant in neonates only), and skeletal muscle (adults and neonates) can increase heat production 40% to 100%.

3. **Measurement**

a. Accurate measurement of core temperature in the SICU is via a thermal sensor–equipped PA catheter or distal esophageal probe in the unconscious patient. Invasive bladder probes and tympanic membrane monitors are designed to measure core temperature.

b. Rectal and oral temperatures are clinical estimates of core temperature.

B. FEVER

1. **Pathophysiology:** In response to noxious stimuli (such as endotoxin, complement activation, immune complexes, tissue injury), activated macrophages or lymphocytes release cytokines (primarily IL-1, IL-2, IL-6, TNF, and interferons), which ultimately raise the hypothalamic thermal set point.

2. **Treatment of fever:** Fever should be treated with drugs affecting prostaglandin synthesis (acetaminophen, NSAID) to reduce the discomfort of associated myalgias or to ameliorate increased metabolic activity that stresses a compromised cardiovascular system.

a. Topical cooling does not reduce fever and actually increases metabolic demand unless the hypothalamic-driven effectors of temperature regulation are blocked; this can be accomplished in extreme instances by sedation and pharmacologic paralysis.

b. Specific treatment should be directed to the underlying infection or damaged tissue.

3. **Complications of fever:** Major complications related to fever are the result of the causative agent or illness and not the elevated temperature.

a. Febrile seizures rarely occur after the age of 6 years and are usually benign.

b. Patients with marginal cardiovascular reserve can suffer serious consequences (stroke, MI, dysrhythmia, CHF) if unable to meet the increased Vo_2 (7% increase in Vo_2 for each 1° C fever) or decreased SVR of pyrexia; aggressive treatment is indicated in these instances.

20

C. HYPERTHERMIA

1. **Examples** include malignant hyperthermia, thyroid storm, dehydration, heat stroke, and hypothalamic injury (trauma, tumor, infarction).

2. **Hyperthermia cannot be distinguished from fever based on the magnitude of pyrexia;** certain clinical situations produce a readily apparent diagnosis, but endocrinologic and hypothalamic disorders require extensive testing.

3. **Treatment** includes therapy directed to the underlying disorder, withdrawal of offending drugs, and adequate hydration.

   a. Clinical features of a drug fever include relative bradycardia with temperature greater than 38.5° C, nontoxic appearance, elevated WBC count (with left shift) and ESR greater than 100 mm/hr, mild elevation of serum transaminases, and eosinophils without eosinophilia. Maculopapular rashes are uncommon.

   b. Specific pharmacotherapy (dantrolene for malignant hyperthermia, propylthiouracil for thyroid storm) is used when indicated (see Chapter 24).

   c. Topical cooling should be used for temperatures higher than 40° C.

D. HYPOTHERMIA

1. **The most common causes of hypothermia** (core body temperature greater than 35° C) in the SICU are general and regional anesthesia, prolonged abdominal surgery, cooling during CPB, sepsis, environmental exposure after burns or trauma, and clinical mismanagement (e.g., 1000 ml of infused crystalloid at ambient temperature or a single unit of PRBCs at 4° C decreases mean body temperature by approximately 0.25° C).

2. **Metabolic causes** include hypoglycemia, hypopituitarism, hypothyroidism, and hypothalamic dysfunction.

3. **The most important problems** stem from dysfunction of excitable tissues with ventricular fibrillation at more than 30° C the most common cause of death. Core hypothermia of 1.5° C triples the incidence of ventricular tachycardia and morbid cardiac arrhythmias. Slow positive deflections in the latter part of the QRS complex (J waves) are diagnostic and may be the first sign of profound hypothermia in the anesthetized patient. Additional complications of perioperative hypothermia include increased incidence of surgical wound infection, coagulopathy, "cold diuresis," and prolonged duration of paralytics.

4. **Passive rewarming** using continuous ECG and core temperature monitoring, 100% oxygen, IV fluids and inspired gases warmed to 39° C, and external heating sources is used if temperature is greater than 30° C and the patient's homeostatic regulatory mechanisms (shivering) are intact.

5. **Active rewarming** using gastric, colonic, or peritoneal lavage with 39° C lactated Ringer's solution or femoral-femoral CPB is used for temperatures less than 30° C, passive rewarming rates of less than 1° C per hour, or when normal physiologic mechanisms are impaired (e.g., arrested cardiac rhythm).

6. **Vasodilatation** secondary to rewarming may result in profound hypovolemia and hypotension.

7. **Hypothermic patients are not dead until warmed beyond 32° C.**

II. SURGICAL INFECTIONS

A. SIGNS AND SYMPTOMS

1. **Signs and symptoms** include fever, leukocytosis, and local signs of infection, such as inflammation, wound drainage, or foul sputum.

2. **The classic signs of infection are usually (but not always) present,** especially in immunocompromised patients. These include fever ($T > 38.5°$ C), tachycardia ($HR > 90$), tachypnea ($RR > 20$), hypoxemia, hypotension, elevated serum glucose, ileus, DIC, altered mental status, and/or hypothermia ($T < 35°$ C)

3. **Risk factors** that increase the likelihood and severity of infections include advanced age, diabetes, malnutrition, immunocompromise (steroids, burns, AIDS), and multiple organ dysfunction syndrome.

B. SYSTEMIC MANIFESTATIONS

1. **Bacteremia:** The presence of viable bacteria in the blood occurs in only 50% of patients with septic shock. Clinical judgment differentiates contamination from diagnostic culture.

2. **Sepsis:** Infection plus signs of systemic response; tachypnea, tachycardia, hyperthermia or hypothermia, and leukocytosis or leukopenia.

3. **Sepsis syndrome:** Sepsis plus evidence of altered organ perfusion.
   a. Pao_2/Fio_2 less than 280 mm Hg
   b. Elevated lactate
   c. Oliguria (<0.5 ml/kg/hr for at least 1 hour)
   d. Altered mental status

4. **Septic shock:** Clinical diagnosis of the sepsis syndrome plus hypotension refractory to fluid administration or pharmacologic intervention (e.g., $SBP < 90$ mm Hg or a 40 mm Hg decrease from baseline for 1 hour despite adequate volume resuscitation).

5. **Systemic inflammatory response syndrome (SIRS):** Systemic response characterized by uncontrolled inflammation followed by a period of immunosuppression.

6. **Multiple organ dysfunction syndrome:** Altered organ function in an acutely ill patient such that homeostasis cannot be maintained without intervention.

7. **Risk factors** for SIRS include use of indwelling catheters, implantation of prosthetic devices, immunodeficient states (HIV, transplant, compromised nutrition, cancer, elderly), immunosuppressive drugs (corticosteroids, chemotherapy), long-term and broad-spectrum use of antibiotics, multisystem trauma, extensive burns, pancreatitis, cardiogenic shock, prolonged operative procedures, and overwhelming infections.

8. **Although commonly associated with gram-negative sepsis,** causative organisms are not identified in 10% to 30% of septic patients and the incidence of gram-positive infections now equals that of gram-negatives.

C. MEDIATORS AND PATHOPHYSIOLOGY OF SEPSIS

1. **Bacterial toxins,** including lipopolysaccharide (LPS) endotoxin from gram-negative bacilli outer membranes, gram-negative formyl peptides and proteases, and exotoxins, enterotoxins, and lipoteichoic acid from gram-positive organisms, have all been implicated in the etiology of sepsis.

2. **Toxins stimulate release** of the macrophage proinflammatory cytokines TNF-α and IL-1, both of which stimulate the proinflammatory interleukins IL-6 and IL-8.

3. **Proinflammatory cytokines** may induce tissue factor expression on endothelial cells, thereby activating the extrinsic pathway of coagulation and contributing to DIC.

4. **Nitric oxide synthetase (NOS)** is induced by inflammatory mediators. NO may mediate the myocardial depression, hypotension, vasodilation, and capillary leak characteristic of septic shock.

III. EVALUATION OF FEVER AND DIAGNOSIS OF SEPSIS

A. EVALUATION OF FEVER

1. **Primary diagnostic goal** is to distinguish between fevers of infectious etiology and those of noninfectious origin. Fever patterns may predict etiology. Etiology determines appropriate treatment.

2. **A variety of febrile medical conditions are excluded** by fevers greater than or equal to 102° F (38.9° C), including myocardial infarct, pulmonary embolism, thrombophlebitis, cholecystitis, GI bleed, pancreatitis, ARDS, and uncomplicated wound infections.

3. **Acute, intermittent fevers** greater than or equal to 38.9° C generally reflect invasive infectious disease or transient bacteremia (e.g., line sepsis, manipulation of the biliary tract). Noninfectious sources include drug fevers and transfusion reactions.

4. **Persistent low-grade fevers** less than 38.9° C are generally noninfectious but may also represent persistent foci of infection (e.g., intraabdominal or CNS abscess, endocarditis).

5. **A substantial proportion of infected patients are not febrile** and may be euthermic or hypothermic (e.g., elderly, burn patients with extensive skin loss, immunosuppressed, chronic antipyretics).

6. **Within 48 hours of surgery or trauma,** the most common causes of fever are atelectasis, clostridial or streptococcal wound infections, infections related to anastomotic leak, and generalized immune activation after major trauma. The presence of a preoperative infection may be the cause of early postoperative fever.

7. **Beyond 48 hours,** temperatures of 38.3° C to 38.5° C should elicit a more extensive evaluation of the patient as to potential infectious sources. Practice parameters for the evaluation of fever in critically ill patients have recently been reviewed by the Society for Critical Care Medicine.

   a. Wounds should be examined, including all sites of transcutaneous catheters.

   b. A thorough head, eyes, ears, nose, and throat (HEENT) examination for signs of otitis, sinusitis, or meningitis is especially important in patients with an intubated nasopharynx or oropharynx.

   c. Thoracic examination should detect areas of pulmonary consolidation, effusions, or bronchospasm.

d. Abdominal examination is used to evaluate cholecystitis, pancreatitis, intraabdominal abscess, or intestinal obstruction.

e. Prostatitis and perirectal abscess are evaluated by rectal examination.

f. Look for signs of thrombophlebitis.

g. Laboratory studies include CBC with differential, urinalysis, and two sets of blood cultures drawn during the febrile episode (greater than or equal to 38.5° C) from separate peripheral sites and central venous catheters.

h. CXR should be obtained.

i. More extensive testing (e.g., abdominal CT scan, ventilation-perfusion scan, lumbar puncture, sinus films, and echocardiogram) are performed as indicated.

B. MANAGEMENT OF THE FEBRILE PATIENT

1. **In the hemodynamically stable patient** without suspicion of sepsis, diagnosis of an infectious etiology is the primary clinical goal. This requires detailed history and physical examination and appropriate laboratory and radiographic studies to rule out noninfectious febrile conditions. We do not routinely start empiric antibiotics without identifying an infectious source.

2. **In the hemodynamically unstable patient** with a presumptive diagnosis of sepsis, resuscitation is the primary clinical goal.

C. DIAGNOSIS AND MANAGEMENT OF THE SEPTIC PATIENT

1. **Sepsis is frequently overdiagnosed** in the critical care environment. Acute myocardial infarct, pulmonary embolism, acute GI bleeding, adrenal insufficiency, and drug and transfusion reactions may all mimic sepsis in terms of fever, leukocytosis, and hemodynamic instability.

2. **Resuscitation** is the first line of therapy of the patient in shock, regardless of cause.

a. Elective intubation should be pursued early in patients with respiratory insufficiency.

b. Pulmonary artery catheters are used routinely by Duke University surgical residents to facilitate diagnosis, volume resuscitation, and selection of specific cardiovascular agents for treatment of shock.

c. Resuscitation parameters are guided by hemodynamic optimization of end-organ perfusion using calculated values of oxygen delivery and consumption and clinical markers of inadequate perfusion (e.g., lactate; see Chapter 2).

d. After resuscitation and stabilization, begin a diagnostic evaluation for infection.

3. **Treatment of sepsis** involves identification of the infectious source, surgical eradication of the infectious focus, and appropriate antibiotic therapy. Several immunomodulation and anticytokine therapies are in clinical trial. Evidence for the use of corticosteroids is contradictory.

4. **Sepsis arises** from untreated infections of the intraabdominal cavity, cardiopulmonary system, urogenital tract, or indwelling central venous catheters. Patients without infectious foci at one of these sites are unlikely to have sepsis.

20

INFECTION AND SEPSIS

5. **When the source of infection is known,** a specific treatment based on the most likely pathogens can begin; however, the source of infection is often not obvious and empiric therapy should be instituted in the unstable patient. Ampicillin, gentamicin, and metronidazole are often started as broad-spectrum empiric therapy after all cultures have been obtained. Consider a loading dose of vancomycin in septic patients whose clinical history suggests methicillin-resistant *Staphylococcus aureus* (MRSA).

a. Fungal sepsis must be considered in patients who manifest septic physiology after 7 to 10 days of antibiotic therapy.

b. Antibiotics alone are insufficient to treat sepsis, and specific surgical therapy is instituted as indicated. This may include exploratory laparotomy in a postoperative patient without a specific diagnosis.

IV. SPECIFIC INFECTIONS

A. INTRAABDOMINAL SEPSIS

Secondary to trauma, spontaneous rupture of a hollow viscus (e.g., diverticulitis, duodenal perforation, inflammatory bowel disease, mesenteric ischemia), or postoperative complications (e.g., anastomotic leak, occult bowel injury).

1. **Diagnosis** requires high index of suspicion based on history and physical examination. Patients may present with localized tenderness and spiking fevers characteristic of enclosed abscesses or vague, generalized complaints of diffuse abdominal pain progressing to frank peritonitis characteristic of free perforations (e.g., acute abdomen). Mortality is 10% to 50%, depending on site of perforation and patient risk factors.

2. **Contrast CT is the diagnostic modality of choice.** Diagnostic studies should not preclude immediate exploration of the patient with clinical signs of an intraabdominal catastrophe. Unstable patients may benefit from resuscitation before operative intervention.

3. **Treatment is primarily surgical** (e.g., CT-guided drainage of abscess cavities or exploratory laparotomy for free perforation).

4. **Microbiology** represents complex polymicrobial disease involving both aerobes and anaerobes. Gram-positive aerobes predominate in the stomach and duodenum; gram-negative anaerobic species are more common in the small bowel and colon. Most common species in community-acquired intraabdominal infections are aerobic *Escherichia coli* and anaerobic *Bacteroides fragilis*. Opportunistic pathogens, such as *Pseudomonas aeruginosa, Serratia marcescens,* and *Acinetobacter* spp., may contribute to infections in chronic ICU patients.

5. **Current recommendations of the Surgical Infection Society** (1992) for single-agent treatment of intraabdominal infections include ticarcillin/clavulanate, cefoxitin, or cefotetan for moderate community-acquired infections and imipenem/cilastatin for severe infections. Combination regimens include clindamycin or metronidazole for anaerobic coverage with an aminoglycoside in young patients with normal renal function or aztreonam in patients with renal compromise.

B. PNEUMONIA: COMMUNITY ACQUIRED, NOSOCOMIAL, AND VENTILATOR ASSOCIATED

1. **Prolonged intubation and underlying lung disease** are associated with an increased risk of bacterial pneumonia in postoperative patients; nosocomial pneumonia is the most common severe, hospital-acquired infection identified in critical care environments (reported death rates of more than 30%).

2. **Although *Streptococcus pneumoniae* and *Haemophilus influenzae* are the most common pathogens** in patients with community-acquired pneumonia (CAP) and early postoperative pneumonias, gram-negative bacilli *(Pseudomonas, Acinetobacter, Klebsiella, Serratia)* are more frequently found in patients with chronic lung disease and late nosocomial infections. *Staphylococcus aureus* (including MRSA) is the most common cause of nosocomial pneumonia. Common atypical pathogens include *Legionella, Mycoplasma,* and *Chlamydia* spp.

3. **Diagnosis of ventilator-associated pneumonia (VAP) is difficult.** Fewer than 50% of patients with fever, leukocytosis, and a pulmonary infiltrate (e.g., clinical pneumonia) will have pneumonia by quantitative culture criteria.

   a. Pulmonary infiltrates are an insensitive predictor of pneumonia. Signs of consolidation are present in only 30% of patients, and "infiltrates" may represent noninfectious pulmonary atelectasis, aspiration, contusion, barotrauma, embolus, infarct, edema, or early ARDS.

   b. Qualitative sputum cultures in intubated patients represent colonization and inflammation of the tracheobronchial tree, are not diagnostic of pneumonia, and do not require treatment.

   c. Quantitative cultures (≥100,000 CFU/ml) obtained by site-directed bronchoscopy, and bronchoalveolar lavage (BAL) is the diagnostic modality of choice. Recent evidence suggests that quantitative analysis of endotracheal aspirates may offer a noninvasive alternative with comparable clinical efficacy.

   d. The use of empiric vs. pathogen-driven antibiotic treatment of VAP is controversial, as is the decision to treat with single vs. combination drug therapy. We routinely start empiric monotherapy with a third-generation cephalosporin (ceftazidime) or combination β-lactam/β-lactamase inhibitor (ticarcillin/clavulanate). Vancomycin is given empirically for a clinical suspicion of MRSA. Antibiotic therapy is stopped or modified based on culture results. Synergistic combination therapy with an aminoglycoside and β-lactam antibiotic (ticarcillin/tobramycin) is used when *Pseudomonas* is suspected or identified.

4. **Effusions greater than 10 mm** on lateral decubitus films should be considered for diagnostic thoracentesis (Gram's stain and culture, cell count with differential, pH, protein, LDH, and glucose).

C. UROSEPSIS AND URINARY TRACT INFECTIONS

1. **Uncomplicated urinary tract infections** are common and rarely cause sepsis. Dysuria, frequency, hesitancy, and inability to void are frequent

symptoms of cystitis; flank pain, fever, and ileus may be due to pyelonephritis. The presence of pyuria, leukocyte esterase, nitrite, and bacteriuria are suggestive of infection, but a positive culture (>100,000 colonies/ml of urine) is definitive.

2. **Obstruction of the urogenital system** with subsequent bacteremia defines urosepsis, and sepsis from a GU source without obstruction is rare. Urinary retention and instrumentation predispose to urinary infections and may contribute to urosepsis.

3. **Treatment** includes adequate urinary drainage (e.g., nephrostomy tubes) and appropriate antibiotics—quinolones or aminoglycosides for common GNRs, combination coverage for *Enterococcus* with ampicillin, and amphotericin or fluconazole for funguria.

D. ENDOCARDITIS

1. **Acute bacterial endocarditis** can present as sepsis; subacute bacterial endocarditis may be a cause of persistent low-grade fevers.

2. **Diagnosis** should be entertained in any patient with unexplained fever and a cardiac murmur. A murmur may be absent with right-sided or mural infections, and a "new onset" murmur is found in only 15% of patients.

3. **Blood cultures are positive in 95% of cases,** excluding fungal endocarditis and patients who have received antibiotics within 2 weeks of presumptive diagnosis.

4. **Diagnosis requires at least three sets of blood cultures** (10 to 15 ml/ culture tube) taken at least 15 minutes apart. Echocardiography should be performed to search for vegetations.

5. **Toxic patients are most likely to have *Staphylococcus aureus,* enterococcus, or Group B streptococcus pathogens.** Empiric therapy is vancomycin and gentamicin. *S. aureus* endocarditis has been associated with central venous catheters and is characterized by rapid onset, high fevers, frequent involvement of normal valves, and absence of classic endocarditis stigmata (e.g., 55% of cases diagnosed at autopsy were not suspected on clinical grounds).

6. **Antibiotic prophylaxis** should be given to all patients at high and intermediate risk (e.g., valvular heart disease, prosthetic valves, previous endocarditis, patent ductus arteriosus [PDA]), VSD, Marfan syndrome, aortic coarctation, tetralogy of Fallot, and mitral valve prolapse with insufficiency) who are undergoing instrumentation of the oral, respiratory, GI, and urinary tracts. Standard prophylaxis includes ampicillin 2 g IV plus gentamicin 1.5 mg/kg 30 minutes before procedure followed by amoxicillin 1.5 gm PO 6 hours later.

E. LINE SEPSIS

1. **Highest infectious risk** with short-term, noncuffed central venous catheters (5 to 10 cases/1000 catheter days) and temporary hemodialysis catheters, intermediate risk with surgically implanted catheters (2 bacteremias/1000 catheter days), and minimal risk from peripheral IV catheters (<0.2 cases/1000 catheter days).

2. **Indwelling central venous catheters should be immediately removed** and cultured in patients with evidence of emboli, vascular compromise, or unexplained sepsis. Central venous catheters placed emergently (e.g., trauma, cardiopulmonary arrest) should be replaced early.
3. **Fever workups** should include simultaneous cultures from a peripheral site and the central venous catheter. A quantitative blood culture drawn from an infected catheter will demonstrate a tenfold or greater concentration of organisms compared with a peripheral quantitative culture. The clinical significance of a positive catheter culture in the absence of a positive blood culture is unknown, and clinical judgment should determine if this represents colonization or infection.
4. **Catheter infections** are suggested by temporal association of clinical bacteremias with line utilization and by multiple blood cultures containing organisms generally considered contaminants (e.g., coagulase-negative *Staphylococcus, Corynebacterium jeikeium, Bacillus* spp., *Candida,* or *Malassezia*).

F. **SOFT TISSUE INFECTIONS**
1. **Infections associated with soft tissue inflammation usually require surgical intervention.**
2. **Signs and symptoms** include fever, leukocytosis, and a specific area of inflammation; the site should be examined for inflammatory reaction, fluctuance, crepitus, and tissue necrosis.
   a. The presence of erythema without fluctuance, drainage, or devitalized tissue is most likely cellulitis. Patients with impaired lymphatic drainage (e.g., saphenous venectomy sites, axillary dissections) are prone to recurrent episodes of cellulitis.
   b. An area of erythema occurring over a vein associated with a palpable cord may represent suppurative thrombophlebitis.
   c. Linear red streaks proximal to an inflammatory site on a distal limb represent lymphangitic spread.
3. **Management** should include antimicrobial agents effective against both staphylococci and streptococci (e.g., penicillinase-resistant penicillins: nafcillin, methicillin, or dicloxacillin).
4. **Failure to improve rapidly** should lead one to suspect a resistant organism, an occult abscess, or a less common pathogen (e.g., *Streptococcus pneumoniae, Haemophilus influenzae,* vibrios, clostridia, or gram-negative bacilli).
5. **Deep inflammation** is characterized by the presence of local inflammation associated with fluctuance, drainage, or sinus tracts.
   a. Needle aspiration with a large-bore needle and a small syringe may be helpful to determine if an undrained collection is present.
   b. If there is no collection, an abscess may not have formed yet or an unconsidered diagnosis may exist.
   c. If a collection is present, surgical drainage is required because an abscess is resistant to the action of antibiotics.

6. **The presence of devascularized skin, deep necrosis, and crepitus** indicates the possibility of a more serious soft tissue infection.
   a. A history of crush injury with devitalized tissue, foreign body, systemic signs of toxemia, muscle necrosis, and gram-positive rods are signs of clostridial myositis (gas gangrene).
   b. Extensive debridement is necessary and often requires limb amputation.
   c. Aggressive circulatory support is needed to maintain tissue perfusion.
   d. Penicillin G 20 to 24 million U/day IV is given.
   e. Hyperbaric O_2 may be helpful; however, treatment by debridement has priority over transfer to hyperbaric O_2 chamber.
7. **The presence of a rapidly spreading infection, mixed organisms on Gram's stain, necrotic fascia, and thrombosis and obliteration of subcutaneous vessels** are signs of necrotizing fasciitis; gram-negative synergistic necrotizing cellulitis is part of a spectrum of necrotizing infections that may present as a necrotizing infection of the abdominal wall. Extensive debridement of necrotic fascia is necessary, but limbs can usually be salvaged. Elevated muscle compartment pressures (>40 mm Hg) contribute to myonecrosis and should elicit early fasciotomy.
8. **The distinction between cellulitis and fasciitis is crucial** because the former is amenable to antibiotic therapy and the latter requires surgical debridement. CT, MRI, and frozen section biopsy can provide information on depth of invasion and diagnosis.

G. **MENINGITIS**
1. **CNS infections rarely cause encephalopathy without focal neurologic findings.**
2. **Patients with focal neurologic findings should undergo a noncontrast CT** to exclude mass lesions (including brain abscesses) and to identify obstructive hydrocephalus that would preclude subsequent lumbar puncture. Patients with suspected brain abscesses should not undergo lumbar puncture because of the risk of herniation and limited bacteriologic yield—antibiotics and aspiration are the treatment of choice.
3. **Ommaya reservoirs and ventriculoperitoneal shunts** should be routinely cultured in patients with suspected CNS infections.
4. **CSF results in patients with bacterial meningitis** include glucose less than 35 mg/dl, a CSF–blood glucose ratio of less than 0.23, a CSF protein level of greater than 220 mg/dl, and greater than 2000 WBCs per microliter. A normal opening pressure, fewer than 5 WBCs, and a normal CSF protein level essentially preclude bacterial meningitis in an immunocompetent adult. The diagnosis of viral encephalitis (e.g., herpes) requires more detailed analysis by virus-specific polymerase chain reaction.

H. **SINUSITIS**
1. **The paranasal sinuses are normally sterile.** Although sinusitis is commonly seen in patients with prolonged nasal intubations (ET or NG tubes), definitive documentation that this site is the source of clinically significant fevers is uncommon.

2. **Gram-negative bacilli constitute 60% of bacterial isolates,** with *Pseudomonas aeruginosa* being the most common. *Staphylococcus aureus* is the most common gram-positive isolate, and 5% to 10% of isolates are fungal. Only 25% of ICU patients with proven sinusitis have purulent nasal discharge.

3. **Opacification or air-fluid levels** on standard sinus radiographs is sensitive but nonspecific. CT scans have a higher diagnostic yield, but sinus puncture and aspiration under aseptic conditions with subsequent microbial analysis is required for definitive diagnosis. Aspiration, removal of devices obstructing the ostia, and pathogen-specific antibiotics are the treatments of choice.

I. **DIARRHEA**

1. **Defined** as more than two stools per day that conform to the container in which they are placed.

2. **Enteral feedings and antibiotics** are the common causes of diarrhea in the SICU, but the differential includes ischemic colitis, inflammatory bowel disease, intraabdominal sepsis, drugs other than antibiotics, and conventional enteric pathogens (SSCY: *Shigella, Salmonella, Campylobacter,* and *Yersinia*). *Entamoeba histolytica, Microsporidium, Mycobacterium avium* complex, and CMV may cause diarrhea in the immunocompromised patient.

3. *Clostridium difficile* is a spore-forming obligate anaerobic bacillus found in the stool of 5% of healthy adults and 10% or more of hospitalized patients without diarrhea who have received antibiotics or chemotherapy. *C. difficile* is the most common enteric cause of fevers in the ICU, and enterotoxin-producing strains are responsible for 10% to 25% of antibiotic-associated diarrheas.

4. **Diarrhea** associated with *C. difficile* should be suspected in patients with fecal leukocytes and an otherwise unexplained fever and leukocytosis who have been exposed to antibiotics (especially cephalosporins, ampicillin, or clindamycin). The absence of fecal leukocytes does not eliminate the diagnosis of *C. difficile.*

5. **Although tissue culture assay for** *C. difficile* is the diagnostic standard, enzyme immunoassay for the enterotoxins A and/or B provides a more rapid diagnosis. Initially, a single stool sample should be evaluated. If this is negative and diarrhea persists, one or two additional cultures should be obtained. Colonoscopy is diagnostic when pseudomembranes are identified but is generally reserved for special situations when other colonic diseases are in the differential.

6. **Standard treatment** consists of cessation of offending antibiotics, supportive therapy, and metronidazole 500 to 750 mg PO tid for 7 to 10 days. Vancomycin is used only for treatment failures, resistant strains, and pregnant patients. Patients should be recultured after therapy to confirm efficacy. Management guidelines for *Clostridium difficile* disease have recently been published.

20

INFECTION AND SEPSIS

V. SPECIFIC PATHOGENS

A. BACTERIAL PATHOGENS

1. Gram-positive cocci

a. *Staphylococcus aureus* is a coagulase-positive, gram-positive commensal colonizing nares, axilla, vagina, pharynx, and areas of damaged skin. Frequently associated with nosocomial pneumonias, bacteremias, wound- and catheter-related infections. Treat preferentially with nafcillin or oxacillin.

b. MRSA has same virulence as *S. aureus* but requires treatment with vancomycin.

c. *S. epidermidis* is often associated with infections of prosthetic materials; because the organism is part of normal skin flora, it may appear as a contaminant in blood cultures. Treat with vancomycin.

d. Streptococci are often a cause of cellulitis and endocarditis; Group A are causative in scarlet fever, erysipelas, and rheumatic fever. Treat with penicillin G.

e. Enterococci are recognized pathogens in endocarditis, meningitis, urinary tract infections, and biliary sepsis. These infections may be treated with ampicillin and gentamicin. Although enterococci are found in 10% to 20% of intraabdominal infections, their virulence remains in question. Vancomycin-resistant strains of *Enterococcus faecium* (VRE) have been identified, and opportunistic enterococcal bacteremias have been identified in surgical patients treated with cephalosporins.

2. Gram-positive rods

a. *Clostridium tetani* and *C. perfringens* are anaerobic bacteria that cause tetanus and gas gangrene, respectively. Treatment requires debridement and high-dose penicillin G.

b. *Corynebacterium diphtheriae* is the causative organism in diphtheria. Prevention is by immunization with diphtheria toxoid, which is usually given with tetanus toxoid. Treat with diphtheria antitoxin and penicillin G.

3. Gram-negative cocci

a. *Neisseria gonorrhoeae* causes gonorrhea. Treat with penicillin.

b. *N. meningitidis* causes meningitis and septic shock. Treat with penicillin.

4. Gram-negative rods

a. *Bacteroides* organisms are anaerobic bacteria of the GI tract, often involved in intraabdominal abscesses; *B. fragilis* is the most eminent. Treat with metronidazole or clindamycin.

b. The *Enterobacteriaceae* family includes *Escherichia coli* and *Klebsiella, Enterobacter, Serratia*, and *Proteus* organisms; they are involved in biliary, urinary, and GI-related infections. Treat with aminoglycosides; alternatively, a second- or third-generation cephalosporin may be used.

c. *Haemophilus influenzae* may cause meningitis, epiglottitis, or pneumonia. Treatment is with aztreonam, imipenem, β-lactam agents combined with a β-lactamase inhibitor, or third-generation cephalosporin (ampicillin-resistant strains now common).

d. *Pseudomonas aeruginosa* is common in nosocomial infections; wound infections typically have greenish exudate with fruity odor. Treat with two synergistic drugs to avoid resistance (usually mezlocillin, aztreonam, or ceftazidime combined with an aminoglycoside).

B. FUNGAL PATHOGENS

1. **Invasive *Candida albicans* infections are the most common (60%).** Predisposing factors for nosocomial candidemia include use of corticosteroids, long-term use of broad-spectrum antibiotics, central venous catheters, dialysis, malnutrition, prolonged illness, and TPN. Systemic colonization may predispose to infection.

2. **Primary diagnostic goal** is to distinguish superficial from invasive infections and to identify disseminated *Candida* characteristic of a systemic fungal infection rather than colonization.

a. Candidal endophthalmitis, characterized by white, fluffy chorioretinal lesions on ophthalmoscopic examination, has been shown to correlate with disseminated fungal infection and is an indication for systemic antifungal therapy.

b. Additional indications for systemic treatment of disseminated *Candida* include organisms isolated from three or more separate sites with negative blood cultures, two positive blood cultures at least 24 hours apart in the absence of a central venous catheter, positive blood cultures more than 24 hours after the removal of a colonized central venous catheter, and a positive peritoneal culture for *Candida.* Approximately half of all patients with disseminated candidiasis will not have positive blood cultures.

c. Disseminated candidiasis may produce maculopapular skin lesions amenable to biopsy.

3. **Treatment** of symptomatic candidal urinary tract infections consists of amphotericin bladder irrigation and/or oral fluconazole for more severe infections.

4. **Prophylaxis** against oral candidiasis is best accomplished with oral nystatin. Oral candidiasis may be treated with either oral nystatin or fluconazole.

5. **Other fungal pathogens** include *Cryptococcus histoplasma, Mucor* organisms, and *Aspergillus* organisms.

6. **The decision to treat a presumed fungal infection is based on the clinical setting in conjunction with culture results.** A consensus conference has recommended empiric treatment of neutropenic patients with persistent fevers for 5 to 7 days despite appropriate antibiotic therapy and no identifiable source of fever after extensive evaluation for nonfungal infection. We routinely treat such high-risk patients with fluconazole 200-400 mg qd and consider empiric antifungal therapy in critically ill patients with candiduria, a single positive blood culture, or isolation of *Candida* from two body sites.

C. VIRAL PATHOGENS

1. **Hepatitis B** is transmitted by blood, blood products, or sexual contact and can result in chronic active hepatitis and cirrhosis. Needle sticks from carriers can be treated by hepatitis B immune globulin and vacci-

20

INFECTION AND SEPSIS

nation. Prevention is best managed by immunization with hepatitis vaccine.

2. **Hepatitis C**

a. Hepatitis C virus (HCV) is a blood-borne infection. Infection rate after needle stick injury is 5% to 10%. Transmission from infected surgeons, human bites, and transplanted organs has been documented.

b. HCV ribonucleic acid (RNA) is detectable by polymerase chain reaction (PCR) within 1 week of exposure but infection is diagnosed by anti-HCV enzyme-linked immunosorbent assay (ELISA). Chronic infection occurs in 85% of exposed patients, and 20% develop cirrhosis within 20 years. HCV is currently the major cause of liver disease requiring transplantation.

c. Patients with persistently elevated serum aminotransferases and histologic evidence of progression to cirrhosis should be treated with α-interferon.

3. **HIV**

a. Needle sticks from seropositive patients carry 1 in 250 to 1 in 300 risk of infection.

b. Exposure to blood of seropositive patients should be managed by serotesting the exposed health care worker and repeated testing 6 weeks, 3 months, 6 months, and 12 months after exposure.

c. Protocols exist for use of zidovudine (AZT) in exposed health care workers (AZT 250 mg PO q4h $\times$ 6 to 7 weeks).

4. **Herpes viruses**

a. CMV is the most important pathogen affecting bone marrow and organ transplant recipients. A seronegative recipient of seropositive tissues has a greater than 50% chance of symptomatic disease.

b. CMV demonstrates both latency and cell-specific replication. Latent virus may be reactivated by any systemic infection with active disease manifest as an acute viral syndrome (fever and myalgias, atypical lymphocytosis, thrombocytopenia) or organ-specific inflammation (e.g., pneumonitis, hepatitis, myocarditis).

c. CMV-mediated immunosuppression may facilitate opportunistic pathogens (e.g., *Aspergillus*), and CMV should be sought as a cofactor in unusual infections.

d. Diagnosis of CMV is by direct observation of inclusion bodies on biopsy of infected tissues, demonstration of antigenemia, or primer-specific PCR of virus from blood.

e. Treatment of clinical CMV involves IV ganciclovir until viremia resolves. Low-dose ganciclovir associated with oral therapy may contribute to resistance.

f. Epstein-Barr virus is present in 20% to 40% of transplant patients and is responsible for posttransplantation lymphoproliferative disease. Treatment is reduction or cessation of immunosuppressive therapy.

g. Herpes simplex causes oral and genital skin eruptions, pneumonitis, and encephalitis. Varicella zoster virus is the causative agent in both chickenpox (primary) and zoster (reactivation). Both can be treated with acyclovir.

VI. PREVENTION AND TREATMENT OF SURGICAL WOUND INFECTIONS

1. **Although wound infections are usually evident by physical examination** (erythema, drainage, and the presence of crepitus), precise definitions of nosocomial surgical site infections have been published by the Centers for Disease Control and Prevention.

2. **Cellulitis** is manifested by a tender, warm, erythematous wound without drainage or fluctuance; treat with antibiotics typically active against gram-positive and gram-negative organisms.

3. **Wound infections associated with drainage or fluctuance should be opened;** drainage and dressing changes are usually all the treatment that is needed, and antibiotics are used only if there is a component of cellulitis or systemic evidence of infection.

4. **Infection over vascular grafts requires expert care;** graft removal and extraanatomic bypass may be required, and the operating surgeon should be notified immediately.

5. **The presence of infection before surgery increases the risk of wound infection,** and elective surgery should be postponed until the infection has been treated.

6. **Antiseptic showers before surgery** and skin preparation with chlorhexidine or povidone iodine perioperatively decrease wound infection rate.

7. **Perioperative prophylactic antibiotics** for elective procedures are chosen according to the pathogen likely to be present in the operative field. For most procedures, cefazolin (1-2 g) is effective. In chronically ill patients, patients colonized with MRSA, and institutions with a high incidence of MRSA, vancomycin (1 g) may serve as an alternative to cefazolin. For colorectal surgery and appendectomy, cefoxitin or cefotetan are preferred because of increased activity towards bowel anaerobes. Third-generation cephalosporins should not be used for routine prophylaxis because their activity against staphylococci is less than that of cefazolin.

8. **Wound infection rates are as follows:**

a. Clean case—no gross contamination (hernia, thyroidectomy); wound infection rate less than 1%

b. Clean-contaminated case—minor contamination (biliary surgery); wound infection rate 2% to 5%

c. Contaminated case—major contamination (gross spillage from unprepared bowel); wound infection rate 5% to 30%

d. Dirty case—contamination from infected source (drainage of appendiceal abscess); wound infection rate greater than 30%

9. **Patient risk factors** include hyperglycemia, steroids, advanced age, malnutrition, renal failure, obesity, perioperative radiation, and chemotherapy with secondary neutropenia.

VII. INFECTION IN THE IMMUNOCOMPROMISED HOST

A. THE IMMUNOCOMPROMISED HOST

1. **The immunocompromised host** is any patient with impaired host defenses who is at increased risk of developing infection; such infections are likely to be of greater severity than in the normal host.

2. **The increasing prevalence of immunocompromised patients** is due to the following:

   a. Advances in cancer chemotherapy

   b. Organ transplantation

   c. Immunosuppressive therapy of nonmalignant disease

   d. Increasing prevalence of AIDS

3. **In the immunocompromised host, infection is the most common immediate cause of death.**

4. **Infection is likely to be due to opportunistic pathogens;** because the host's ability to mount an inflammatory response is impaired, signs of serious systemic infection may be nonspecific or absent.

B. DEFECTS IN THE IMMUNE RESPONSE

1. **Granulocytopenia**

   a. Absolute granulocyte count less than 500/ml or defect in phagocytosis; incidence or severity of infection related to absolute granulocyte count and rapidity of onset of granulocytopenia

   b. Etiology includes the following:

      (1) Leukemia, lymphoma, collagen-vascular disease

      (2) Cytotoxic chemotherapy or radiation therapy for malignant disease

      (3) Immunosuppressive therapy for autoimmune disease and posttransplantation (corticosteroids, azathioprine)

   c. Common pathogens include the following:

      (1) Gram-positive: *Staphylococcus aureus, Staphylococcus epidermidis*

      (2) Gram-negative: *Escherichia coli, Klebsiella pneumoniae, Pseudomonas aeruginosa*

      (3) Fungal: *Candida albicans*, *Aspergillus* and *Mucor* organisms

      (4) Viral: herpes viruses, especially CMV

2. **Cellular immune dysfunction**

   a. Etiology

      (1) Lymphoma

      (2) AIDS

      (3) Autoimmune disease

      (4) Organ transplant recipients (corticosteroids, immunosuppressive therapy)

   b. Common pathogens

      (1) Bacterial: *Listeria monocytogenes, Salmonella* organisms, *Nocardia asteroides, Legionella* organisms, mycobacteria

      (2) Fungal: *Cryptococcus neoformans, Candida* organisms, *Histoplasma capsulatum, Coccidioides immitis*

      (3) Viral: VZV, CMV, HSV

(4) Parasitic: *Pneumocystis carinii, Toxoplasma gondii, Giardia lamblia, Entamoeba histolytica, Cryptosporidium enteritis, Strongyloides stercoralis*

3. Humoral immune dysfunction

a. Etiology

(1) Multiple myeloma, chronic lymphocytic leukemia, sickle cell disease

(2) Chemotherapy

b. Common pathogens

(1) *Streptococcus pneumoniae*

(2) *Haemophilus influenzae*

C. EVALUATION OF THE IMMUNOCOMPROMISED PATIENT

1. Evaluation of potential infection in the immunocompromised host is similar to evaluation in the normal patient, with some exceptions.

a. The subtle and atypical nature of symptoms and signs demands a high index of clinical suspicion, willingness to intervene early, and persistence in search for potential causative organisms by rigorous and repeated septic workups.

b. Minimal symptoms demand complete evaluation.

2. Nonspecific signs (clinical deterioration leukocytosis, leukopenia, hypothermia, hypotension, glucose intolerance, low-grade pyrexia) may require full septic workup.

3. Identification of infectious agent must be prompt and precise.

4. Consider early use of invasive diagnostic procedures (transbronchial or open-lung biopsy).

D. THERAPY

1. Required information for therapeutic intervention

a. Presence of immunologic deficiencies in the compromised host

b. Infections the patient is susceptible to on basis of impaired host defenses

2. General principles

a. Drainage or debridement of localized collections of infected material

b. Specific antibiotics

c. Reconstruction of deficient antimicrobial defenses (FFP for complement deficiencies, immune serum globulin for IgG deficiency, reduction or cessation of immunosuppressive therapy, colony-stimulating factor, WBC transfusion)

3. Empiric antibiotic therapy

a. Broad-spectrum regimen against potential major gram-positive and gram-negative pathogens

b. Use of synergistic antibiotic combinations rather than single-agent or nonsynergistic combinations reduces morbidity and mortality (e.g., vancomycin + ticarcillin + amikacin, ceftazidime + amikacin)

c. Amphotericin B for a febrile, neutropenic patient who is unresponsive to antibacterial treatment

4. Prevention of infection

a. Avoid damage to physical barriers (repeated venipuncture, indwelling venous or urinary catheters, prolonged intubation).

b. Bolster host defenses (immune serum globulin, hyperimmune varicella-zoster immune globulin, vaccination against *Pneumococcus, Haemophilus,* and *Meningococcus* organisms).

c. Maintain optimal nutritional status.

d. Avoid acquisition of new potential pathogens (sterility, isolation).

e. Use prophylaxis for specific infections with high incidence in certain populations (trimethoprim-sulfamethoxazole and aerosolized pentamidine for protection against *Pneumocystis carinii* pneumonia in patients with AIDS).

VIII. ANTIBIOTICS

A. PRINCIPLES OF ANTIMICROBIAL THERAPY

1. Mechanisms of action

a. Bacteriostatic: Prevention of growth and multiplication of bacteria (bacteria not killed); infection cleared by host defenses.

b. Bactericidal: Bacterial killing; mandatory in immunocompromised host.

2. Use of multiple antibiotics

a. Possible or proven multiple organisms (e.g., gram-negative septicemia)

b. Prevention of emergence of resistant strains (e.g., *Pseudomonas* organisms, mycobacteria)

3. Antimicrobial synergy

a. Potentiation at a biochemical level

b. Assistance to cellular penetration (e.g., action of penicillin at cell wall level interferes with the ability of *Enterococcus faecalis* to resist penetration by aminoglycosides)

c. Protection (e.g., clavulanic acid—broad-spectrum enzyme inhibitor—protects amoxicillin against degradation by β-lactamase)

d. Antibiotic incompatibilities: interference with action of β-lactam antibiotics on cell wall synthesis by bacteriostatic agents (tetracyclines)

4. Monitoring of serum levels

a. Guide to drug dosage (ensure therapeutic levels, minimize complications)

b. Mandatory if renal function impaired

c. Most accurate dosing regimen provided by individualized pharmacokinetics: steady-state levels achieved after fifth dose
   (1) Peak levels measured 1 hour after IV or IM administration
   (2) Trough levels measured immediately before next dose

d. Important for agents with known toxicity, dose-related complications, narrow therapeutic range
   (1) Aminoglycosides
   (2) Vancomycin
   (3) Ketoconazole
   (4) Chloramphenicol

B. COMPLICATIONS OF ANTIBIOTIC THERAPY

1. Antibiotics: may induce hepatic enzyme activity, which increases metabolism of concurrently administered drugs

2. Hypersensitivity reactions

a. Most frequently seen with β-lactam agents

b. A 6% cross-sensitivity with cephalosporins

3. Suppression of normal flora and superinfection

a. Candidiasis or other fungal infection

b. *Clostridium difficile* (pseudomembranous) enterocolitis

4. Neurotoxicity: aminoglycosides

5. Encephalitic reactions: high-dose penicillin, cephalosporins, nalidixic acid

6. Peripheral neuropathy: isoniazid, chloramphenicol, metronidazole, nitrofurantoin

7. Neuromuscular blockade: aminoglycosides

8. Marrow toxicity

a. Sulfonamides

b. Chloramphenicol: aplastic anemia (non−dose-dependent with 50% mortality)

c. Penicillins: hemolytic anemia, granulocytopenia

C. SPECIFIC AGENTS

1. Aminoglycosides

a. Activity

   (1) Bactericidal against most aerobic and facultative anaerobic gram-negative bacilli

   (2) Moderate activity against gram-positive cocci

   (3) No activity against anaerobes

b. Adverse reactions

   (1) There is a narrow therapeutic margin, and monitoring of serum levels is required.

   (2) Nephrotoxicity is rare on initial administration; adjustment of dosage intervals allows use in established renal failure.

   (3) Ototoxicity is a vestibular or auditory dysfunction resulting from seventh cranial nerve injury.

   (4) A neuromuscular blockade is an anticholinesterase effect.

c. Drug interactions

   (1) Cephalosporins: synergistic nephrotoxicity

   (2) Diuretics: may potentiate ototoxicity and nephrotoxicity as a result of volume contraction

   (3) Penicillin: inactivation of aminoglycosides (clinical significance unknown)

d. Specific agents

   (1) Gentamycin, tobramycin: similar spectrum; gentamycin slightly more nephrotoxic

   (2) Amikacin: active against many strains that are resistant to gentamycin or tobramycin

   (3) Netilmicin: less nephrotoxic and ototoxic, but may cause hepatic toxicity

2. **Penicillins**
   a. Bactericidal against majority of the following:
      (1) Gram-positive cocci
      (2) Gram-negative cocci
      (3) Gram-positive bacilli
   b. Adverse reactions
      (1) Hypersensitivity: fever, rash, serum sickness, anaphylaxis
      (2) Neurotoxicity: convulsions, encephalitis, encephalopathy
      (3) Nephrotoxicity: interstitial nephritis
      (4) Hematologic: display of Coombs'-positive hemolytic anemia
      (5) Hypercalcemia: After high dosage with renal insufficiency
   c. Drug interactions
      (1) Aminoglycosides are inactivated by penicillin.
      (2) Probenecid, aspirin, and indomethacin may block renal tubular secretion of penicillin and lead to high serum levels.
   d. Specific agents
      (1) Penicillin G: most active against streptococci
      (2) Ampicillin: Enterococcus organisms, *Haemophilus influenzae*
      (3) Methicillin: penicillinase-resistant; may be associated with interstitial nephritis
      (4) Nafcillin: penicillinase-resistant; less nephrotoxic than methicillin; may be associated with neutropenia, phlebitis
      (5) Oxacillin: penicillinase-resistant; may be associated with hepatotoxicity
      (6) Azlocillin, mezlocillin, piperacillin (uriedo-penicillin): broad spectrum against gram-negative organisms; activity against *Escherichia coli, Proteus* and *Enterobacter* organisms, and many strains of *Pseudomonas* organisms; mezlocillin and piperacillin also active against some strains of *Klebsiella* and *Serratia* organisms
      (7) Carbenicillin, ticarcillin (carboxypenicillin): highly active against gram-negative organisms, including *Pseudomonas*; may be associated with hepatitis, hypokalemia, and decreased platelet aggregation

3. **Cephalosporins**
   a. First generation: effective against gram-positive and some gram-negative bacteria
   b. Second generation: increased gram-negative but less gram-positive activity
   c. Third generation: main effect on gram-negative bacteria
   d. Adverse reactions: large safety margin and high therapeutic margin
      (1) Hypersensitivity: cross-sensitivity in penicillin-allergic patients is 6% to 9%; use avoided in patients with history of anaphylactic penicillin hypersensitivity
      (2) Nephrotoxicity: interstitial nephritis
      (3) Neurotoxicity: convulsions, confusion
      (4) Hematologic: Coombs'-positive anemia, thrombophlebitis, inhibition of platelet aggregation, suppression of vitamin K−dependent clotting factors

4. **Vancomycin**
a. Activity: bactericidal against all gram-positive bacteria, including methicillin-resistant staphylococci and *Clostridium* (pseudomembranous colitis) organisms
b. Adverse reactions
   (1) Ototoxicity: associated with high serum levels
   (2) Nephrotoxicity: infrequent
   (3) Hypotension: associated with rapid infusion
   (4) Hypersensitivity
c. Dose: 20 to 30 mg/kg/24 hr (1 g IV q12h)
d. Monitored serum levels
   (1) Peak: 35 mg/ml
   (2) Trough: 10 mg/ml

5. **Metronidazole**
a. Activity against anaerobic bacteria, *Trichomonas* and *Giardia* organisms, and *Entamoeba histolytica*
b. Adverse reactions
   (1) Nausea, vomiting
   (2) Headache, ataxia, vertigo, neuropathy, seizures
c. Dose: 30 mg/kg/24 hr (500 mg IV q6h)

6. **Clindamycin**
a. Activity: gram-positive bacteria and gram-negative anaerobes
b. Adverse reactions
   (1) Diarrhea in 20% to 30%
   (2) Hepatotoxic
   (3) Pseudomembranous colitis
c. Dose: 30 to 40 mg/kg/24 hr (600 to 900 mg IV q8h)

7. **Chloramphenicol**
a. Activity: gram-negative bacteria, including species resistant to conventional agents (rickettsial disease, psittacosis, lymphogranuloma venereum)
b. Adverse reactions: bone marrow suppression (aplastic anemia)
c. Dose: 0.25 to 1 g PO q6h (500 mg); 0.5 to 1.0 g IV q6h
d. Monitored serum levels
   (1) Peak: 20 mg/ml
   (2) Trough: 2 mg/ml

8. **Erythromycin**
a. Activity: bacteriostatic (bactericidal in high doses) against gram-positive bacteria; good substitute for penicillin in allergic patient
b. Adverse reactions
   (1) Nausea, vomiting, epigastric discomfort, diarrhea
   (2) Cholestatic jaundice (>10-day course, repeated courses)
   (3) Thrombophlebitis
c. Dose: 0.25 to 1 g PO or IV q6h

9. **Imipenem-cilastatin**
a. Broad spectrum of activity against *Pseudomonas, Serratia*, and *Enterobacter* organisms; enterococcus; anaerobes

20

INFECTION AND SEPSIS

b. May cause seizures, nausea, vomiting

c. Dose: 0.5 to 1 g IV q6-8h

10. Quinolones

a. Active against most aerobic gram-positive and gram-negative bacteria, mycobacteria, *Mycoplasma* organisms, chlamydia

b. Useful for UTI, enteric infection

c. May cause nausea, vomiting, dizziness, seizures

d. Dose

(1) Norfloxacin 400 mg PO q12h

(2) Ciprofloxacin 200 to 300 mg IV q12h; 750 mg PO q8-12h

11. Trimethoprim/sulfamethoxazole (TMP/SMX)

a. Active against *Pneumocystis* and *Shigella* organisms and gram-negative bacilli except *Pseudomonas* organisms

b. May cause nausea, vomiting, blood dyscrasias

c. Dose: 10 to 20 mg/kg/24 hr in 2 to 4 divided doses (based on trimethoprim component)

d. Available for injection: TMP 80 mg and SMX 400 mg/5ml

12. Aztreonam

a. Bactericidal against gram-negative aerobes, including *Pseudomonas* organisms

b. May cause nausea, vomiting, phlebitis

c. Dose: 1 to 2 g IV q6-8h

13. Tetracyclines

a. Bacteriostatic against a variety of gram-positive and gram-negative bacteria, rickettsia, *Mycoplasma* organisms, chlamydia

b. High incidence of bacterial resistance limits use

c. May cause hepatotoxicity, GI upset, thrombophlebitis

d. Dose: 250 to 500 mg PO q6h; 500 mg IV q12h (5 mg/ml infusion; 2 ml/hr)

14. Amphotericin B

a. Active against most fungi, including *Histoplasma*, *Coccidioides, Candida, Aspergillus, Blastomyces, Cryptococcus, Sporotrichum*, and *Phycomycetes* organisms

b. Adverse reactions

(1) Nephrotoxicity is dose-related; most patients experience a 30% decrease in GFR with standard treatment; volume loading reduces renal toxicity.

(2) Chills, fever, headache, anorexia, weight loss, nausea, vomiting (50% to 80%)

(3) Thrombophlebitis, anemia, hypersensitivity

(4) Arachnoiditis, auditory neurotoxicity

c. Systemic: total dose of amphotericin B usually 6 mg/kg; should not usually exceed 8 mg/kg (total dose of 3 to 5 g prescribed for more severe or persistent infections)

(1) Dilution in D5W to concentration of 10 mg/dl; stable for 24 hours

(2) Slow IV infusion over 6 hours, monitoring BP, pulse, respiratory rate, and temperature q30min during treatment

(3) Test dose (1 mg) given over 30 minutes with observation for 1 hour, monitoring for fever, hypotension, tachycardia

(4) First day: 0.25 mg/kg IV over 6 hours; increase dose by 0.1 mg/kg/day to dose of 0.5 to 0.7 mg/ kg/day

(5) Discontinuation of treatment or dose reduction if temperature is greater than 38.9° C; systolic BP less than 100 mm Hg, fall in systolic BP of more than 30 mm Hg; pulse greater than 130

(6) May ameliorate febrile or hypotensive reaction by premedicating with 125 mg hydrocortisone IV 30 minutes before treatment; may also be beneficial to use diphenhydramine and acetaminophen

d. Amphotericin B bladder irrigation

(1) Amphotericin B 50 mg in 1 L NS infused through Foley catheter over 8 hours as continuous bladder irrigation

(2) Irrigation is usually continued for 7 to 10 days

(3) After cessation of bladder irrigation, urine is cultured for fungal culture

15. Flucytosine

a. Active against *Candida* and *Cryptococcus* organisms

b. May cause diarrhea, colitis, allergic rash, neutropenia, thrombocytopenia, hepatotoxicity

c. High incidence of resistance when used as single agent; used in combination with amphotericin B to reduce dose of latter

d. Dose

(1) Amphotericin B reduced to 0.3 mg/kg/day IV

(2) Flucytosine 375 mg/kg q6h PO

16. Fluconazole

a. Indications: oral, pharyngeal, and esophageal candidiasis; cryptococcosis; and coccidioidal meningitis

b. Adverse reactions: hepatic toxicity; monitoring of LFTs recommended

c. Recommended dose for oral pharyngeal candidiasis: 200 mg PO loading dose followed by 100 mg PO q6h

d. Doses of up to 400 mg/day for severe esophageal candidiasis or cryptococcal meningitis

e. Parenteral administration (doses per PO administration) is by IV infusion: maximum rate 200 mg/hr

17. Nystatin

a. For use in oral candidiasis

b. Dose: nystatin liquid 5 ml PO q6h (swish and swallow); nystatin tablets one or two PO q6h

18. Ketoconazole

a. Active against *Candida, Coccidioides, Histoplasma, Blastomyces,* and *Paracoccidioides* organisms, dermatophytes

b. May cause hepatotoxicity, hepatic necrosis, pruritus, dizziness, somnolence

c. Dose: 400 mg/day PO

19. Acyclovir

a. Active against HSV-1, HSV-2, VZV, EBV, inactive against human CMV

20

INFECTION AND SEPSIS

b. Dose
    (1) IV: 5 to 10 mg/kg q8h
    (2) PO: 50 to 200 mg PO q4-8h (suppression therapy)
    (3) Topical: 5% ointment, four to six applications per day

20. Ganciclovir
a. Activity against CMV
b. Dose: 5 mg/kg q12h IV × 14 to 21 days, then 5 mg/kg/day maintenance

SUGGESTED READINGS

Astiz ME, Rackow EC: Septic shock, *Lancet* 351:1501, 1998.

Cunha BA: Fever in the critical care unit, *Crit Care Clin* 14:1, 1998.

de Vera ME, Simmons RL: Antibiotic-resistant enterococci and the changing face of surgical infections, *Arch Surg* 131:338, 1996.

Fekety R: Guidelines for the diagnosis and management of *Clostridium difficile*, *Am J Gastroenterol* 92:739,1996.

Fishman JA, Rubin RH: Infection in organ-transplant recipients, *N Engl J Med* 338:24, 1998.

Henderson VJ, Hirvela ER: Emerging and reemerging microbial threats, *Arch Surg* 131:330, 1996.

Levy SB: Multidrug resistance—a sign of the times, *N Engl J Med* 338:1376, 1998.

Lowy FD: *Staphylococcus aureus* infections, *N Engl J Med* 339:520, 1998.

Natanson C, Hoffman WD, Suffredini AF, et al: Selected treatment strategies for septic shock based on proposed mechanisms of pathogenesis, *Ann Intern Med* 120:771, 1994.

O'Grady NP, Barie PS, Bartlett J, et al: Practice parameters for evaluating new fever in critically ill adult patients, *Crit Care Med* 26:392, 1998.

Sessler DI: Mild perioperative hypothermia, *N Engl J Med* 336:1730, 1997.

VENTILATOR MANAGEMENT

R. Anthony Perez-Tamayo

I. INDICATIONS FOR VENTILATORY SUPPORT
A. CONDITIONS THAT REQUIRE VENTILATORY SUPPORT
1. Failure of ventilation
a. Level of consciousness compromising ventilation/airway protection
b. Secretions in excess of patient's clearance
c. Inadequate muscle strength
d. Excessive work of breathing
e. Upper airway obstruction
2. Inadequate oxygenation
a. ARDS, pulmonary edema, pneumonia
b. Atelectasis or consolidation unresponsive to more conservative therapy
B. INDICATIONS FOR ENDOTRACHEAL INTUBATION
1. Failure of airway adjuncts
a. Oral airways
b. Positioning
c. Reversal of sedation
2. Inadequate bag-mask-valve ventilation
3. Required prolonged ventilatory support
4. Patients with compromised airways
a. Maxillofacial fractures
b. Massive hemoptysis
c. Supraglottic obstruction
d. Airway protection in high aspiration risk
   (1) Excessive secretions
   (2) Massive upper GI bleeding
5. Elective intubation under controlled circumstances preferable to emergent intubation
C. SUMMARY OF CRITERIA FOR INTUBATION
1. Inadequate ventilation
a. RR greater than 35 bpm
b. $Paco_2$ greater than 50 mm Hg
c. Respiratory acidosis, pH less than 7.25
2. Inadequate oxygenation
a. Pao_2 less than 60 mm Hg
b. O_2 saturation less than 85%
c. Pao_2/Fio_2 less than 250
3. Inadequate airway protection
a. Glasgow Coma Scale score lower than 9
b. Secretions requiring suction frequency greater than once per hour

II. TRACHEOSTOMY
A. INDICATIONS FOR TRACHEOSTOMY
1. Upper respiratory obstruction

2. **Uncontrolled respiratory tract secretions,** even with adequate ventilation
3. **Inadequate strength or vital capacity** (neurologic or obstructive)
4. **Anticipated mechanical ventilatory support** longer than 3 weeks
5. **Mental status inadequate to protect airway over long term**

B. **ADVANTAGES OVER TRANSLARYNGEAL INTUBATION**
   1. **Upper airway obstruction bypassed**
   2. **Reduction of ventilatory dead space (V_d)**
   3. **Reduction of breathing work**
   a. Larger-bore airway
   b. Shorter tube
   4. **Improved access to lower respiratory tract for pulmonary toilet**
   5. **More secure airway**
   6. **Restoration of glottic function**
   7. **Patient comfort**
   8. **Easier to wean patient from ventilator** (see section IX, C)
   9. **Lower incidence of chronic laryngeal injury**
   10. **Reduced rates of nosocomial pneumonia in tracheostomy patients have not been consistently demonstrated**

C. **COMPLICATIONS OF TRACHEOSTOMY**
   1. **Mortality 1.5%**
   2. **Morbidity 5.9%**
   a. Early complications: displacement of tracheostomy tube, infection, perioperative hemorrhage
   b. Late complications: tracheoinnominate artery fistula, dysphagia, subglottic stenosis, tracheoesophageal fistula

III. ELEMENTS OF MECHANICAL VENTILATION

A. **VOLUME-CYCLED VENTILATION**
   1. **The ventilator delivers a programmed, machine-generated, tidal volume** (V_T) at a programmed, machine-generated flow, regardless of chest wall compliance, potentially resulting in high airway pressures and barotrauma.
   2. **Limit in volume-cycled ventilation = flow.** Set flow rate will not be exceeded or altered.
   3. **Cycle in volume-cycled ventilation depends on volume.**
   a. Inspiratory phase = length of time it takes set flow to deliver programmed V_T.
   b. Expiratory phase begins when V_T is delivered and lasts as long as it takes V_T to be passively exhaled.
   4. **Reliable minute-ventilation under conditions of changing compliance.**

B. **PRESSURE-CYCLED VENTILATION**
   1. **On inspiration,** patient airways exposed to programmed, machine-generated pressure for a programmed length of time. V_T therefore indirectly determined by programmed pressure and inspiratory time interacting with total compliance.

2. Limit in pressure-cycled ventilation = airway pressure.
a. Set pressure will not be exceeded.
b. By setting pressure limit, barotrauma reduced.
c. Inspiratory flow automatically provided by servomotor mechanism to achieve set pressure and sustain it for set inspiratory time.
3. Cycle in pressure-cycled ventilation depends on set inspiratory time.
a. Inspiratory phase = set inspiratory time.
b. Expiratory phase begins when inspiratory time over and lasts as long as it takes indirectly determined V_T to be passively exhaled.
4. Minute-ventilation varies with changing compliance.
C. CONTROL
1. Breath initiated by machine
2. Used when patient cannot initiate breath
3. Would be uncomfortable for awake patient because of dyssynchrony between patient and machine breaths
D. ASSIST
1. Breath initiated by patient
2. Patient initiates breath by attempting to inhale
a. Negative inspiratory pressure triggers breath
b. Amount of negative inspiratory pressure necessary to trigger breath = sensitivity
3. Greater synchrony, greater comfort for patient

IV. STANDARD VENTILATOR SETTINGS
A. RATE
1. Frequency of ventilator cycling
a. In some ventilator modes, patient can generate breaths above this set rate
b. Machine rate is the minimum rate possible, therefore often used as a "backup" to ensure a lower limit to ventilation
2. Higher rates may not allow sufficient time for passive exhalation, resulting in breath-stacking, higher airway pressures, and so-called autoPEEP
B. TIDAL VOLUME
1. Volume-cycled ventilators: set directly (10 ml/kg)
2. Pressure-cycled ventilators: indirectly controlled function of inspiratory pressure and compliance
3. For jet ventilation: V_T is 3 to 4 ml/kg
C. INSPIRATORY FLOW RATE
1. Increases in IFR
a. Shorten inspiration
b. Provide longer period for exhalation
2. Importance of lung compliance
a. Lungs with normal compliance are relatively insensitive to IFR.
b. With diminished compliance, high IFR results in excessive PIP.
D. INSPIRATORY TIME
1. In volume-cycled ventilation, determined by set IFR and set V_T.
2. In pressure-cycled ventilation, inspiratory time directly programmed.

21

VENTILATOR MANAGEMENT

3. Normal ratio of inspiratory to expiratory time (I:E ratio) is 1:2 to 1:3.

a. Expiratory time = time it takes V_T to be passively exhaled.

b. Expiratory time depends on total compliance and airway resistance.

E. PEAK INSPIRATORY PRESSURE

1. Pressure-cycled ventilator: pressure to which airways are exposed during inspiratory time

2. Volume-cycled ventilator: pressure at which overpressure alarm sounds

F. Fio_2

1. Fio_2 is the fraction of oxygen in inspired air (room air = 0.21).

2. Adjust Fio_2 to provide for Pao_2 of 60 to 90 mm Hg and Sao_2 greater than 90%.

3. Fio_2 may be directly and safely reduced using Pao_2:Fio_2 ratio:

$$\text{Desired } Fio_2 = (\text{actual } Fio_2/\text{actual } Pao_2) \times \text{desired } Pao_2$$

4. An Fio_2 in excess of 0.5 subjects the patient to the risk of oxygen toxicity.

G. POSITIVE END-EXPIRATORY PRESSURE

1. PEEP maintains positive airway pressure at end expiration.

a. Counterbalances airway closing forces

b. Increases functional residual capacity (FRC) by recruiting alveoli

c. Maintains small airway patency at end expiration

2. Five centimeters H_2O = physiologic PEEP provided by glottic closure.

3. Supraphysiologic levels used to improve oxygenation in pulmonary edema (see section VI, C)

H. PRESSURE SUPPORT

1. Allows inspiratory support of patient-initiated breaths

2. PS of 5 to 10 cm H_2O overcomes resistance of typical endotracheal tube

3. Stepwise reduction in PS commonly used as a weaning mode (see section VI, A)

I. SENSITIVITY

1. Inspiratory force the patient must generate to trigger an inspiratory cycle

2. If too high (excessively insensitive), may waste energy attempting to initiate breaths

3. If set too low (too sensitive), may trigger breaths too easily and result in hyperventilation

V. PRIMARY VENTILATOR MODES

A. VOLUME CONTROL VENTILATION

1. Otherwise known as controlled mechanical ventilation (CMV)

2. V_T set, IFR set, RR set

3. Breath initiated by machine

4. Ventilator delivers calculated minute-ventilation

a. Determined by the preset V_T and rate

b. Independent of patient's breathing

5. **No air flow is provided between ventilator breaths**
6. **CMV is appropriate when the patient is unable to initiate breaths**
   a. Paralyzing agents
   b. Anesthesia
   c. Neurologic disease
7. **No patient effort, respiratory muscles at risk of atrophy**

B. VOLUME ASSIST VENTILATION
1. **V_T set, IFR set, minimum RR typically set as backup**
2. **Patient triggers breath** when initial negative pressure on inhalation exceeds programmed sensitivity
3. **Each triggered breath delivers full set V_T**
4. **This mode is usually combined with control as volume assist-control**
   a. If patient rate is slower than machine backup rate, no assisted breaths occur, and mode is essentially volume control.
   b. If machine rate close to zero, few control breaths occur, and mode is essentially volume assist.
5. **Patient's only effort is triggering breath; respiratory muscles at risk for atrophy**

C. PRESSURE CONTROL VENTILATION
1. **Inspiratory pressure set, inspiratory time set, RR set**
2. **Breath initiated by machine**
3. **Sufficient inspiratory pressure and time is provided** to generate satisfactory V_T as permitted by total chest and lung compliance. Automatic control of servomotor delivers whatever flow necessary to achieve set pressure and sustain it for set inspiratory time.
4. **Rate set given the achieved V_T to deliver desired minute ventilation**
5. **Same patient population as volume control**
6. **No patient effort; respiratory muscles at risk of atrophy**

D. PRESSURE ASSIST VENTILATION
1. **Inspiratory pressure set, inspiratory time set, RR set as backup**
2. **Patient triggers breath** when initial negative pressure on inhalation exceeds programmed sensitivity
3. **With each triggered breath,** patient airways exposed to programmed inspiratory pressure
   a. As patient inhales, chest expands, airway pressure goes down, servomotor automatically increases flow to drive airway pressure up to set inspiratory pressure, and sustain it for set inspiratory time.
   b. The stronger the patient's inhalational effort, the lower the inspiratory pressure needed to achieve desired V_T.
4. **This mode is usually combined with control as pressure assist-control**
   a. If patient rate is slower than machine backup rate, no assisted breaths occur, and mode is essentially pressure control.
   b. If machine rate close to zero, few control breaths occur, and mode is essentially pressure assist.
5. **The greater the patient effort, the lower the risk of respiratory muscle atrophy**

VI. SECONDARY VENTILATOR MODES

A. PRESSURE SUPPORT

1. **Inspiratory pressure set, RR set as backup**
2. **Instead of a programmed inspiratory time,** the length of the inspiratory cycle is terminated when inspiratory flow falls to two thirds of maximum.
3. **Patient triggers breath when initial negative pressure on inhalation exceeds programmed sensitivity.**
4. **With each triggered breath,** patient airways exposed to programmed inspiratory pressure.
   a. As patient inhales, chest expands, airway pressure goes down, and servomotor automatically increases flow to drive airway pressure up to set inspiratory pressure and sustain it until flow falls below two thirds of maximum.
   b. The stronger patient's inhalational effort, the lower the inspiratory pressure needed to achieve desired V_T.
   c. A patient who is not strong enough to achieve desired V_T, even with higher levels of PS, may benefit from the extra support with pressure assist-control and its set inspiratory time.
5. **PS can be used in conjunction with any of the primary modes, or alone.** Most commonly it is used with a pressure control backup.
6. **PS is a form of partial support,** with each breath partially assisted.
   a. Often used as a weaning tool.
   b. Gradual decrease in PS increases patient responsibility for ventilation and promotes respiratory muscle strength.
   c. The greater the patient effort, the lower the risk of respiratory muscle atrophy.
7. **V_T will vary with patient strength and total compliance.** Greater supervision is therefore required because minute ventilation is not guaranteed.

B. SYNCHRONIZED INTERMITTENT MANDATORY VENTILATION

1. **Machine V_T set, machine IFR set, minimum RR set.**
2. **Patient can breathe above the minimum set RR.**
   a. The patient is responsible for the V_T and frequency of these breaths.
   b. These breaths can be augmented with the addition of pressure support.
3. **Machine breaths are intermittent and synchronized.**
   a. Machine initiates breath if patient has not in a certain time.
   b. Machine will not deliver breath during inhalation or exhalation of patient-generated breath.
4. **SIMV is another form of partial support.**
   a. SIMV often used for weaning.
   b. Gradual decrease in machine RR; increases patient's share of total minute ventilation.
   c. The greater the patient effort, the lower the risk of respiratory muscle atrophy.

C. SUPRAPHYSIOLOGIC POSITIVE END-EXPIRATORY PRESSURE

1. **Used to improve oxygenation in cases of pulmonary edema** (e.g., ARDS, CHF).
   a. Recruits alveoli and keeps open diseased small airways, increasing FRC.

   b. Also thought to redistribute edema fluid within diseased alveoli, improving oxygen diffusion.

2. Complications stem from increased airway and intrathoracic pressure.

   a. Barotrauma

   (1) Acute injury, such as alveolar rupture and pneumothorax

   (2) Chronic lung injury, manifested by fibrosis and decreased compliance

   b. Diminished cardiac output

   (1) RV preload decreased as intrathoracic pressure exceeds caval pressure

   (2) RV afterload increased as intrathoracic pressure increases pulmonary vascular resistance

   (3) LV preload diminished

3. With each increment in PEEP (typically, but not necessarily 5 cm H_2O increments), assessments should be made of blood gases, total compliance, and cardiac output.

   a. Improved oxygenation allows decreased Fio_2.

   b. Compliance monitors potential for barotrauma—paralysis and sedation may be necessary to improve compliance.

   c. Drops in cardiac output treated with fluid replacement followed by inotropes as necessary.

4. Invasive cardiac monitoring is strongly recommended with PEEP greater than 10 cm H_2O.

D. INVERSE RATIO VENTILATION

1. Diminishes the impact of airway pressure by spreading it out over a longer inspiratory time.

   a. IRV is a response to a criticism of PEEP, that airflow in PEEP preferentially goes to healthier alveoli, injuring them by overdistention, rather than opening diseased alveoli

   b. IRV thought to better distribute volume throughout diseased and healthy alveoli

   c. Lower peak airway pressures

2. IRV is instituted by prolonging inspiratory time and adjusting RR (normal I:E ratio is 1:3).

   a. Phase I: inspiratory time prolongation, expiratory time sufficient for exhalation to return to FRC

   b. Phase II: inspiratory time prolongation to extent that expiratory time insufficient to return to FRC, air-trapping/auto-PEEP occurs

3. IRV is very uncomfortable.

   a. Generally requires paralysis and sedation

   b. Paralysis potentiates respiratory and other muscle atrophy

E. CONTINUOUS POSITIVE AIRWAY PRESSURE/BiPAP

1. Form of partial assist

   a. Does not require intubation, can be administered via mask

   b. Can help prevent need for intubation

2. Positive pressure provided throughout inhalation and exhalation

   a. Physiologically equivalent to PEEP plus pressure support

   b. Maintains small airway patency by improving FRC

21

VENTILATOR MANAGEMENT

c. Helps treat somnolence-related upper airway obstruction (e.g., sleep apnea)

3. May be contraindicated in patients with a normal FRC

a. Possibility of lung overexpansion

b. Decreased compliance

c. Increased work of breathing because of opposition posed to exhalation by positive expiratory pressure

d. Diminished gas exchange

4. Used postoperatively to hasten return of FRC to preoperative levels

5. BiPAP is a form of CPAP in which different levels of airway pressure are set for inspiration vs. expiration (expiratory PAP typically much lower than inspiratory PAP)

F. HIGH-FREQUENCY JET VENTILATION

1. Provides ventilation at reduced peak airway pressures

a. Lower incidence of pulmonary barotrauma

b. Higher cardiac output

c. Lower ICP

2. Methods

a. Jet injector lumen endotracheal tube

b. 14-gauge needle injector

c. Sliding venturimeter; provides the greatest VT

3. Setup of ventilator

a. RR = 50 to 300 cycles/min

b. V_T of 3 to 4 ml/kg, adjusted using ventilator driving pressures

c. High ventilator driving pressures (5 to 50 psig), but low airway pressures

4. Tip of endotracheal tube positioned 10 cm proximal to the carina to prevent preferential single-lung ventilation

5. Established indications

a. Bronchopleural fistula

(1) Peak airway pressure less than opening pressure of bronchopleural fistula

(2) Will limit air leak and allow healing

b. Bronchoscopy or laryngoscopy

c. Infants who are hypoxic on standard ventilatory modalities

d. Excessive peak airway pressure on standard ventilator modes (relative indications)

6. Potential complications

a. Inadequate minute ventilation

b. Inadequate humidification

c. Tracheal mucosal injury secondary to high shear forces

VII. ADJUNCTS TO MECHANICAL VENTILATION

A. PRONE POSITION

1. Inexpensive and effective adjunct therapy for pulmonary edema/ARDS

a. Theoretically redistributes pulmonary edema away from dependent lung segments

b. Ventilation-perfusion mismatch thereby improved
c. Between 70% and 80% of patients respond with Po_2 improvements up to 50 mmHg
d. Improved oxygenation allows decreased Fio_2 and airway pressures

2. Method

a. Patient typically, but not necessarily, sedated and paralyzed
b. Turned supine 1 hour q12h for dressing and bedding changes and family visits
c. Po_2 worsens when supine, but benefit rapidly restored once prone again

3. Complications

a. Hemodynamic instability with prone position
b. Padding and posture important to prevent complications such as decubitus and blindness

B. NITRIC OXIDE THERAPY

1. Nitric oxide (NO) = endothelial-derived relaxing factor, potent vasodilator

a. Inhaled NO preferentially delivered to alveoli with better ventilation
b. Resulting local vasodilation improves ventilation-perfusion match

2. Method

a. Start at 1 ppm
   (1) Pulmonary artery hemodynamic response can be seen at low doses
   (2) Hemodynamic response thought to predict oxygenation response (not conclusively demonstrated)
b. Increase to 5 ppm, then by 5-ppm increments, to a maximum of 40 to 60 ppm

3. Complications

a. Response rate 30% to 40% in septic patients, 50% to 60% in nonseptic ARDS patients
b. Systemic hypotension can occur, especially with worsened shunting in sepsis
c. Patients can become NO dependent
d. Pregnant personnel should avoid room because of teratogenicity

VIII. TROUBLESHOOTING

A. HYPERCAPNIA

1. Ventilator malfunction

a. Disconnection
b. Inadequate V_T because of circuit capacitance or air leak

2. Inadequate V_T

a. Bronchospasm—bronchodilators
b. Mucus plugging—suction/bronchoscopy
c. Atelectasis—increase airway pressure/PEEP/V_T
d. Tension pneumothorax
e. Incorrect ventilator settings
f. Inadequate compensation for dead space

21

VENTILATOR MANAGEMENT

3. Increased physiologic dead space

a. PE

b. Diminished cardiac output with inadequate perfusion

4. Increased CO_2 production

a. Fever

b. Rigors—paralytics potentially therapeutic

c. Rewarming

d. Hypermetabolic state

e. Excessive carbohydrate-to-fat caloric ratio

B. HYPOXIA AND SUDDEN RESPIRATORY DECOMPENSATION

1. Disconnect from the ventilator and hand ventilate with 100% Fio_2

2. Physical examination

a. Evaluate for adequate bilateral ventilation.

b. Evaluate hemodynamic status.

3. Laboratory evaluation

a. Obtain ABG and mixed venous blood gas.

b. Obtain CXR.

    (1) Check endotracheal tube position.

    (2) Exclude pneumothorax.

    (3) Assess lung fields for edema, consolidation, or Westermark's sign.

4. Treatment

a. Low resistance to manual ventilation

    (1) Hemodynamically stable: exclude ventilator malfunction, consider PE, subjective dyspnea

    (2) Hemodynamically unstable: exclude pneumothorax, PE, sepsis

b. High resistance to manual ventilation

    (1) Obstructed endotracheal tube: replace/reposition

    (2) If no obstruction, should consider one of the following: bronchial mucus or thrombus plugging, bronchospasm, or pulmonary edema

C. ALARMS

1. Low pressure (disconnect alarm)

a. Excellent monitoring of disconnection

b. Most common failure: alarm deactivated for endotracheal suctioning

2. Low exhaled volume

a. If exhaled V_T is not equal to inhaled V_T, air leak or disconnection exists

b. Alarm set to 90% to 100% of VM_T to account for circuit capacitance

3. Maximum PIP

a. Alarm set 15% above PIP

b. Triggering of alarm

    (1) Lack of synchronization with the patient's breathing

    (2) Inadequate exhalation time resulting in breath-stacking

    (3) Malpositioned endotracheal tube

4. O_2 concentration of inspired gases

a. Set at Fio_2, plus or minus 0.10

b. Alarm signals ventilator failure or failure of oxygen source

5. **End-tidal CO_2**
a. The gold standard for verifying tracheal intubation
b. Low end-tidal CO_2
    (1) Disconnection
    (2) Extubation
    (3) Esophageal intubation
c. On-line assessment of P_{CO_2}
    (1) Usually 4 to 6 mm Hg lower than measured Pa_{CO_2}.
    (2) Values may be 10 to 12 mm Hg lower with large V_D.

IX. WEANING FROM MECHANICAL VENTILATION
A. METHODOLOGY
1. Maximize patient responsibility for minute ventilation
a. Use partial support modes (SIMV, PS, SIMV + PS) to gradually increase patient effort
b. Progress during day, rest at night
2. RR most reliable guide to wean
a. Monitor V_T
b. Distinguish anxiety from air hunger
B. CRITERIA FOR SUCCESSFUL EXTUBATION
1. Oxygenation: Po_2 greater than or equal to 60 mm Hg with Fio_2 less than 0.50
2. Mental status
a. Responsive to commands
b. Ability to cough (intact gag reflex)
3. Strength
a. Muscular paralysis is reversed.
b. Sustained head lift (>5 seconds)
c. Bilateral hand grip
4. Respiratory mechanics
a. V_T greater than 4 ml/kg
b. RR equal to 8 to 25 breaths/min
c. RR/V_T ratio less than 100 breaths/min
d. Negative inspiratory force less than -25 cm H_2O
5. Ventilator support compatible with extubation
a. PEEP equals 5 cm H_2O
b. Pressure support equals 10 cm H_2O
c. Fio_2 less than 0.50
C. DIFFICULT-TO-WEAN PATIENTS
1. Patient factors
a. Treat underlying pathology (e.g., pulmonary edema, pneumonia).
b. Acidosis (pH near 7.3) may be required to effect adequate respiratory drive.
c. Reduce excessive ventilation demands by holding carbohydrates to less than 33% of caloric intake.
d. Theophylline increases diaphragmatic contractility.

21

VENTILATOR MANAGEMENT

e. Use CPAP/BiPAP to maintain FRC off ventilator.
f. Excess Fio_2 results in resorption atelectasis.
g. Build respiratory muscle strength with trials of reduced settings/tracheostomy collar/CPAP.

2. Airway factors
a. Excessive work required by small endotracheal tubes
b. Functional internal diameter limited by partial obstruction of the endotracheal tube
c. Excessive V_D
    (1) Tracheostomy reduces V_D by 100 to 150 ml.
    (2) This will favorably improve V_D/V_T.
d. Tracheostomy makes extubation/reintubation unnecessary for trial off ventilator

---

X. MECHANICAL VENTILATION COMPLICATIONS

A. DISCONNECTION
1. Most frequent mechanical complication
2. Easily diagnosed if appropriate alarms have not been disabled

B. INFECTION
1. Intubation inhibits normal airway defenses.
a. Mucociliary elevator
b. Macrophages
c. Nasotracheal filtering/humidification
2. Gram-negative rod colonization of the normally sterile trachea less than 72 hours after intubation.
3. Hypoxia, hyperoxia, and acidosis of critical illness further impede host resistance.
4. Sinusitis occurs in 2% to 5% of patients with nasotracheal intubation.
a. Sinus films
b. May require CT for adequate visualization
c. Treatment
    (1) Change route of intubation
    (2) Antibiotic
    (3) Drain sinuses in resistant cases
5. Pneumonia
a. Risk raised twentyfold by mechanical ventilation
b. Usually gram-negative rods
c. Sources of pathogens
    (1) Oropyarngeal colonization
    (2) Aspiration
    (3) Contaminated ventilatory circuitry
    (4) Hematogenous spread
d. Treatment
    (1) Pulmonary toilet
    (2) Antibiotics based on culture and sensitivity

C. BAROTRAUMA

1. **Hyperventilation of normal tissue in presence of large regions of low compliance**

a. Atelectasis

b. Contusion

c. Pneumonia

d. High-risk conditions

   (1) COPD

   (2) Mucous plugging

   (3) Bronchoscopy

   (4) CPR

2. **Alveolar rupture**

a. Air dissecting along perivascular tissue planes

   (1) Pneumomediastinum

   (2) Subcutaneous emphysema

b. Pneumothorax from disruption of parietal pleura

3. **Solutions**

a. Spontaneous assisted ventilation will result in lowest peak airway pressures.

b. Muscular paralysis will improve the chest wall compliance portion of total lung compliance.

c. Jet ventilation will allow adequate gas exchange at a lower PIP.

D. TRACHEAL AND LARYNGEAL STENOSIS

1. **Endotracheal tubes cause mucosal ulceration and chronic inflammation**

2. **Resultant problems**

a. Fibrosis

b. Tracheomalacia

c. Stenosis

d. Tracheoesophageal fistulas

3. **Solutions**

a. Use thin-walled, low-pressure, high-volume cuffs.

b. Maintain cuff pressure less than 20 to 25 mm Hg.

E. DISUSE ATROPHY

1. **Maximize spontaneous ventilatory effort.**

2. **After prolonged ventilatory support, gradual reduction in support.**

3. **Maintain positive nitrogen balance** to avoid catabolism of respiratory muscles.

4. **Periodic exercise** (lower settings, CPAP, tracheostomy trials) with rest.

21

VENTILATOR MANAGEMENT

SUGGESTED READINGS

Burns SM, Clochesy JM, Hanneman SK, et al: Weaning from long-term mechanical ventilation, *Am J Crit Care* 4:4-22, 1995.

Dries DJ: Weaning from mechanical ventilation, *J Trauma* 43:372-384, 1997.

Loiacono J, Cunneen CC: Mechanical ventilation of the postoperative patient, *Chest Surg Clin North Am* 7:801-815, 1997.

MacIntyre NR: New modes of mechanical ventilation, *Clin Chest Med* 17:411-421, 1996.

Minei JP, Barie PS: Current management of acute respiratory distress syndrome, *Adv Surg* 31:167-188, 1997.

Pinsky MR: The hemodynamic consequences of mechanical ventilation: an evolving story, *Intensive Care Med* 23:493-503, 1997.

NUTRITION

J.E. (Betsy) Tuttle-Newhall

I. NUTRITIONAL ASSESSMENT

A. CLASSIFICATION OF MALNUTRITION

1. Simple starvation (marasmus)

a. Malnutrition resulting from insufficient energy intake without the catabolic stress of illness (e.g., anorexia nervosa).

b. Usually occurs over several months to years of semistarvation.

c. Metabolic priority is to preserve visceral proteins at the expense of fat stores.

d. Over time, plasma insulin falls, which stimulates lipolysis, ketogenesis, amino acid metabolism, gluconeogenesis, and decreased protein synthesis.

e. Brain shifts to metabolism of ketones and free fatty acids to preserve visceral proteins.

f. Decreased basal metabolic rate.

2. Protein calorie malnutrition (kwashiorkor)

a. Malnutrition is related to the body's response to infection and inflammation.

b. Rapidly occurs in response to injury and infection (associated with the hormonal and cytokine storm of catabolic stress).

c. Metabolic priority is to maintain a physiologic defensive posture by mobilizing visceral protein stores.

d. As part of the catabolic response to injury, counterregulatory hormones are produced that lead to hyperglycemia, insulin resistance, and protein catabolism.

e. Increased metabolic rate.

f. Counterregulatory hormones promote protein breakdown and subsequent nitrogen wasting in the urine. Degree of catabolism can be related to amount of nitrogen lost.

g. Nutritional support will modify protein losses, not totally prevent them. Correction of the underlying catabolic stress is required for anabolic metabolism.

B. PATIENTS AT RISK FOR MALNUTRITION

1. Preexisting nutritional deficit present at the time of admission

a. Nonvolitional weight loss of more than 10% of usual body weight

b. High risk disease for nutritional complications (malignancy, AIDS, renal failure with dialysis, hepatic failure)

2. History of intestinal malabsorption

a. Intestinal fistula

b. Inflammatory bowel disease

c. Pancreatic exocrine insufficiency

3. Postoperative inanition

a. Prolonged postoperative ileus

b. Postoperative small bowel obstruction

   c. Inanition greater than 5 to 7 days in patients with normal nutritional stores

4. Hypermetabolic states or need for specialized nutrition

   a. Sepsis or ARDS

   b. Multiple trauma or major burns

   c. Short gut syndrome

C. NUTRITIONAL ASSESSMENT OF THE SURGICAL PATIENT

1. History

   a. Dietary habits

   b. Stability of weight

   c. Presence of chronic or acute illness

2. Physical

   a. Fat and muscle wasting

   b. Peripheral edema, ascites

   c. Excessive hair loss

3. Anthropometrics

   a. Triceps skinfold thickness to determine the degree of body fat

   b. Arm muscle circumference to measure lean body mass

   c. Values obtained are compared with standards and calculated as a percentage of those standards

   d. Very sensitive in addition to history in determining energy stores

4. Biochemical indicators of nutritional status

   a. Albumin

     (1) Oldest and most common laboratory measurement of serum protein stores.

     (2) Low levels at the time of admission have been associated with increased morbidity and mortality, as well as decreased survival.

     (3) A poor indicator of nutritional stability in hospitalized patients because it falls as part of the stress response to illness.

     (4) Long half-life (more than 20 days) makes it a poor indicator of nutritional recovery in simple starvation.

   b. Transferrin

     (1) Best known as binding and transport protein of ferric iron.

     (2) Short half-life (10 days), but also falls as part of the stress response to illness.

     (3) May fall with prolonged inanition, but certain conditions may alter levels that do not reflect nutritional stability (malignancy, anemia, hepatic dysfunction, renal failure).

   c. Prealbumin (transthyretin)

     (1) Best known as a transport protein of thyroxine and vitamin A.

     (2) Prealbumin depends on presence of adequate calories and proteins for normal serum concentration.

     (3) Short half-life (2 to 3 days), small body pool, and early response to nutritional deficits make this more sensitive than albumin or transferrin to both nutritional deficits and nutritional repletion; however, it still falls as part of the stress response to illness.

(4) Limitations occur in interpreting prealbumin in patients with chronic renal failure, hyperthyroidism, and protein-losing enteropathies.

5. Urinary measures of nutritional status

a. Creatinine height index (CHI)

(1) Creatinine excretion is proportional to the amount of lean tissue and is based on measured urinary creatinine excretion compared with normal gender- and height-matched controls.

(2) CHI is calculated as follows:

$$CHI = \frac{\text{actual 24-hour creatinine excretion}}{\text{expected 24-hour creatinine excretion}} \times 100$$

(3) Less than 80% indicates a moderate loss of muscle mass. Less than 60% represents severe muscle mass depletion and in itself has been associated with significant morbidity.

(4) Limitations occur in patients with varying creatinine excretion, the elderly, and the very thin or morbidly obese.

b. Nitrogen balance

(1) A 24-hour urine collection can be used to determine nitrogen excretion.

(2) Protein is the body's major substrate that contains nitrogen, and the waste associated with nitrogen metabolism can be used to determine degree of catabolism and lean tissue stores.

(3) Nitrogen balance can be calculated as follows:

$$\text{Nitrogen balance} = \frac{\text{dietary protein (g)}}{6.25} - (\text{UNN} + 4)$$

UUN = urine urea nitrogen
4 represents nitrogen loss in stool and skin

(4) A positive balance is indicative of adequate protein and calorie support, as well as anabolic metabolism and lean tissue accrual.

(5) Sequential nitrogen collections at intervals of 5 to 7 days with stable nutritional support can guide re-nutrition.

(6) Nitrogen excretion can also be reflective of catabolic stress, and indexes have been created, such as the catabolic index
(CI = UUN − [(0.5 × dietary protein) × 0.16] + 3 g).

(a) This index represents degree of lean tissue loss during catabolic illness.

(b) Less than 0 indicates no stress, between 0 and 5 indicates moderate stress, and greater than 5 indicates severe stress.

(7) Nitrogen studies are limited in patients with renal dysfunction, although a conversion formula is available for rises in creatinine. They are also limited by adequacy of the urine collection and patient compliance if used in the outpatient setting.

(8) CHI can be used as a measure of quality control to determine if the collection is adequate.

22

NUTRITION

D. ENERGY AND SUBSTRATE REQUIREMENTS FOR HOSPITALIZED PATIENTS

1. **In normal physiologic states,** a mixed fuel system of carbohydrates, protein, and fat is required for metabolic homeostasis
2. **Although the rate of metabolism increases with catabolic stress,** the basal energy expenditure (BEE), the external energy requirements may be very small.
3. **Key point:** BEE is dependent on amount of lean tissue present; it is dependent on gender and age
4. **Energy requirements**
   a. Harris-Benedict equation
      (1) Not very helpful in hospitalized patients because it is based on data from healthy male volunteers
      (2) Formula:

$$\text{Males} : 66 + 13.7W \text{ (kg)} + 5H \text{ (cm)} - 6.8A \text{ (years)} = BEE$$
$$\text{Females} : 65 + 9W \text{ (kg)} + 1.8H \text{ (cm)} - 4.7A \text{ (years)} = BEE$$

   Grossly underestimates or overestimates some patients with catabolic stress. Stress factors developed are "best guess" scenario.
   b. Energy requirements for hospitalized patients:

Kcal/kg	Condition
35-40	Severe burns
30-35	Severe blunt trauma
25-30	Sepsis/penetrating trauma
25	Uncomplicated surgical patient
20-25	Morbid obesity

   (Should be less for elderly/females)
   c. Sequential (after 5 to 7 days of stable nutritional support) urine nitrogen studies can assess adequacy of calorie support by effect on degree of nitrogen wasting or anabolism.
   d. Indirect calorimetry (metabolic cart).
      (1) Measures resting energy expenditure (REE) by calculating respiratory quotient.

$$RQ = Vco_2/Vo_2$$

      (2) RQ gives an indication of the balance of fuel substrates being metabolized.
      (3) Different substrates have different RQ values:
         (a) Oxidation of fat = 0.71
         (b) Protein = 0.82
         (c) Carbohydrate = 1
         (d) Adequate mixed fuel support should provide an RQ = 0.85
      (4) RQ greater than 1 indicates overfeeding with predominantly glucose calories and indicates lipogenesis and increased CO_2 production.

(5) Maximum oxidation rate for glucose is 4 mg/kg/min. Excess provision of glucose calories to SICU patients can lead to hyperglycemia, increased CO_2 production, and hepatic steatosis.

(6) Indirect calorimetry may be helpful in ventilated patients who are difficult to wean or have a preexisting history of COPD to determine appropriate calorie support.

e. Approximate caloric values of these metabolic fuel sources:

   (1) Fat = 9 kcal/g

   (2) Carbohydrate

      (a) 4 kcal/g enterally

      (b) 3.4 kcal/g intravenously

   (3) Protein = 4 kcal/g

f. Protein

   (1) Protein needs during critical illness double from RDA (0.8 g/kg) to 1.5 g/kg.

   (2) Normal healthy individuals have approximately 100 g of surplus protein in reserve. When depleted after 24 to 48 hours, gluconeogenesis occurs at the expense of skeletal and visceral proteins.

   (3) Dextrose infusion alone has no protein-sparing effect.

   (4) Patients with severe catabolic stress require "stress doses" of protein even if renal function is compromised. Breakdown products of protein may require more frequent dialysis, but in the patient with renal dysfunction, the nitrogen-wasting metabolism of catabolic stress is the same.

g. Carbohydrates

   (1) They are the primary fuel in normal nutrition.

   (2) Maximal degradation rate is 4 mg/kg/min.

   (3) In diabetic patients and patients with increased peripheral insulin resistance from stress, serum glucose levels should be aggressively controlled to levels below 180 mg/dl to maintain nitrogen homeostasis and limit infectious complications.

h. Fat

   (1) Endogenous fat is the major energy reserve for nonstressed starvation.

   (2) In catabolic stress, the protein-sparing effect of stored fat is lost.

   (3) Lipids should be administered as no more than 30% of total calories in the stressed patient.

   (4) The infusion of long-chain triglycerides has been associated with decreased function of the reticuloendothelial system and may be immunosuppressive if given as a bolus IV infusion.

   (5) Specialized fats such as ω-3 fatty acids or medium-chain triglycerides (MCTs) may aid in the metabolic management of the critically ill SICU patient.

i. Refeeding

   (1) Refeeding syndrome can occur in the patient with severe nutritional deficits. It is the phenomenon of metabolic consequences resulting

22

NUTRITION

from physiologic intolerance of infusions of large volumes of glucose or sodium-containing solutions.

(2) Danger is related to increasing insulin levels in the patient who is severely malnourished.

(3) Insulin has powerful antinatriuretic properties and can, in the face of a large glucose load, cause dramatic sodium and free-water retention.

(4) Severe hypophosphatemia, hypomagnesemia, and hypokalemia can also occur.

(5) In patients with severe malnutrition, initial feeding should limit volume, sodium, and dextrose calories; weight gain should be monitored closely, as well as serum electrolytes during the first week.

II. ENTERAL ALIMENTATION

A. INDICATIONS

1. **Existing nutritional deficit**
2. **High risk for hospital-acquired malnutrition** (severe catabolic stress or postoperative prolonged ileus)
3. **Traumatic injury or burns**
4. **ARDS**
5. **Severe pancreatitis** ("jejunal brake theory" feed distal to the ligament of Treitz limits pancreatic exocrine secretion as part of a negative feedback loop)
6. **Low-output enterocutaneous fistulas**

B. CONTRAINDICATIONS

1. **Absolute contraindications**
a. Complete intestinal obstruction
b. Failure of enteral support
c. Shock or presence of pressors
2. **Relative contraindications**
a. Severe pancreatitis
b. Malabsorption syndromes (can be fed with specialized nutritional formulas, i.e., MCTs or low fat)
c. Ileus (small bowel activity returns almost immediately postoperatively; gastric motility is delayed)

C. ADVANTAGES OF ENTERAL FEEDING

Physiologic: Enteral feeding allows maintenance of the intestinal structure via trophic effects of intestinal nutrients.

1. **Intestinal integrity of the intestinal mucosa** is preserved.
2. **Risk of sepsis secondary to bacterial translocation** is decreased.
3. **GI hormonal function** is generally maintained.
4. **Usual pattern of nutrient absorption** into the portal circulation is preserved.
5. **Formulations** more nutritionally complete than intravenous options.
6. **Less expensive** than intravenous hyperalimentation.
7. **No specialized personnel** required for administration.
8. **Options available** for metabolic management via specialized nutritional formulas.

D. METHODS OF DELIVERY FOR ENTERAL NUTRITION

1. Stomach

a. Small-bore feeding placed in the stomach or gastrostomy tube

b. Advantages

(1) Tube placement is simple.

(2) Delivery of food into the stomach simulates normal GI function.

(3) High osmolar loads are tolerated.

(4) Bolus feeding is tolerated and can assist with long-term placement of the patient if necessary.

c. Disadvantages

(1) The infusion of food into the stomach increases the risk of aspiration.

(2) Frequent measurement of gastric residuals is mandatory.

(3) Success of feeding may be limited in the patient with severe catabolic stress because gastric emptying is severely delayed and large residuals may limit feedings.

2. Small intestine

a. Nasoduodenal or jejunostomy tube

b. Advantages

(1) Access for immediate postoperative feedings

(2) Significantly reduced risk of aspiration

(3) Enables use of enteral nutrition in patients who are not candidates for gastric feeding

(4) Patients with altered mental status, including comatose patients

(5) Patients with gastroparesis can be fed long-term

(6) Patients with proximal enterocutaneous fistulas (tube placed distal to fistula)

c. Disadvantages

(1) Continuous feeding is necessary; bolus feeding to the small intestine is tolerated poorly.

(2) Needle jejunostomy tubes are prone to obstruction.

(3) Nasoduodenal tubes or needle catheters cannot be used for medications.

(4) Nasoduodenal tubes are prone to dislodgment.

E. ENTERAL FORMULAS

Can be divided into three groups: standard, predigested, and specialized.

1. Standard formulas

a. Nutritionally complete with all vitamins and micronutrients in RDA quantities

b. Generally 1 kcal/ml

c. Contain 50% to 55% calories from carbohydrates, 15% to 20% from protein, and 30% from fat

d. Protein is provided in intact form

e. Fats are usually long-chain fats

(1) MCTs can be included in combination.

(2) MCTs can be absorbed directly into the portal vein and are not lymphatic dependent for transport. They are 100% used for energy and cannot be stored as fat.

22

NUTRITION

    f. Concentrated formulas
- (1) Usually 1.5 to 2.0 kcal/ml
- (2) Used in patients with fluid restriction concerns
- (3) Renal solute load may be higher (unless specially formulated for patients with renal dysfunction)

    g. High-protein formulas
- (1) These are most commonly used in a SICU setting to provide the 1.5 g/kg/day protein supplementation.
- (2) 20% of calories are from protein sources.

    h. Fiber supplemented: used in the SICU setting in the patient with diarrhea

2. Elemental
a. Refers to formulas with protein in a predigested form and low fat content
b. Indicated in patients with impaired digestion or known malabsorption (AIDS, enterocutaneous fistula, short gut)
c. 1 kcal/ml
d. Proteins are given as dipeptides, tripeptides, or amino acids and are easily absorbed
e. These formulas are very expensive, and some are hyperosmolar
f. Once tolerance to goal has been reached, transition to a standard formula can occur

3. Disease specific
a. Immune modulating
- (1) Arginine, glutamine, and ω-3 fatty acids have been found to be modulators of nonspecific inflammation in the setting of catabolic illness
- (2) Glutamine
  - (a) Primary fuel source of a number of rapidly dividing cells
    - (i) Enterocytes and colonocytes
    - (ii) Lymphocytes
  - (b) Increased uptake and metabolism during stress
  - (c) Experimental evidence that absence from the diet results in progressive intestinal atrophy with the following:
    - (i) Breakdown of the mucosal barrier
    - (ii) Bacterial translocation
    - (iii) Sepsis
  - (d) Generally present in only small quantities in most enteral formulations
    - (i) The instability of glutamine in solution precludes its routine addition to most enteral formulas.
    - (ii) Glutamine supplements are available in the form of L-glutamine powder; the recommended daily dose is 6 to 8 g/day.
    - (iii) Three commercially available formulas have these specific additives.
    - (iv) Recommend their use in patients with ARDS, sepsis, or pancreatitis.

b. Hepatic formulas
   (1) These enteral formulas contain large amounts of branched-chain amino acids (BCAAs; e.g., valine, leucine, isoleucine) and low amounts of the aromatic amino acids (AAA; e.g., phenylalanine and tryptophan).
   (2) Their use in patients with hepatic failure is based on the theoretic concept that encephalopathy is based on an imbalance between the AAA and BCAA.
   (3) Multiple clinical trials have shown little benefit from BCAA supplementation in patients with hepatic failure and encephalopathy in terms of survival; however, most data are from a nontransplantable patient population. BCAA will allow nutritional support while limiting encephalopathy.
   (4) Provision of adequate calories and protein, with bowel decontamination therapy for encephalopathy, has been shown to minimally improve mortality rates.
c. Pulmonary formulas
   (1) These are designed to be high in fat to limit CO_2 production.
   (2) The carbohydrate content may not be enough to meet caloric needs.
   (3) Too much enteral fat can lead to gas bloating or diarrhea.

F. ADMINISTRATION OF ENTERAL NUTRITION

1. Stomach

a. Intermittent (bolus) feeding
   (1) Begin with approximately 100 ml of half-strength hyperosmolar formula or 100 ml of full-strength isotonic formula administered q4h.
   (2) If tolerated for the first three or four feedings, hyperosmolar formulas may be advanced to three-fourths and full strength at 8- to 12-hour intervals.
   (3) Once full-strength feedings are tolerated, then the volume should be advanced by 50 to 100 ml every 8 to 12 hours as tolerated, until full support is achieved.
   (4) Gastric residuals must be checked before each intermittent feeding.
   (5) The tube must be flushed with 25 to 50 ml of water after each feeding.
b. Continuous infusion
   (1) Initiate with half-strength hyperosmolar or full-strength isotonic formula.
      (a) Begin at rate of 50 ml/hr.
      (b) Increase rate by 25 ml/hr every 8 hours as tolerated until appropriate rate is achieved.
   (2) Hyperosmolar formulas are increased to three-fourths and then full-strength at 8-hour intervals.
   (3) Residuals should be assessed every 4 hours.
   (4) The tube should be flushed regularly with water.

2. Small intestine

a. Route most likely to be used in the critically ill

22

NUTRITION

b. Must administer infusions continuously and not intermittently
   (1) Initiate feedings with 10 to 20 ml/hr with standard formula.
   (2) Increase rate by 10 ml/hour every 8 hours as tolerated until the appropriate rate is achieved.
   (3) No medications should be given as crushed tablets.
   (4) Frequent flushing with water is imperative (small-bore tube clogs easily).

G. MONITORING
1. Physical examination
a. Abdominal examination for distention
b. Daily weights
2. Accurate recording of total input and output
3. Laboratory studies
a. Serum electrolytes with calcium, magnesium, and phosphorus
b. Glucose
   (1) Causes of hyperglycemia
       (a) High carbohydrate levels in enteral formulas
       (b) Diabetes
       (c) Glucose intolerance associated with major illness or sepsis
   (2) Treatment of hyperglycemia
       (a) Treat underlying condition.
       (b) Use insulin as necessary.

H. COMPLICATIONS OF ENTERAL FEEDING
1. Diarrhea
a. Occurs in 60% to 70% of critically ill patients receiving enteral alimentation.
b. Etiology in this subset of patients is variable; key is to rule out opportunistic infection.
c. Treatment includes the following:
   (1) Search for the cause.
   (2) Treat the underlying conditions.
   (3) Diet-related causes may be managed by decreasing the infusion rate or osmolality or changing to formula with less fat.
2. Aspiration pneumonia: less likely with feeding tube beyond the ligament of Treitz
3. Tube misplacement
4. Tube dislodgment

III. PARENTERAL NUTRITION
A. CONTRAINDICATION
Functional GI tract
B. INDICATIONS
1. Failure of enteral support
2. Severe short gut (either anatomic or functional)
3. Need for aggressive metabolic support in the form of electrolyte or acid-base substrates

C. ADVANTAGES

1. **Provides satisfactory nutrition** for patients with nonfunctioning or absent intestinal tracts
2. **Can be tailored** to meet the specific needs of patients with a variety of disorders
3. **May allow fluid restriction** while maintaining adequate nutritional support

D. DISADVANTAGES

1. **Mandates central venous access** either by central line or peripheral infusion catheter (PIC)—centrally placed
2. **Promotes atrophy of the intestinal tract**
3. **Not a physiologic method of nutrient delivery**
4. **Expense**

E. COMPONENTS OF TPN FORMULATIONS

1. **Volume requirements**
a. Should include maintenance requirements plus ongoing losses.
b. In patients who are critically ill, volume formulation should be calculated daily to potentially respond to patient's changing needs.

2. **Acid-base requirements**
a. Na or K come in either Cl or acetate.
b. Patients with metabolic acidosis from renal tubular acidosis (RTA) or as diarrhea can have their base requirements met by the TPN formulation.
c. Patients with severe metabolic alkalosis can potentially have their disorder corrected by adding Cl substrate or HCl as 1N in non—fat-containing bags.
d. HCl must be given centrally, in nonfat bags and no more than 100 mEq in a 24-hour period to avoid overcorrection.

3. **Electrolyte requirements**
Approximate daily requirements are the following:
    (1) Sodium: 1 to 2 mEq/kg/day
    (2) Potassium: 1 to 2 mEq/kg/day
    (3) Chloride: 1 to 2 mEq/kg/day
    (4) Calcium: 0.2 to 0.3 mEq/kg/day
    (5) Magnesium: 0.25 to 0.35 mEq/kg/day
    (6) Phosphate: 7 to 9 mmol/1000 kcal/day

4. **Protein and substrate needs**
a. Protein
    (1) Determine the protein requirement (usually 1.5 g/kg/day)
    (2) Administered as amino acids
    (3) Patients with severe catabolic stress use protein as an energy source
b. Carbohydrate
    (1) The most common source in TPN is dextrose (caloric value 3.4 kcal/g).
    (2) The dextrose concentration of commercially available base solution is 70%.
    (3) In patients with underlying diabetes or stress-related insulin resistance, start at 2 mg/kg/min with 10 to 20 units insulin per bag. Control glucose with aggressive sliding scale to keep less than 180 mg/dl.

22

NUTRITION

(4) Once insulin-to-dextrose ratio is calculated, may increase to 4 mg/kg/min with additional insulin in TPN as needed.

c. Fat
(1) Efficient source of calories
(2) Provides essential fatty acids
(3) Fat emulsions available in concentrations of 10% (1.1 kcal/ml) and 20% (2.2 kcal/ml)
(4) Should not constitute more than 30% of daily caloric requirements
(5) May be immunosuppressive and has been reported when given to patients with ARDS as a rapid bolus to cause a decrease in Po_2

d. Vitamins
(1) Fat- and water-soluble vitamin supplements must be added to TPN solutions.
(2) Formulations for adults do not contain vitamin K. Add vitamin K directly to TPN solution, 1 to 2 mg/day, or administer SQ or IM 5 to 10 mg/week.

e. Trace element recommended daily supplementation: zinc, copper, manganese, chromium, selenium

f. Other additives
(1) Albumin: 25 g/day in TPN solution to correct low-colloid oncotic pressure; very controversial
(2) Heparin (1000 U/L): to decrease the risk of catheter thrombosis
(3) Insulin: for patients with glucose intolerance

g. Glutamine
(1) Presently not in TPN solutions
(2) Glutamic acid has been added to some solutions
(3) Lability of glutamine has precluded its addition to solutions
(4) May be added to TPN in future

F. MONITORING
1. Accurate assessment of daily input and output
2. Daily weights
3. Physical examination
a. Decreased fat and muscle wasting
b. Decreased ascites and peripheral edema
c. Improved anthropometric measures over time
4. Laboratory studies
a. Daily
(1) Serum electrolytes and BUN
(2) Serum glucose q6h if indicated
b. Twice weekly
(1) Serum electrolytes (Ca, P, and Mg)
(2) Blood studies (Hgb, Hct, WBC)
c. Weekly
(1) Liver function tests (transaminases, bilirubin, and alkaline phosphatase)

(2) Triglyceride level (provides indication of patient's ability to tolerate lipid infusion)

(3) Nitrogen balance

G. DISCONTINUING TPN

1. TPN infusion is associated with increased serum insulin levels.

a. Sudden cessation of TPN is occasionally associated with hypoglycemia.

b. Hypoglycemia can occur in as few as 15 minutes.

2. Methods of tapering TPN include the following:

a. Elective taper

(1) If patient receiving more than 500 g of glucose per day, decrease glucose by 250 g per day to 500 g per day.

(2) When 500 g/day of glucose is attained, discontinue TPN and administer 5% dextrose at 75 to 125 ml/hour for 6 to 8 hours.

(3) Remove TPN catheter.

b. Emergent taper

(1) Indications

(a) Catheter sepsis

(b) Emergency surgery

(2) Procedure

(a) Administer 5% dextrose (with 1/4 or 1/2NS and potassium) at the same rate TPN was infused before cessation.

(b) Restart TPN when appropriate.

H. COMORBID CONDITIONS INFLUENCING PARENTERAL NUTRITION

1. Renal failure

a. Concentrated solutions of carbohydrate, fat, and amino acids may be used so that total volume of infusion is decreased.

b. Dialysis should be used liberally so that full nutritional support may be maintained.

2. Hepatic failure

a. Patients with mild liver failure are capable of tolerating TPN solutions, but it is not the method of choice for nutritional support.

b. Patients with moderately severe hepatic dysfunction have depressed levels of branched-chain amino acids and may benefit from formulas with increased levels.

3. Cardiac failure

a. Patients are unable to tolerate large volume loads.

b. Use concentrated solutions of carbohydrate, fat, and amino acids.

4. Pulmonary failure: Patients with chronic obstructive lung disease would probably benefit from decreased respiratory quotient and increase fat and decrease carbohydrate calories.

5. Glucose intolerance

a. Blood glucose levels must be under control before the initiation of TPN.

b. TPN should be advanced slowly in these patients over a period of a few days.

c. Blood glucose levels must be monitored closely.

d. Administer insulin.

22

NUTRITION

SUGGESTED READINGS

Grant JP: *Handbook of total parenteral nutrition,* ed 2, Philadelphia, 1992, WB Saunders.

Shikora SA, Blackburn GL, editors: *Nutrition support: theory and therapeutics,* New York, 1997, Chapman & Hall.

Wilmore DW: *The metabolic management of the critically ill,* New York, 1977, Plenum Press.

Zaloga G: *Nutrition and critical care,* St Louis, 1993, Mosby.

ANESTHESIA AND ANALGESIA

Eugene W. Moretti

I. PHYSIOLOGIC EFFECTS OF ANESTHESIA IN THE CRITICALLY ILL

A. AIRWAY CONSIDERATIONS OF THE CRITICALLY ILL

Endotracheal intubation is required to provide a patent airway when patients are at risk for aspiration, when airway maintenance by mask is difficult, and for prolonged controlled ventilation.

1. Laryngospasm

a. Reflexive closure of the vocal cords most commonly caused by an irritative stimulus, that is, secretions, vomitus, and blood.

b. Treatment includes administration of 100% oxygen with positive pressure under a good mask fit, which should break the spasm.

c. If that is unsuccessful, continue to ventilate with 100% oxygen and administer 10 to 20 mg of succinylcholine IV.

2. Laryngoedema

a. Any irritant stimulus, for example, oversized endotracheal tube, head and neck surgery, or allergic reactions, can produce an inflammatory response, producing edema in the larynx or trachea.

b. Occurring most commonly in children, it may present as dyspnea, stridor, tachypnea, tachycardia, and/or suprasternal retractions.

c. Treatment is humidified, cool, moist oxygen and racemic epinephrine by aerosol.

d. Steroids may be effective, but this has not definitely been proven.

3. Aspiration

a. Aspiration of gastric contents from vomiting or regurgitation may cause bronchospasm, hypoxemia, atelectasis, tachypnea, tachycardia, and hypotension.

b. Severity of symptoms depends on volume and pH of gastric material aspirated.

c. Conditions that predispose to aspiration include gastric outlet obstruction, gastroesophageal reflux, small bowel obstruction, hiatal hernia, pregnancy, severe obesity, and recent food ingestion.

d. Management includes a chest x-ray, ventilatory support, and possibly bronchoscopy.

e. Antibiotics are controversial and probably not indicated in a previously healthy patient.

B. CARDIOVASCULAR EFFECTS OF ANESTHESIA (Table 23-1)

1. Inhalational anesthetics (halothane, enflurane, isoflurane, desflurane, sevoflurane)

a. Produce dose-dependent myocardial depression and systemic vasodilatation.

b. Heart rate tends to be unchanged, although desflurane has been associated with hypertension and tachycardia at induction.

TABLE 23-1

CARDIOVASCULAR EFFECTS OF ANESTHETIC AGENTS

Agents	Cardiac Output	SVR	Heart Rate	Blood Pressure	Miscellaneous
Inhalation	Decreased	Decreased or N/C	Increased or N/C	Decreased	Agent-specific variation
Nitrous oxide	N/C	N/C	N/C	N/C	
Barbiturates	N/C	Decreased	Increased	Decreased	
Benzodiazepines					
Propofol	Decreased	Decreased	N/C	Decreased	
Etomidate	N/C	Mild Reduction	N/C	N/C or slight decrease	
Ketamine	Increased	Increased	Increased	Increased	
Narcotics	Decreased or N/C	Decreased or N/C	Decreased*	Decreased	
Local anesthetics	Decreased	Decreased	Decreased	Decreased	Highly arrhythmogenic. Cocaine would have opposite effects in all four categories.

*Meperidine increases HR.

c. They also sensitize the myocardium to the arrhythmogenic effects of catecholamines (halothane > enflurane > isoflurane > desflurane > sevoflurane).

d. Particular concern should be exhibited with infiltration of epinephrine-containing solutions (not to exceed 2 mg/kg of epinephrine subcutaneously infiltrated over 20 minutes).

2. Nitrous oxide

a. A mild myocardial depressant and a mild sympathetic nervous system stimulant.

b. Heart rate and blood pressure are usually unchanged, but pulmonary vascular resistance may increase.

3. Local anesthetics

a. Used for regional anesthetic techniques (e.g., epidural, spinal, and peripheral nerve blocks).

b. Includes esters, such as procaine, and amides, such as lidocaine and bupivacaine.

c. Cardiovascular toxicity becomes evident as decreased ventricular contractility, decreased conduction, and loss of peripheral vasomotor tone, which may lead to cardiovascular collapse.

d. The intravascular injection of bupivacaine or etidocaine may result in cardiovascular collapse that is refractory to therapy because of the high degree of tissue binding displayed by these agents.

e. Management includes oxygen, cardioversion, bretylium, and CPR.

C. CNS EFFECTS

General anesthesia induces an unconscious state believed to be brought about by irregular descending depression of the reticular activating system. The stage or plane of anesthesia was described after observation of patient responses during induction with diethyl ether. However, it is now a widely held view that induction with modern agents is sufficiently rapid that these stages are not seen. These stages are of some benefit insofar as they describe progression from an awake to an anesthetized state.

1. Stage I: Induction period—gradually increasing amnesia, analgesia.

2. Stage II: Onset of unconsciousness—unpredictable reactions, involuntary movements, irregular respirations, persistence of reflexes, loss of all volitional responses.

3. Stage III: Surgical anesthesia—progressive obtundation, gradual loss of protective reflexes, progressive hypoventilation and generalized paralysis.

4. Stage IV: Medullary paralysis—respiratory arrest, myocardial depression, obtundation of catecholamine release, flaccid paralysis.

D. ANESTHESIA AND BODY TEMPERATURE

1. Under anesthesia, the patient becomes pokilothermic (i.e., temperature changes are determined by the difference between metabolic heat production and heat loss to the environment). Heat production is reduced during general anesthesia as shivering is inhibited.

2. **Malignant hyperthermia:**
a. A hypermetabolic syndrome occurring in genetically susceptible patients after exposure to an anesthetic triggering agent (most commonly volatile anesthetics and succinylcholine).
b. The syndrome is thought to be due to a reduction in the reuptake of calcium by the sarcoplasmic reticulum necessary for termination of muscle contraction.
c. Clinical signs include unexplained tachycardia, hypercapnia, tachypnea, acidosis, muscle rigidity, hypoxemia, ventricular arrhythmias, hyperkalemia, fever (a very late sign), myoglobinuria, and a large gradient between mixed venous and arterial carbon dioxide tension.
d. It usually occurs in the OR but may be delayed for up to 24 hours after an anesthetic.
e. Management includes enlistment of help, discontinuance of triggering agent, 100% oxygen, dantrolene 2.5 mg/kg IV (repeat to total of 10 mg/kg), sodium bicarbonate administration guided by pH and P_{CO_2} measurement, insulin and glucose for hyperkalemia, initiation of cooling, maintenance of urine output greater than 2 ml/kg/hr by mannitol 25 g and furosemide 20 mg IV along with copious IV fluid administration, and ICU observation for 48 to 72 hours to observe for recrudescence, DIC, and ATN.
f. Call the Malignant Hyperthermia Hotline (800-644-9737) with any questions.

II. INDUCTION

Induction produces an unconscious patient with depressed reflexes who is entirely dependent on the anesthesiologist for maintenance of homeostatic mechanisms and safety.

A. INDUCTION TECHNIQUES

Guided by patient's medical condition, anticipated airway management (e.g., risk of aspiration, difficulty of intubation), and patient preferences.

1. **IV induction**
a. Preceded by the administration of oxygen via face mask.
b. A potent short-acting hypnotic is administered IV with unconsciousness occurring soon thereafter.
c. Additional agents may be administered, and the patient may continue to breathe spontaneously or with assistance.

2. **Inhalational induction**
a. Often used to maintain spontaneous ventilation, usually used in children.
b. After preoxygenation, inhalational anesthetics are added at low concentration and then increased 0.5% every 3 to 4 breaths until the depth of anesthesia is adequate for an IV placement or airway manipulation.
c. As an alternative, a single vital-capacity breath inhalation induction can be achieved using a high concentration of a less pungent agent (e.g., sevoflurane).

3. Rapid-sequence induction

a. Used in patients who are at risk for aspiration (e.g., patients who have recently eaten; pregnant patients; those with bowel obstruction, morbid obesity, or symptomatic reflux).

b. After preoxygenation for 3 to 5 minutes (four vital capacity breaths of 100% oxygen may accomplish the same thing when time is of the essence).

c. An assistant places firm downward pressure on the cricoid cartilage, effectively compressing and occluding the esophagus (Sellick maneuver).

d. This reduces the risk of passive regurgitation of gastric contents into the pharynx.

e. There should be no attempt to ventilate the lungs by mask.

f. Intubation should be performed within 30 to 60 seconds.

g. Cricoid pressure is maintained until successful endotracheal intubation is verified.

h. If intubation techniques are unsuccessful, cricoid pressure should be maintained continuously during all following intubation attempts while mask ventilation is in progress.

B. INDUCTION AGENTS

Induction agents produce a state of unconsciousness via depression of the CNS (Table 23-2).

1. Barbiturates—thiopental, thiamylal, methohexital

a. Indications and mode of action

(1) Ultrashort onset of action (30 seconds)

(2) Depress reticular activating system, augment inhibitory tone of CNS GABA pathways, depress release of CNS excitatory neurotransmitters

(3) Produce no analgesia

b. Pharmacology

(1) Early reawakening (5 to 10 minutes) as a result of tissue redistribution

(2) Metabolized to inactive products by the liver, excreted by the kidneys

(3) Long elimination half-life

c. Side effects

(1) Dose-dependent decrease in BP, myocardial contractility; minimal effect on HR

TABLE 23-2

INDUCTION AGENTS

	Induction Dose (mg/kg)	Onset (sec)	Duration (min)
Thiopental	3-6	10-20	5-15
Methohexital	0.7-1.0	20-40	5-10
Propofol	2-2.5	<40	5-10
Ketamine	1-2.5 IV (IM = 5-10)	<30	5-15
Etomidate	0.1-0.4	30-60	3-10
Midazolam	0.05-0.350	30-60	15-80

    (2) Dose-dependent decrease in respiratory rate, tidal volume; occasionally apnea

  d. Dosage and administration (induction): 3 to 4 mg/kg thiopental, 0.7 to 1 mg/kg methohexital

2. Ketamine

a. Indications and mode of action

    (1) Produces analgesia, amnesia, "dissociative" anesthesia (eyes open, normal muscle tone)

    (2) Useful for short, painful procedures in ICU setting

    (3) Mode of action not well defined; theorized to involve antagonism at the N-methyl-D-aspartate (NMDA) receptor

b. Pharmacology: similar to phencyclidine

c. Side effects

    (1) Mildly depresses respiration; less likely to produce apnea than barbiturates

    (2) Activates the sympathetic nervous system, causing increased HR, BP; ideal for hypovolemic patients; contraindicated in patients with CAD

    (3) Causes cerebral vasodilation and increased intracranial pressure; contraindicated in patients with increased intracranial pressure or space-occupying lesions

    (4) Stimulates oral secretions, necessitating pretreatment with an antisialagogue

    (5) Often associated with restlessness, agitation, and hallucinations during emergence, which may be treated or prevented with benzodiazepines

d. Dosage and administration

    (1) Induction: 1 to 2 mg/kg IV or 5 to 10 mg/kg IM

    (2) Sedation: 0.2 mg/kg IV (titrated to effect)

3. Etomidate

a. Indications and mode of action

    (1) Ultrashort onset of action (30 seconds)

    (2) Appears to augment inhibitory tone of GABA pathways in the CNS

b. Pharmacology

    (1) An imidazole-containing hypnotic, unrelated to other anesthetic agents

    (2) Early reawakening (3 to 5 minutes) as a result of tissue redistribution

c. Side effects

    (1) Minimal effects on BP, HR, myocardial contractility; ideal for compromised patients

    (2) Dose-dependent depression of respiratory rate, tidal volume (less than barbiturates)

    (3) Reduces cerebral blood flow and metabolism; ideal for patients with increased ICP, but may activate seizure foci, precipitate myoclonus

    (4) Occasionally associated with postoperative nausea and vomiting

    (5) May suppress adrenal corticosteroid synthesis, particularly after prolonged infusion

d. Dosage and administration (induction): 0.3 mg/kg IV

4. Propofol
a. Indications and usage
  (1) Increases activity at inhibitory GABA synapses
  (2) Useful as induction agent or for continuous anesthesia or sedation
  (3) Produces no analgesia
b. Pharmacology
  (1) Rapid onset of action (30 to 45 seconds); conscious sedation with low dosages
  (2) Early reawakening as a result of tissue redistribution
c. Side effects
  (1) Dose-dependent decrease in respiratory rate, tidal volume; occasionally apnea
  (2) Dose-dependent decrease in BP, myocardial contractility; minimal effect on HR
d. Dosage and administration
  (1) Induction: 2 to 2.5 mg/kg IV
  (2) Continuous infusion for maintenance of anesthesia: 100 to 200 μg/kg/min
  (3) Continuous infusion for sedation: 3 to 4 mg/kg/hr
  (4) 1% isotonic oil-in-water emulsion containing egg lecithin, glycerol, and soybean oil; high associated venous irritation; caution with use in patients with lipid disorders, pancreatitis, or history of allergy to egg products

III. BENZODIAZEPINES
Diazepam, midazolam, lorazepam
A. INDICATIONS AND MODE OF ACTION
1. **Produce dose-dependent sedative, amnestic, muscle relaxant, and anticonvulsant effects**
2. **Produce no analgesia,** often used in combination with opioids for effects ranging from control of mild postoperative pain/anxiety to maintenance of general anesthesia
3. **Bind to specific receptors in the CNS,** enhance inhibitory tone of GABA pathways
B. PHARMACOLOGY
1. **Rapid conversion of midazolam to inactive metabolites** in the liver (relatively short duration)
2. **Conversion of diazepam and lorazepam to active metabolites** (longer duration of action)
C. SIDE EFFECTS
1. **Produce mild depression in BP and cardiac output;** may be more pronounced when given rapidly or with a narcotic, particularly in hemodynamically compromised patients.
2. **Mild, dose-dependent depression in respiratory rate and tidal volume;** may be more pronounced in elderly or debilitated patients, particularly if administered with a narcotic.

TABLE 23-3

BENZODIAZEPINES

	Sedation Dose (mg)	Onset (min)	Infusion Rate	Elimination $t_{1/2}$
Midazolam	0.5-1	1-2	20-300 µg/kg/hr	15-80 min
Diazepam	4-8	< 2	—	20 hr
Lorazepam	0.5	1-5	—	6-10 hr
Reversal Agent	**Reversal Dose***	**Overdose***	**Onset**	**Duration**
Flumazenil	0.2-1.0 mg IV q20min at 0.2 mg/min	3-5 mg IV at 0.5 mg/min	1-2 min	1-2 hr (dose dependent

Reversal Dose is for reversal of benzodiazepine sedation; Overdose is for reversal of benzodiazepine overdose.

3. **Variable response between patients;** requires careful monitoring.
4. **Associated with birth defects** when administered during pregnancy, especially first trimester.
5. **Avoid in patients receiving valproate;** may precipitate psychotic episode.

D. **DOSAGE AND ADMINISTRATION**

See Table 23-3.

E. **BENZODIAZEPINE REVERSAL—FLUMAZENIL**

1. **Competitive antagonist,** shorter acting than the benzodiazepines that it antagonizes
2. **Use cautiously in patients on long-term therapy or patients treated for seizures**
3. **Dosage:** 0.3 mg IV bolus, repeated q30-60sec up to 5 mg
4. **Repeated administration** may be necessary because of short duration of action

IV. NARCOTICS

Morphine, meperidine, fentanyl, hydromorphone

A. **INDICATIONS AND MODE OF ACTION**

1. **Dose-dependent analgesia and sedation;** anesthesia in high-dose administration
2. **Act at specific opioid (endorphin) receptors** in the brain and spinal cord

B. **PHARMACOLOGY**

Primarily metabolized by the liver, excreted by the kidneys

C. **SIDE EFFECTS**

1. **Minimal cardiovascular effects,** although may cause bradycardia (central vagal stimulation) and/or peripheral vasodilation (sympathetic depression and/or histamine release)
2. **Dose-dependent respiratory depression,** particularly decreased respiratory rate and diminished response to hypercapnia; apnea with large doses
3. **Smooth muscle stimulation,** resulting in increased GI secretions and decreased motility, precipitating gastric retention, biliary colic, constipation, urinary retention

4. **Nausea and vomiting** resulting from direct stimulation of the chemoreceptor trigger zone
5. **Dose-dependent muscle rigidity,** particularly of thoracic and abdominal musculature
6. **Dose-dependent pupillary constriction** (miosis), often useful for monitoring effect of agent

D. **DOSAGE AND ADMINISTRATION**

1. **Intravenous dosages** of commonly used agents are summarized in Table 23-4.
2. **Patient-controlled anesthesia** is a popular method of postoperative pain control in which individual bolus administration of narcotics is provided upon demand by the patient via an intravenous pump system, incorporating preset incremental dosage amounts and maximum numbers of doses per unit time. The initial "loading" dose often facilitates delivery of adequate analgesia, and dosage parameters are titrated based upon utilization and symptomatology.

E. **NARCOTIC REVERSAL—NALOXONE**

1. **Competitive antagonist** to narcotics at opioid receptors
2. **Dose-dependent reversal** of narcotic effects
3. **Peak CNS effects within 1 to 2 minutes;** diminished effects within 30 minutes
4. **May precipitate abrupt onset of pain** with associated hypertension or tachycardia
5. **Dosage:** 0.04 mg IV bolus repeated q2-3min to reach desired effect; may be given IM
6. **Crosses the placenta;** may decrease neonatal respiratory depression caused by narcotics

V. NEUROMUSCULAR BLOCKING AGENTS

A. **INDICATIONS AND MODE OF ACTION**

1. **Act via interference with normal acetylcholine neuromuscular transmission**
2. **Cause generalized paralysis,** facilitating endotracheal intubation and/or mechanical ventilation, decreasing systemic Vo_2, and optimizing surgical conditions
3. **Must be used in conjunction with other agents** providing analgesic and/or amnestic effects
4. **Use requires mechanical ventilation**

B. **DEPOLARIZING AGENTS—SUCCINYLCHOLINE**

1. **Pharmacology**
a. Binds and activates the acetylcholine receptor, leading to normal postjunctional depolarization
b. Degraded much more slowly than acetylcholine; requires plasma cholinesterase activity
c. Leads to muscle fasciculation followed by relaxation
2. **Side effects**
a. May cause transient increases in HR and BP as a result of vagolytic effects

TABLE 23-4

NARCOTICS

	Relative Potency	Analgesic Dose	Maintenance Dose	Demand Dose	PCA Lockout Interval	PCA 4-Hour Limit	Loading Dose
Morphine	1	0.05-0.2 mg/kg	0.02 mg/kg/hr	0.02 mg/kg	8 min	30 mg	0.05 mg/kg q10min t max of 3 doses
Fentanyl	100	1-2 µg/kg	0.2 µg/kg/hr	0.2 µg/kg	6 min	300 µg	0.5 µg/kg q10min to max of 3 doses
Meperidine	0.1	0.5-2 mg/kg	†				
Hydromorphone	5	0.01-0.04 mg/kg	0.004 mg/kg/hr	0.004 mg/kg	8 min	6 mg	0.01 mg/kg q10min to max of 3 doses

Reversal Agent	Reversal Dose	Onset	Duration	Miscellaneous
Naloxone	0.04-0.4 mg doses IV q2-3min	2-3 min	20-60 min (dose dependent)	‡

*Dosages are guidelines and should be adjusted for individual patient variation.
†Because of normeperidine (major metabolite of meperidine) toxicity and the possibility of seizures, it is not recommended to use meperidine in a PCA system.
‡For narcotic-induced pruritus, can be given as 0.4 mg in 1 L of IV fluid that is run at the patient's maintenance rate.

b. May cause transient increases in intraocular and intragastric pressures (fasciculation)

c. **May cause an elevation of serum potassium levels up to 0.5 mEq/L resulting from sustained depolarization; should be avoided in patients with renal insufficiency or hyperkalemia**

d. May lead to prolonged neuromuscular blockade in patients with the following:

(1) Low levels of plasma cholinesterase: patients with burns, shock, cardiac failure, liver insufficiency, starvation, and hypothyroidism, and patients in third trimester of pregnancy

(2) Pharmacologic inhibition of cholinesterase resulting from anticholinesterases, echothiophate eyedrops, phenelzine (monoamine oxidase inhibitor), organophosphate compounds

(3) Atypical plasma cholinesterase—4% of population heterozygous, 1/2800 homozygous

C. **NONDEPOLARIZING AGENTS—PANCURONIUM, VECURONIUM, CIS-ATRACURIUM, ROCURONIUM**

1. **Competitive inhibition with acetylcholine** (bind receptor, no postjunctional depolarization)

2. **Action terminated** by redistribution and subsequent metabolism of agent

3. **Two pharmacologic classes**—steroid derivatives and benzylisoquinolines

4. **Leads to relaxation without fasciculation,** posttetanic potentiation, and the presence of fade following tetanic or train-of-four stimulation

5. **Vary on rate of onset, duration of action, cardiovascular side effects, and metabolism**

D. **DOSAGE AND ADMINISTRATION**

See Table 23-5.

E. **REVERSAL OF NEUROMUSCULAR BLOCKADE**

1. **Recovery after administration of succinylcholine cannot be reversed pharmacologically** but typically occurs within 10 to 15 minutes (except situations noted above).

2. **Action of nondepolarizing agents may be reversed** by administration of anticholinesterases, which cause a transient increase in acetylcholine available for competition at neuromuscular junction.

3. **Anticholinesterase administration causes peripheral side effects** (bradycardia, salivation) resulting from effects of acetylcholine on muscarinic receptors (should be attenuated with atropine or glycopyrrolate).

VI. INHALATION ANESTHETIC AGENTS

A. **INDICATIONS AND MODE OF ACTION**

1. **Typically used for maintenance of general anesthesia** rather than induction, although often used as induction agents in pediatric patients.

2. **Generally not used in the ICU setting,** but effects must be considered in postoperative patients.

3. **Interaction with cellular membranes in CNS,** although exact mechanisms are not clear.

23

ANESTHESIA AND ANALGESIA

TABLE 23-5

NEUROMUSCULAR BLOCKING AGENTS

	Dose (mg/kg)*	Onset (min)	Duration (min)	Elimination
DEPOLARIZING				
Succinylcholine	1-2	1-1.5	5-10	Plasma cholinesterase
NONDEPOLARIZING				
Pancuronium	0.08-0.10	3-5	80-100	70%-80% renal
Vecuronium	0.1-0.12†	2-3	25-30	80% biliary
Cis-atracurium	0.15-0.20‡	1.5-2	50-60	Hoffmann
Rocuronium	0.6-1.2	1-1.5	40-150	Hepatic
ANTICHOLINESTERASES				
Edrophonium	0.5-1	1	40-65	Administer in with atropine (7-10 μg/kg) or glycopyrrolate (3-5 μg/kg)
Neostigmine	0.03-0.06	7	55-75	Administer in with atropine (15-30 μg/kg) or glycopyrrolate (7-15 μg/kg)

*Repeat doses of 20% to 25% initial dose may be given every 45 to 60 minutes to maintain relaxation.

†Vecuronium dose for continuous infusion is 1 μg/kg/min.

‡Cis-atracurium dose for continuous infusion is 1 to 2 μg/kg/min.

Neuromuscular blockers given by infusion should be titrated to maintain a one-twitch response to train-of-four nerve stimulator monitoring.

B. PHARMACOLOGY

1. **The rate of absorption/elimination** is a function of the agent's solubility in blood; decreased solubility leads to increased rates of absorption/elimination.
2. **Elimination is predominantly via exhalation,** although hepatic metabolism contributes for the more blood-soluble agents.
3. **Dosages** are expressed as minimal alveolar concentration or the percent atmospheric pressure at which movement in response to skin incision is inhibited in 50% of patients.

C. SPECIFIC AGENTS

1. Nitrous oxide

a. Relatively low solubility, high rate of absorption/elimination
b. Dose-dependent analgesia, but high minimal alveolar concentration precludes ability to obtain surgical anesthesia
c. Often used in combination with other inhalational agents, increasing alveolar concentration of second gas at lower total inspired volumes
d. Causes mild myocardial and respiratory depression, sympathetic activation
e. May increase pulmonary vascular resistance in adults
f. May limit Fio_2 during administration and cause diffusion hypoxia after cessation of administration resulting from rapid diffusion from blood into alveoli

g. Should be avoided in the presence of closed gas-containing spaces (e.g., pneumothorax, obstructed bowel, occluded middle ear, air embolus) because of expansion caused by diffusion of nitrous oxide into closed spaces in exchange for nitrogen

2. Volatile agents (halothane, enflurane, isoflurane, sevoflurane, desflurane)

a. Liquids at standard temperature and pressure with potent evaporative vapors

b. Produce unconsciousness and amnesia at relatively low inspired concentrations

c. Rate of absorption/elimination inversely proportional to solubility in blood: halothane > enflurane > isoflurane > desflurane > sevoflurane

d. Tend to increase cerebral blood flow and decrease cerebral metabolism

e. Produce dose-dependent myocardial depression and systemic vasodilation

f. May sensitize the myocardium to arrhythmogenic effects of catecholamines

g. Produce dose-dependent respiratory depression (decreased tidal volume)

h. Tend to cause bronchodilation but may be bronchial irritants/precipitate bronchospasm (desflurane and isoflurane with greatest irritant effect)

i. Tend to decrease hepatic perfusion; rarely associated with hepatitis (halothane)

j. Tend to decrease renal perfusion; rarely associated with nephrotoxicity as a result of release of fluoride ions (enflurane and sevoflurane)

k. Even trace amounts of volatile agent can diminish the ventilatory response to hypoxia

VII. REGIONAL ANESTHESIA

A. SPINAL (SUBARACHNOID) ANESTHESIA

1. Indications and mode of action

a. Surgical anesthesia (either used alone or in combination with general anesthesia) is occasionally useful for postoperative pain management.

b. The effect of a direct blockade of spinal nerves is greater on smaller fibers (pain) than on larger fibers (motor, proprioception).

2. Pharmacology

a. Agents most commonly used include lidocaine, bupivacaine, tetracaine (with or without epinephrine), either as isobaric, hyperbaric, or hypobaric solutions

b. May use morphine or fentanyl for postoperative pain control

3. Side effects

a. Hypotension: related to degree of sympathetic blockade

b. Dyspnea: caused by proprioceptive blockade or apnea with direct C3-C5 blockade; delayed respiratory depression occasionally after narcotic administration

c. Nausea and vomiting: caused by hypotension or unopposed vagal stimulation

d. Headache: usually 24 to 48 hours postoperatively as a result of continued CSF leak; usually managed conservatively, occasionally requiring "blood patch"

e. Urinary retention: sacral blockade with atonic bladder necessitating use of a Foley catheter

f. Infection: rare

B. EPIDURAL ANESTHESIA

1. Indications and mode of action

a. Surgical anesthesia and/or postoperative pain control

b. Administered as single dose, multiple injections, or continuous infusion

c. Catheter may be left in place for several days

   (1) If narcotic only epidural, no limitations on ambulation.

   (2) If local anesthetic is used in a lumbar epidural, patient must remain in bed because of possibility of motor weakness.

   (3) For thoracic epidurals, theoretically, no limitation on ambulation, but be wary of orthostatic hypotension, especially if local anesthetic is used.

d. Acts at spinal nerve roots located laterally in epidural space

e. Caudal blocks: administration of anesthesia into caudal space, the direct extension of the epidural space below the sacral hiatus

2. Pharmacology

a. Chloroprocaine and bupivacaine are used most commonly.

b. Narcotics are often used for postoperative pain control.

3. Side effects

a. Similar to subarachnoid anesthesia

b. Epidural hematoma: uncommon, but may require urgent laminectomy when severe; epidural anesthesia relatively contraindicated in patients requiring systemic anticoagulation

c. Dural puncture: can be managed by conversion to spinal anesthesia or replacement at higher level; may result in inadvertent total spinal anesthesia if unrecognized

d. Direct spinal cord injury, nerve root trauma, anterior spinal cord ischemia (uncommon)

e. Dosage and administration: summarized in Tables 23-6 and 23-7

C. REGIONAL NERVE BLOCKS

1. Useful for surgical anesthesia and/or postoperative pain control

2. Require accurate identification of peripheral nerve anatomy and infiltration with local agent

3. Brachial plexus blocks for upper extremity

4. Femoral, sciatic, or lumbar plexus blocks for lower extremity

5. Paravertebral blocks for thoracic, breast, and hernia surgery

D. LOCAL INFILTRATION

1. Surgical anesthesia for localized procedures

2. Most effective when administered according to anatomic distribution of cutaneous nerves

TABLE 23-6

EPIDURAL DOSING AND ADMINISTRATION

	Concentration	Rate of Infusion	Comment
LOCAL ANESTHETICS			
Bupivacaine	0.06-0.25%	2-10 ml/hr	Sympathetic effects occur with higher concentrations; motor and proprioceptive weakness may occur; tachyphylaxis develops with continuous epidural use
Ropivacaine	0.1-0.4 %	2-10 ml/hr	Same precautions as bupivacaine; less potential risk of cardiac toxicity
NARCOTICS			
Hydromorphone	10-50 μg/ml	2-6 ml/hr	Spreads well in the epidural space
Morphine	50-100 μg/ml	2-6 ml/hr	Spreads well in the epidural space, but with slow onset
Fentanyl	2.5-10 μg/ml	2-10 ml/hr	Systemic effects of opioids will occur; the catheter site should be close to dermatomal level of pain
Meperidine	2.5 μg/ml	2-6 ml/hr	Potential for neurotoxicity due to normeperidine accumulation

For breakthrough pain, Fentanyl 0.5 to 1 μg/kg diluted to 10 μg/ml provides a rapid onset; however, because of risk of respiratory depression, use a lower dose if opioids are already being systemically infused.

Lidocaine 2%, 2 to 4 ml will define if epidural catheter is in place by a well-demarcated band of local anesthesia; however, there is a risk of sympathetic blockade and hypotension.

Combinations of local anesthetics and opioids are used for synergism (e.g., bupivacaine 0.25% with fentanyl 2.5 μg/ml).

E. LOCAL ANESTHETIC AGENTS

1. Indications and mode of action

a. Temporary local or regional anesthesia

b. Blockade of local nerve action potential propagation via specific interaction of ionized moiety with receptors on intracellular portion of axonal $Na+$ channels, inhibiting $Na+$ ion influx

2. Pharmacology

a. Composed of aromatic ring (hydrophobic) and a tertiary amine (hydrophilic) connected by either ester or amide linkage

b. All weak bases; degree of ionization relevant to lipid solubility and ability to cross axonal membrane (directly correlates with potency, rate of onset)

c. Duration of effect related to degree of protein binding, mechanism of metabolism

TABLE 23-7

PATIENT-CONTROLLED EPIDURAL ANESTHESIA

	Loading Dose	Continuous Infusion	Demand Dose	Lockout	Maximum Dose
Morphine*	2-3 mg	0.2% at 0.4 mg/hr	0.2 mg	10-15 min	1-2 mg/hr
Bupivacaine	0.625%, 4 ml	3-10 ml/hr†	2-4 ml	10-20 min	12 ml/hr

*Only preservative-free morphine should be used in the epidural space.
†Depends on the level of catheter (i.e., thoracic or lumbar).

d. Esters rapidly degraded by plasma cholinesterase to inactive products including *p*-aminobenzoic acid (may cause allergic reactions)
e. Amides degraded by *n*-dealkylation and hydrolysis, primarily in the liver—toxicity possibly more likely in patients with hepatic insufficiency
f. Adjuvant agents
   (1) Epinephrine: prolongs duration of anesthesia, decreases systemic toxicity and bleeding, increases intensity of nerve block; must be avoided in areas with poor collateral blood flow (nose, digits, penis)
   (2) Sodium bicarbonate: raises the pH, increasing concentration of non-ionized base; increases rate of onset of blockade, and decreases pain associated with local infiltration

3. Side effects
a. Allergic reactions: rare; must be differentiated from common responses (syncope, vasovagal)
b. Systemic reactions: usually caused by accidental intravascular injection or overdose
c. CNS toxicity: restlessness, lightheadedness, tinnitus, metallic taste, circumoral numbness, muscle twitching, loss of consciousness, generalized seizure, apnea, coma
   (1) Treatment consists of stopping administration of the drug and ventilation with 100% O_2. Use anticonvulsant therapy as indicated with diazepam or thiopental.
   (2) Intubation and neuromuscular blockade may be necessary when other therapies fail.
d. Cardiovascular toxicity: decreased conduction, depressed contractility, loss of peripheral vasomotor tone, cardiovascular collapse
   (1) Treat with 100% O_2, volume replacement, and inotropic agents as needed.
   (2) Intravascular injection of bupivacaine is particularly toxic and may require prolonged CPR until effects of the drug have subsided.

VIII. MISCELLANEOUS AGENTS

A. KETOROLAC

1. Indications and mode of action
a. Parenteral NSAID recently approved in United States
b. Adjunct to narcotic agents for management of acute pain
c. Inhibition of cyclooxygenase; decreased prostaglandin synthesis

2. Pharmacology
a. Onset of action approximately 10 minutes, duration 4 to 8 hours
b. Metabolized in the liver; excreted by the liver and kidneys
c. Dosage: IM/IV: 30 to 60 mg, then 15 to 30 mg q6h; PO: 10 mg q4-6h

3. Side effects—similar to other NSAIDs
a. Gastric irritation and ulceration
b. Renal dysfunction
c. Platelet dysfunction

23

ANESTHESIA AND ANALGESIA

B. HALOPERIDOL
1. Indications and mode of action
a. Antipsychotic/tranquilizer often used in ICU setting for sedation
b. Butyrophenone, which reduces dopaminergic activity in the CNS
c. Also possesses anticholinergic and α-adrenergic effects
2. Pharmacology
a. Onset of action: peak effect less than 20 minutes
b. Dosage: 0.5 to 2 mg IV
3. Side effects
a. Neuroleptic malignant syndrome
b. Extrapyramidal reactions
c. May lower seizure threshold
d. Potentiates anesthetics, opiates

SUGGESTED READINGS

Morgan GE Jr, Mikhail MS: *Clinical anesthesiology,* ed 2, Norwalk, Conn, 1996, Appleton & Lange.

Stoelting RK, Diedorf SF: *Anesthesia and co-existing disease,* ed 3, Edinburgh, 1993, Churchill Livingstone.

Stoelting RK, Miller RD: *Basics of anesthesia,* ed 3, Edinburgh, 1994, Churchill Livingstone.

MEDICATIONS AND DRIPS

Shahab A. Akhter

Drug (Trade Name)	Dosage
Acebutolol (Sectral)	Start 200 mg PO q12h, can increase to 600-1200 mg daily, given in divided doses
Acetaminophen (Tylenol)	Regular strength: 325-650 mg PO q4-6h prn
•	Extra strength: 500-1000 mg PO q4-6h prn
	Liquid: 30 ml PO q4-6h prn
Acetaminophen/ propoxyphene (Darvocet-N 50, Darvocet-N 100)	2 N 50 tablets or 1 N 100 tablet PO q4h prn
Acetazolamide (Diamox)	500 mg PO or IV q8h
Acetylcysteine (Mucomyst)	3-5 ml of 20% solution in nebulizer q6-8h or prn
	For acetaminophen overdose: 140 mg/kg loading dose PO or via NG tube, then 17 doses of 70 mg/kg PO or via NG tube q4h
Acetylsalicylic acid (Aspirin)	Acute MI: 160 mg PO non–enteric coated, then 325 mg PO q24h enteric-coated aspirin
	TIA treatment/stroke prevention: 325 mg PO q6-24h
Acyclovir (Zovirax)	Herpes zoster in immunocompromised host:
	Mild cases: 800 mg PO 5 times daily
	Severe cases: 10-12 mg/kg IV q8h
Adenosine	Initial: 6 mg IV; if no response: 12 mg IV, may be repeated one additional time
Albumin	25 g IV initially, then as indicated
Albuterol (Salbutamol)	Nebulizer: 0.25-0.5 ml of 0.5% solution in 3 ml NS
	MDI: 2 inhalations q4-6h
	Regular-acting: 2-4 mg PO q6-8h
	Long-acting: 4-8 mg PO of long-acting tablets q12h
Allopurinol (Zyloprim)	Initial: 100 mg PO q24h
	Usual: 200-300 mg PO q24h
Alprazolam (Xanax)	Initial: 0.25-0.50 mg PO q8h
	Maximum: 4-6 mg PO q24h
Aluminum carbonate (Basaljel)	15-30 ml or 2-4 tablets PO qac and qhs
Aluminum hydroxide (Alternagel)	1-2 tsp PO prn between meals and qhs
Aluminum hydroxide (Amphojel)	30-60 ml or 600 mg PO qac
Aluminum phosphate (Phosphaljel)	15-30 ml PO q2h between meals and qhs
Amantadine (Symmetrel)	100 mg PO q12h to 300-400 mg PO q24h
Amikacin	Load: 7.5 mg/kg IV
	Maintenance: 5 mg/kg q8h or 7.5-10 mg/kg q12h IM or IV

Drug (Trade Name)	Dosage
Amiloride (Midamor)	5-10 mg PO q12-24h
Aminocaproic acid (Amicar)	5 g IV load, then 1 g/hr IV for 6-24h
Aminophylline	Load: 5-6 mg/kg IV over 30 min
	Maintenance: 0.5-0.6 mg/kg/hr IV (250 mg/50 ml D5W)
Amiodarone (Cordarone)	Load: 150 mg IV over 10 min then 360 mg IV over next 6h
	Maintenance: 540 mg IV over next 24h
	Breakthrough VT/VF: 150 mg IV over 10 min
	800-1600 mg PO q24h for 1-3 wks, then 400-800 mg PO q24h for 1-3 wks, then 200-400 mg PO q24h
Amitriptyline (Elavil)	Initial: 25 mg PO qhs, increase 25 mg weekly
	Maintenance: up to 150 mg PO qhs
Amlodipine (Norvasc)	Initial: 5 mg PO q24h, up to 10 mg PO q24h
Amoxicillin (Amoxil)	250-500 mg PO q8h
Amoxicillin/clavulanate (Augmentin)	250-500 mg PO q8h
Amphotericin B	Systemic illness: 1 mg IV test dose over 30 min, then 0.20-0.25 mg/kg IV on first day; may increase by 0.1-0.2 mg/kg q24h to 0.5-1 mg/kg/d
	Bladder irrigation: 15-50 mg in 1 L sterile water-continuous irrigation over 24 hrs for 3-5 days
Ampicillin	250-1000 mg PO q8h 30 min before meals or 0.5-2 g IM or IV q6h
Ampicillin/sulbactam (Unasyn)	1.5-3 g IV or IM q6h
Amrinone (Inocor)	Initial: 0.75 µg/kg IV bolus over 2-3 min
	Maintenance: 5-10 µg/kg/min (500 mg/100 ml NS)
Anistreplase (APSAC, Eminase)	30 unit IV bolus over 2-5 min
Astemizole (Hismanal)	10 mg PO q24h
Atenolol (Tenormin)	50-200 mg PO q24h
	Acute MI: 5 mg IV over 5 min, repeat in 10 min, then PO therapy
Atropine	Cardiac arrest: 1 mg IV q3-5min up to 3 mg or 1-2 mg diluted in 5 ml NS via endotracheal tube
	Nonarrest: 0.5-1 mg IV, may repeat q5min up to maximum total dose of 2-3 mg
Azathioprine (Imuran)	Initial 3-5 mg/kg PO or IV, maintenance 1-3 mg/kg q24h
Azithromycin (Zithromax)	500 mg PO on day 1, then 250 mg PO q24h
Aztreonam	1 g IV q8h
Beclomethasone nasal inhaler	1-2 inhalations each nostril q12h

Drug (Trade Name)	Dosage
Beclomethasone oral inhaler	2-4 inhalations PO q6h
Benazepril (Lotensin)	10 mg PO q24h, maximum of 20 mg PO q12h
Benztropine (Cogentin)	0.5-1 mg PO or IM qhs, maximum 1-2 mg PO q8h
Bepridil (Vascor)	200-400 mg PO q24h
Bicarbonate (Sodium Bicarbonate)	PO: 300-600 mg q8-12h IV drip: 2 ampules (88 mEq) in 1 L 0.45% NS IV bolus: 1 mEq/kg
Bisacodyl (Dulcolax)	5-10 mg PO, 10 mg PR, enema 37.5 ml
Bretylium (Bretylol)	VF: 5 mg/kg IV, then 10 mg/kg, can repeat up to total 35 mg/kg VT: 5-10 mg/kg IV, can repeat in 10-30 min Maintenance: 1-2 mg/min IV (500 mg/250 ml D5W)
Bromocriptine mesylate (Parlodel)	1.25 mg PO q12h, may increase by 2.5 mg q24h up to 50 mg PO q12h
Bumetanide (Bumex)	PO: 0.5-2 mg q24h IV: 0.5-1 mg over 1-2 min, can repeat q2-3h up to maximum 10 mg q24h
Bupropion (Wellbutrin)	100 mg PO q12h, may increase to 100 mg PO q8h
Buspirone (BuSpar)	5 mg PO q8h up to 20 mg PO q8h
Calcium carbonate (Os-Cal)	250-500 mg PO q8h
Calcium chloride	1 amp (13.6 mEq) of 10% solution IV
Captopril (Capoten)	Initial: 6.25 mg PO Usual: 25-50 mg PO q8-12h
Captopril/hydrochlorothiazide (Capozide)	1 tablet PO q8-12h 1 hr before meals
Carbamazepine (Tegretol)	Start 200 mg PO q12h, may increase up to 400 mg PO q8h
Cefaclor (Ceclor)	250-500 mg PO q8h
Cefadroxil (Duricef)	1-2 g PO daily in 1 or 2 divided doses
Cefazolin (Ancef, Kefzol)	1-2 g IV q8h
Cefixime (Suprax)	200 mg PO q12h or 400 mg PO q24h
Cefoperazone (Cefobid)	2 g IV q12h to 4 g IV q6h
Cefotaxime (Claforan)	1-2 g IM or IV q8-12h up to 2 g IV q4h
Cefotetan (Cefotan)	1-3 g IM or IV q12h
Cefoxitin (Mefoxin)	1-2 g IV q6-12h
Ceftazidime (Fortaz)	1-2 g IM or IV q8-12h
Ceftizoxime (Cefizox)	1-2 g IV q8-12h
Ceftriaxone (Rocephin)	1-2 g IM or IV q12-24h
Cefuroxime (Zinacef)	750-1500 mg IV q8h
Cephalexin (Keflex)	250-500 mg PO q6h

Drug (Trade Name)	Dosage
Charcoal (Activated Charcoal)	50-100 g PO or via NG tube q2-6h for 24 hrs
Chlordiazepoxide (Librium)	Alcohol withdrawal: 50-100 mg PO q1-2h prn Prophylaxis: 50-100 mg PO q6h for 24h then 25-50 mg PO q6h for 24-48 hrs then 25 mg PO q6h for 24 hrs
Chlorothiazide (Diuril)	0.5-1 g q12-24h PO or IV
Chlorpromazine (Thorazine)	10-25 mg PO q4-6h or 25-50 mg IM q3-4h prn
Chlorpropamide (Diabinese)	100-250 mg PO q24h
Cimetidine (Tagamet)	300 mg PO or IV q6h, 400 mg PO q12h, or 800 mg PO qhs
Ciprofloxacin (Cipro)	200-400 mg IV q12h or 250-750 mg PO q12h
Cisapride (Propulsid)	10 mg PO 15 min before meals and qhs
Clarithromycin (Biaxin)	250-500 mg PO q12h
Clindamycin (Cleocin)	600 mg IM or IV q8h
Clonazepam (Klonopin)	0.5 mg PO q8h, may increase until seizures controlled up to maximum 20 mg daily
Clonidine (Catapres)	0.1 mg PO q12h, may increase by 0.1 mg q24h up to 1.2 mg PO q12h Patch: One TTS-1 weekly for 2 wks, may increase by 0.1 mg q24h up to 0.6 mg
Cobalamin (Vitamin B)	100-1000 µg IM q24h for 7 days, then 1-2 doses per month until Hct normal
Codeine	15-60 mg PO, SQ, or IM q4-6h
Colchicine	2 mg IV over 2-5 min, may repeat once after 6 hrs
Cortisone (Cortone Acetate)	25-300 mg PO or IM q24h
Cromolyn sodium (Intal)	Inhale 2 puffs q6h
Cyclobenzaprine (Flexeril)	5-20 mg PO q8h
Cyclosporine A	1-4 mg/hr IV drip or 5-10 mg/kg PO q24h given in divided doses (follow levels)
Dapsone	100 mg PO q24h
Desipramine (Norpramin)	100-200 mg PO q24h
Desmopressin (DDAVP)	0.3 µg/kg in 50 ml NS IV over 15-30 min
Dexamethasone (Decadron)	10 mg IM or IV then 6 mg IM or IV q6h
Diazepam (Valium)	Acute seizure: 5-10 mg IV, may repeat q10-15min to maximum 30 mg Anxiety: 2-10 mg IM or IV
Diazoxide (Hyperstat)	1-3 mg/kg IV up to maximum 150 mg per injection q4-24h
Dicloxacillin	250 mg-1 g PO q6h
Digoxin (Lanoxin)	Atrial fibrillation: 0.25-0.5 mg IV initially then 0.25 mg IV q6-8h to total 1-1.5 mg; then 0.125-0.25 mg IV or PO q24h

Drug (Trade Name)	Dosage
Diltiazem (Cardizem)	0.25 mg/kg IV over 2 min; if response inadequate: 0.35 mg/kg IV over 2 min; maintenance: 5-15 mg/hr Regular pills: 30-90 mg PO q6-8h Cardizem SR: 60-180 mg PO q12h Cardizem CD: 180-300 mg PO q24h
Diphenhydramine (Benadryl)	25-50 mg PO q6h (or qhs for insomnia)
Diprivan (Propofol)	Induction of anesthesia: 40 mg IV q10sec until induction onset Sedation: 5 μg/kg/min IV and titrate
Dipyridamole (Persantine)	75-100 mg PO q8h
Disopyramide (Norpace)	100-200 mg PO q6-8h
Dobutamine (Dobutrex)	Start 2 μg/kg/min IV up to 20 μg/kg/min (500 mg/250 ml D5W)
Docusate sodium (Colace)	50-100 mg PO tid
Dopamine (Intropin)	2.5-20 μg/kg/min IV (400 mg/250 ml D5W)
Doxazosin (Cardura)	1 mg PO q24h, up to 16 mg PO q24h
Doxycycline (Vibramycin)	100 mg PO or IV q12h
Enalapril (Vasotec)	5-40 mg PO q24h or 1.25 mg IV q6h (0.625 mg IV in renal failure or if taking diuretics)
Epinephrine	Status asthmaticus: 0.3-0.5 mg IV (of 1:10,000 solution); may repeat q5-10min; or 0.3-0.5 mg (of 1:1,000 solution) SQ, may repeat q20-30min up to three doses. Cardiopulmonary resuscitation: 1 mg (of 1:10,000 solution) IV push; may repeat q3-5min; may give 2-2.5 mg dose via ETT if no IV access IV drip: 0.7-7 μg/min (1 mg/250 ml D5W)
Erythromycin (E-Mycin)	500 mg-1 g IV q6h or 250-500 mg PO q6-q12h
Erythropoietin (Epogen)	50-100 units/kg IV or SQ given 3 times per wk
Esmolol (Brevibloc)	Load: 500 μg/kg IV over 1 min, then 50-200 μg/kg/min IV
Ethambutol	15 mg/kg PO q24h up to 25 mg/kg q24h
Famotidine (Pepcid)	20 mg IV q12h or 40 mg PO qhs
Felodipine (Plendil)	Start 5 mg PO q24h up to 20 mg PO q24h
Fentanyl citrate (Sublimaze)	Load: 50-100 μg IV over 1-2 min Maintenance: 1-4 μg/kg/h
Ferrous sulfate (Iron)	325 mg PO tid
Flecainide (Tambocor)	50-100 mg PO q12h up to maximum 400 mg PO daily in divided doses q12h
Fluconazole (Diflucan)	Load: 400 mg IV or PO, then 200 mg IV or PO q24h
Fludrocortisone (Florinef)	50-200 μg PO q24h
Flumazenil (Romazicon)	0.2-0.5 mg IV over 1 min, up to total dose of 5 mg
Fluoxetine (Prozac)	Start 20 mg PO q24h up to 68-80 mg PO q24h

MEDICATIONS AND DRIPS

Drug (Trade Name)	Dosage
Fosinopril (Monopril)	Start 10 mg PO q24h up to 20-40 mg PO q24h
Furosemide (Lasix)	Initial: 10-20 mg PO or IV up to total 600 mg daily
Gabapentin (Neurontin)	300 mg PO on day 1, 300 mg PO q12h on day 2, then 300 mg PO q8h on day 3 up to 600 mg q8h
Gentamicin (Garamycin)	Load: 2 mg/kg IV then 1-1.67 mg/kg q8h IV or IM
Glipizide (Glucotrol)	Start 5 mg PO q24h up to 40 mg daily
Glucagon	1 mg (1 unit) SQ, IM, or IV
Glyburide (DiaBeta, Micronase)	Start 2.5-5 mg PO q24h up to 20 mg PO daily
Guanethidine (Ismelin)	10-50 mg PO q24h
Haloperidol (Haldol)	0.5-5 mg PO q8-12h; 2-5 mg IM "Sundowning": 0.5-5 mg PO or IM q4-6h prn
Heparin	DVT prophylaxis: 5000 units SQ q12h Acute MI/thrombotic events (DVT, PE): 5000-unit IV bolus, then 1000 units/hr and titrate to PTT levels (25,000 units/250 ml D5W)
Hydralazine (Apresoline)	20-40 mg IM or IV
Hydrochlorothiazide (HCTZ)	12.5-100 mg PO q24h
Hydrochlorothiazide/ amiloride (Moduretic)	1-2 tablets PO q24h
Hydrochlorothiazide/ triamterene (Dyazide)	1 or 2 capsules PO q24h after meals
Hydrochlorothiazide/ triamterene (Maxzide)	1 tablet PO q24h
Hydrocortisone (Solu-Cortef)	7.5-120 mg IM or IV q12h; 20-240 mg PO q24h
Hydromorphone (Dilaudid)	2-4 mg PO q4-6h prn; 1-2 mg SQ or IM q4-6h prn
Hydroxyzine (Vistaril, Atarax)	50-100 mg PO q6h
Ibuprofen (Advil, Motrin)	200-800 mg PO q6h prn
Imipenem (Primaxin)	250-500 mg IV q6h or 500-750 mg IM q12h
Indapamide (Lozol)	2.5 mg PO q24h
Indomethacin (Indocin)	25-50 mg PO q8h
Ipratropium (Atrovent)	2-4 inhalations via MDI q6h
Isosorbide dinitrate (Isordil)	10-40 mg PO q6h
Isosorbide mononitrate (Imdur)	Start 30-60 mg PO q24h up to 120 mg PO q24h
Isradipine (DynaCirc)	Initial: 2.5 mg PO q12h Maintenance: 2.5-10 mg PO q12h
Itraconazole (Sporanox)	200 mg PO q24h up to 300-400 mg PO q24h
Ketoconazole (Nizoral)	200-1200 mg PO q24h
Ketorolac (Toradol)	10 mg PO q4-6h prn (5-14 days); 30-60 mg IM or IV initially, then 15-30 mg IM or IV q6h for 48-72 hrs

Drug (Trade Name)	Dosage
Labetalol (Normodyne, Trandate)	20 mg IV over 2 min; may then give 40-80 mg IV q10min to maximum 300 mg
Lactulose	30-45 ml PO q1h until diarrhea occurs, then 30-45 ml PO q6-8h; 300 ml with 700 ml water PR q4-6h
Lansoprazole (Prevacid)	Duodenal ulcer: 15 mg PO q24h for 4 wks
	Erosive esophagitis: 30 mg PO q24h for up to 8 wks
Lidocaine (Xylocaine)	Cardiac arrest: 1-1.5 mg/kg IV; may repeat in 3-5 min up to maximum 3 mg/kg
	Maintenance: 2-4 mg/min IV
	Ventricular tachycardia: 1-1.5 mg/kg IV bolus then 2-4 mg/min IV; a second bolus of 0.5 mg/kg IV may be given 10 min after first bolus (2 g/500 ml D5W)
Lisinopril (Prinivil, Zestril)	Start 10 mg PO q24h up to 40 mg PO q24h
Lisinopril/ hydrochlorothiazide (Zestoretic)	1 tablet PO q24h
Lithium carbonate (Lithonate)	Load: 30 mg/kg PO in three divided doses
	Maintenance: 900 mg-1.5 g PO daily divided q6-8h
Lomefloxacin (Maxaquin)	400 mg PO q24h
Lomotil	2 tablets or tsp PO q6-8h
Loperamide (Imodium)	4 mg PO after each unformed stool up to maximum 16 mg PO daily
Loratadine (Claritin)	10 mg PO q24h
Lorazepam (Ativan)	1-2 mg IV; 1-4 mg IM or PO q8-12h
Losartan (Cozaar)	Start 50 mg PO q24h, up to 100 mg PO q24h
Lovastatin (Mevacor)	Start 20 mg PO q24h, up to 80 mg PO q24h
Magnesium oxide (Mag-Ox 400)	1-2 tablets PO q24h
Magnesium sulfate	1-2 g (8-16 mEq magnesium) IV
Mannitol	25-75 g or 1 g/kg of 20% solution IV; may repeat q6h prn
Meclizine (Antivert)	25 mg PO q6-8h
Meperidine (Demerol)	50-150 mg IM, SQ, or PO q3-4h prn
Metaproterenol (Alupent)	PO: 20 mg q6-8h
	Nebulizer: 0.3 ml of 5% solution in 2.5 ml NS
	MDI: 2-3 inhalations q3-4h
Metformin (Glucophage)	Start 500 mg PO q12h up to 2500 mg PO daily in divided doses q8h
Methadone	Pain: 2.5-10 mg PO, IM, or SQ q3-4h
	Detoxification: Start 15-20 mg PO, IM, or SQ q24h, up to 40 mg q12h
Methimazole (Tapazole)	5-20 mg PO q8h
Methyldopa (Aldomet)	Start 250 mg PO q8-12h for 48 hrs; maximum 3 g PO daily

24

MEDICATIONS AND DRIPS

Drug (Trade Name)	Dosage
Methylprednisolone (Solu-Medrol)	60-125 mg IV q6-12h, acute organ rejection 500 mg IV qd
Metoclopramide (Reglan)	10 mg PO, IV, or IM q6h given 30 min before meals
Metolazone (Zaroxolyn)	5-20 mg PO q24h
Metoprolol (Lopressor)	Acute MI: 5 mg IV q5min up to 15 mg HTN: 50-100 mg q12h
Metronidazole (Flagyl)	500 mg IV q6-8h; *Clostridium difficile*: 250 mg PO or IV q8h for 7 days
Mexiletine (Mexitil)	200-400 mg PO q8h
Mezlocillin (Mezlin)	3 g IV q4h or 4 g IV q6h
Midazolam (Versed)	1-10 mg IV over 5 min for sedation
Misoprostol (Cytotec)	200 μg PO q6h with food
Moricizine (Ethmozine)	200-300 mg PO q8h
Morphine (Morphine Sulfate)	Initial: 2 mg IV q10min, 5-10 mg SQ or IM q4h
Nadolol (Corgard)	Start 20-40 mg PO q24h up to 240 mg PO q24h
Naloxone (Narcan)	0.4 mg (1-ml ampule) IV, IM, or SQ; may repeat q2-3min up to 10 mg
Naproxen (Naprosyn)	250-500 mg PO q12h
Nicardipine (Cardene)	Start 5 mg/hr IV up to 15 mg/hr; 20-40 mg PO q8h
Nifedipine (Procardia, Adalat)	10-40 mg PO q8h
Nimodipine (Nimotop)	60 mg PO q4h
Nitrofurantoin (Macrodantin)	50 mg PO q6h
Nitroglycerin (IV)	Start: 20 μg/min IV up to 400 μg/min in increments of 20 μg/min (50 mg/250 ml D5W)
Nitroglycerin paste (Nitropaste)	1-3 inches topically q4-6h
Nitroglycerin patch (Nitro-Dur)	Start 0.2-0.4 mg/hr up to 0.8 mg/hr, applied q24h
Nitroglycerin spray (Nitrolingual)	0.4 mg (1 sprayed dose) under tongue q5min up to 3 doses as needed
Nitroglycerin sublingual tablets	1 tablet SL q5min prn up to 3 tablets
Nitroprusside (Nipride)	Start 0.3-0.5 μg/kg/min IV up to 10 μg/kg/min (50 mg/250 ml D5W)
Nizatidine (Axid)	Active ulcer: 300 mg PO qhs or 150 mg PO q12h Maintenance: 150 mg PO qhs
Norepinephrine (Levophed)	2-12 μg/min IV (4 mg/250 ml D5W)
Norfloxacin (Noroxin)	400 mg PO q12h
Ofloxacin (Floxin)	200-400 mg PO or IV q12h
Omeprazole (Prilosec)	20 mg PO q24h for 4-8 wks
Ondansetron (Zofran)	0.15 mg/kg IV over 15 min, may repeat q4h

Drug (Trade Name)	Dosage
Oxacillin	1-2 g IM or IV q4-6h
Oxazepam (Serax)	10-30 mg PO q6-8h
Oxybutynin (Ditropan)	5 mg PO q6-12h
Pancrelipase (Pancrease)	1-3 capsules with each meal
Pancuronium (Pavulon)	Start: 0.04-0.10 mg/kg IV push
	Maintenance: 0.01-0.02 mg/kg IV push every hr
Paroxetine (Paxil)	Start 20 mg PO q24h up to 50 mg PO q24h
Penicillin	Pneumococcal pneumonia: Procaine PCN G 600,000 units IV q6h
	Aspiration pneumonia: Procaine PCN G 2 million units IV q4h
	Streptococcus pneumoniae or *Neisseria meningitidis* meningitis: PCN G 2 million units IV q2h
Pentamidine (NebuPent, Pentam)	Acute therapy: 4 mg/kg/day IV for 14 days
Pentobarbital (Nembutal)	Load: 100 mg IV
	Maintenance: 1-3 mg/kg IV given hourly prn
Pentoxifylline (Trental)	400 mg PO q8h
Percocet	1-2 tablets PO q4-6h prn
Percodan	1 tablet PO q6h prn
Perphenazine (Trilafon)	Acute psychosis: 5-10 mg IM or IV
Phenobarbital	Initial: 10 mg/kg IV up to maximum 20 mg/kg
Phenylephrine (Neo-Synephrine)	Start 100-200 µg/min IV up to 500 µg/min IV (10 mg/250 ml D5W)
Phenytoin (Dilantin)	Load: 15-20 mg/kg IV then 100 mg PO q6-8h or 300-400 mg PO q24h
Phosphorus (K-Phos, Neutra-Phos)	1-2 tablets PO q6-12h
Pindolol (Visken)	Start 5 mg PO q12h up to 60 mg PO daily
Piperacillin	3-4 g IV q4-6h
Potassium chloride (K-Dur, Slow-K)	20-100 mEq IV or PO daily
Pravastatin (Pravachol)	Start 10-20 mg PO qhs up to 40 mg PO qhs
Prazosin (Minipress)	Start 1 mg PO q8-12h up to 20 mg PO daily
Prednisolone (Delta-Cortef)	5-60 mg PO daily in 2-4 divided doses
Prednisone	Highly variable; usually start 40-60 mg PO q24
Procainamide (Procan SR, Pronestyl)	Load: 17 mg/kg over 45 min
	Maintenance: 2-4 mg/min IV; Pronestyl: 500-1000 mg PO q4-6h; Procan SR: 500-1000 mg PO q8h
Prochlorperazine (Compazine)	5-10 mg IM or PO q6-8h prn up to 40 mg maximum in 24 hrs
Promethazine (Phenergan)	12.5-25 mg PO, PR, IM, or IV q4-6h prn
Propafenone (Rythmol)	Start 150 mg PO q8h for 3-4 days, up to 150-300 mg PO q8h

Drug (Trade Name)	Dosage
Propoxyphene (Darvon)	65-100 mg PO q4h prn
Propranolol (Inderal)	20-40 mg PO q6-12h
Propylthiouracil (PTU)	Start 100-150 mg PO q6-8h, then 50-300 mg PO daily in divided doses given q8h
Pyrazinamide (PZA)	25 mg/kg PO q24h
Pyridoxine (Vitamin B_6)	10-250 mg PO q24h
Quinapril (Accupril)	Start 10 mg PO q24h, then up to 80 mg PO daily in 1 or 2 divided doses
Quinidine (Quinidine Sulfate)	Load: 600 mg PO, then 200-400 mg PO q6h
Ramipril (Altace)	Start 2.5 mg PO q24h, up to 20 mg PO daily given q12-24h
Ranitidine (Zantac)	Acute therapy: 50 mg IV q8h, 150 mg PO q12h, 300 mg PO q24h
	Maintenance: 150 mg PO q24h
Rifampin (Rifadin, Rimactane)	600 mg PO or IV q24h
Simvastatin (Zocor)	Start 5-10 mg PO q24h, up to 40 mg PO q24h
Sodium polystyrene sulfonate (Kayexalate)	15-30 g PO in 50 ml of 20% sorbitol or 50 g in 200 ml of 20% sorbitol PR; may repeat q4-6h up to 5 doses in 24 hrs
Sotalol (Betapace)	Start 80 mg PO q12h; may be titrated upward q2-3d up to maximum 240-320 mg in divided doses q12h
Spironolactone (Aldactone)	25-50 mg PO q6-8h
Spironolactone/hydrochlorothiazide (Aldactazide)	25-200 mg (of each component) PO qd
Streptokinase (Kabikinase, Streptase)	Acute MI: 1.5 million units IV over 1 hr
Streptomycin	1 g IM q24h
Succinylcholine	1 mg/kg IV
Sucralfate (Carafate)	1 g PO q6-12h
Sulfasalazine (Azulfidine)	3-4 g PO daily given in divided doses q6-12h
Sulindac (Clinoril)	150-200 mg PO q12h
Temazepam (Restoril)	15-30 mg PO qhs prn
Tetracycline (Achromycin)	250-500 mg q6h; 500-1000 mg IV q12h
Theophylline (Theo-Dur)	Highly variable: Start 300-400 mg PO or 5 mg/kg PO daily; may increase 25% q3d up to 900 mg PO daily
Thiamine (Vitamin B_1)	100 mg PO, IM, or IV daily; usually for 3 days
L-Thyroxine (Synthroid)	Start 25-50 μg PO q24h; may increase in 25 μg doses every 2-3 wks
Ticarcillin (Ticar)	3 g IV or IM q4h
Ticarcillin/clavulanate (Timentin)	3.1 g IV q4-6h

Drug (Trade Name)	Dosage
Ticlopidine (Ticlid)	250 mg PO q12h
Timolol (Blocadren)	Start 10 mg PO q12h, then up to 30 mg PO q12h
Tissue plasminogen activator	Acute MI: 15 mg IV bolus, then 0.75 mg/kg IV over 30 min, then 0.5 mg/kg over 1 hr
	Pulmonary embolus: 100 mg IV over 2 hrs
Tobramycin	Load: 2 mg/kg IV
	Maintenance: 1-1.67 mg/kg IM or IV q8h
Tocainide (Tonocard)	Start 400 mg PO q8h, then up to 2400 mg PO daily
Tolazamide (Tolinase)	Start 100-250 mg PO q24h; up to 1000 mg PO daily
Triamcinolone (Azmacort)	2 inhalations q6-8h
Triamterene (Dyrenium)	100 mg PO q12h
Triazolam (Halcion)	0.125-0.250 mg PO qhs
Trimethobenzamide (Tigan)	250 mg PO q6-8h; 200 mg IM or PR q6-8h
Trimethoprim/ sulfamethoxazole (Bactrim, Septra)	1 double strength (DS) tablet PO bid or 8-10 mg/kg/ day TMP with 40 mg/kg/day SMTHX IV q8h
Tylenol with codeine	Tylenol Nos. 1, 2, or 3: 1-2 tablets PO q4-6h prn,
	Tylenol No. 4: 1 tablet PO q4-6h prn
Vancomycin	1 g IV q12h; adjust for renal function impairment
	Pseudomembranous colitis: 125-500 mg PO q6h
Vasopressin (Pitressin)	Initial: 0.2-0.4 units/min IV (100 units/250 ml D5W)
	Maintenance: 0.2-0.6 units/min IV
Vecuronium (Norcuron)	Intubation: 0.08-0.10 mg/kg IV
	Continuous infusion: Start 0.001 mg/kg/min IV and adjust as indicated
Verapamil (Calan, Calan SR)	Regular: 40-160 mg PO q8h
	Long-acting: 120-240 mg PO q12-24h
	IV: 2.5-5 mg over 2 min; may repeat dose as indicated
Vicodin	1-2 tablets PO q4-6h prn
Vitamin K	Acute therapy: 10 mg SQ for 3 days
	Chronic therapy: 10 mg SQ or IM monthly or 5-10 mg PO q24h
Warfarin (Coumadin)	Extremely variable; may start 10 mg PO q24h for 3 days, then 2-10 mg PO q24h
Zolpidem (Ambien)	10 mg PO qhs; 5 mg PO qhs in elderly patients

24

MEDICATIONS AND DRIPS

INDEX

INDEX

INDEX